FROM THE GREENWICH HULKS
TO OLD ST PANCRAS
A HISTORY OF TROPICAL DISEASE
IN LONDON

FROM THE GREENWICH HULKS TO OLD ST PANCRAS
A History of Tropical Disease in London

G. C. COOK

Consultant Physician,
Hospital for Tropical Diseases, London

Vice-President and President-Elect,
Royal Society of Tropical Medicine & Hygiene

THE ATHLONE PRESS
London & Atlantic Highlands

First published 1992 by
THE ATHLONE PRESS LTD
1 Park Drive, London NW11 7SG
and 165 First Avenue,
Atlantic Highlands, NJ 07716

© *G.C. Cook 1992*

This Publication is Sponsored by the Hospital for
Tropical Diseases from their Trustees Funds

British Library Cataloguing in Publication Data
A catalogue record for this book is available
from the British Library

ISBN 0 485 11411 9

Library of Congress Cataloging in Publication Data

Cook, G.C. (Gordon Charles)
From the Greenwich Hulks to old St. Pancras: a
history of tropical disease in London / by G.C. Cook.
p.   cm.
Includes bibliographical references and index.
ISBN 0-485-11411-9 (cloth)
1. Tropical medicine--England--London--History.
I. Title.
[DNLM: 1. Tropical Medicine--history. WC 11.1 C771f]
RC962.G7C66   1992
616.9'883'09421--dc20

Typeset by
Bibloset

Printed and bound in Great Britain by
The University Press, Cambridge

Contents

List of Plates   vi

Preface   xi

1. 'Tropical' disease in England before 1900   1

2. Disease in the tropics and the British pioneers   13

3. The Seamen's Hospital Society   33

4. Emergence of Dr Patrick Manson on the London medical scene   68

5. The Manson-Chamberlain collaboration   80

6. A controversial beginning for the new discipline: a major
    dispute within the medical establishment   101

7. Foundation of the London School of Tropical Medicine (LSTM)
    and a 'rival' institution at Liverpool   147

8. The Albert Dock years: 1899 – 1920   163

9. Removal to central London   218

10. The London School of Hygiene and Tropical Medicine, and
    the Ross Institute and Hospital for Tropical Diseases   242

11. The Second World War (1939–1945) – and after   267

12. Removal to Old St Pancras; the itinerant saga continues   287

Appendix 1   300

Appendix 2   304

References   306

Index   325

List of Plates

Plate 1: Dr Thomas Sydenham: engraving of a portrait by Mary Beale; reproduced from the first edition of *Observationes Medicae* (1676).

Plate 2: Dr John Snow, the Yorkshire-born London anaesthetist (he twice administered anaesthetics to Queen Victoria during childbirth) whose epidemiological researches led to the recognition that the *Vibrio cholerae* was a communicable organism many years before the 'germ theory' was established.

Plate 3: Dr Edward Jenner, whose use of safe vaccination against smallpox paved the way to the extinction (nearly two hundred years later) of one of the world's most lethal viruses on 26 October 1977.

Plate 4: Plaque in the main entrance hall of the London School of Hygiene and Tropical Medicine recording the extinction of smallpox in 1977.

Plate 5: Sir Edwin Chadwick, who recognised that the 'fever' (typhus) was closely associated with overcrowding and insanitary housing conditions. This gave rise to his 1842 report which was largely responsible for Parliament's passing of the 1848 Public Health Act.

Plate 6: Sir James McGrigor: for 36 years Director-General of the Army Medical Department, he made significant contributions to the health of the soldier in the West Indies.

Plate 7: Examples of illustrations in Sir James Annesley's *magnum opus* (see text) which was published in 1828. (a) invasive hepatic amoebiasis, (b) hydatidosis involving the liver.

Plate 8: Sir Joseph Fayrer: a major figure in the Indian Medical Service.

Plate 9: Dr David Livingstone: missionary, explorer and also a pioneer in the documentation of disease (including trypanosomiasis) in southern and central Africa.

Plate 10: Mary Slessor: she made major contributions to health education in eastern Nigeria over a 39-year period.

Plate 11: Sir William McGregor: an outstanding administrator whose medical training enabled him to improve conditions in several parts of the tropics.

Plate 12: Sir John Pringle: although he did not serve in the tropics he made major contributions to army health.

Plate 13: James Lind: his monographs included the treatment of scurvy, the health of seamen, and advice to Europeans in hot climates.

Plate 14: Miss Florence Nightingale: she revolutionised Army nursing and also made major public health contributions in India and at Scutari.

Plate 15: The first of the hospital ships - HMS *Grampus* which was used from 25 October 1821 to 30 October 1831. She was moored just upstream from the Royal Hospital, Greenwich.

Plate 16: The second of the hospital ships - HMS *Dreadnought* - which was in use from 31 October 1831 to 25 January 1857.

Plate 17: The interior of a ward in the *Dreadnought* hospital ship.

Plate 18: The third and last of the hospital ships - HMS *Caledonia* (renamed *Dreadnought*) - which was used from 26 January 1857 to 13 April 1870. [*Illustrated London News* 1870; 28 May : 548]

Plate 19: The Dreadnought Hospital, Greenwich in 1870, shortly after its opening; this building had formerly been used as the Infirmary of the Greenwich Hospital.

Plate 20: The Greenwich Hospital in a painting of 1771; the artist is unknown.

Plate 21: The Royal Hospital, Greenwich in 1841, with HMS *Dreadnought* anchored on Greenwich Reach. The artist was William Parrott [reproduced by permission of the Guildhall Library, City of London].

Plate 22: The foundation stone of the Albert Dock Hospital - laid on 15 July 1889 - which remains in place at the rebuilt hospital today.

Plate 23: Cromlet Hill, Oldmeldrum, Aberdeenshire (approximately 18 miles north of Aberdeen), which was Manson's birthplace. A plaque commemorating Manson (inset) was placed by the London School of Hygiene & Tropical Medicine in July 1955.

Plate 24: Dr Patrick Manson at the age of 31 years; this photograph was probably taken whilst he was on leave in Britain, from Amoy.

Plate 25: Dr Patrick Manson around the time he returned to London (1890).

Plate 26: Wall plaque commemorating Manson, at the Albert Dock Hospital; this remains in place to this day.

Plate 27: Plaque at 50, Welbeck Street, W1 where Manson lived after leaving 21, Queen Anne Street. This was unveiled on 11 February 1985.

Plate 28: The Right Honourable Joseph Chamberlain, Secretary of State for the Colonies (1895–1903) with Mrs Chamberlain. She was Chamberlain's first wife – who died in childbirth when their son Austen was born; he subsequently married twice more.

Plate 29: (a) The Royal Victoria Hospital, Netley (viewed from Southampton Water) which was opened after the Crimean War in 1863 (reproduced by permission of the Royal Army Medical Corps). The hospital was later to be used in both World Wars; after the second of these it became increasingly run down, and in 1966 the Army decided to demolish it. The last patients were treated there in 1979. A close co-operation with the Army Medical College and the Indian Medical Service existed until 1902; shortly afterwards the RAMC College at Millbank, London, was opened. (b) The sole remaining part of the Royal Victoria Hospital - the chapel - in 1991.

Plate 30: The Royal Army Medical College, Millbank, which was opened in 1907.

Plate 31: Plaques commemorating: (i) Mr Joseph Chamberlain (1836–1914), and his son (ii) Sir Austen Chamberlain (1863–1937) - which remain to this day displayed on the wall of the 'Chamberlain ward' of the present Hospital for Tropical Diseases, London (chapter 12).

Plate 32 The Dreadnought Seamen's Hospital, Greenwich, photographed early in the twentieth century. [reproduced by permission of the Guildhall Library, City of London]. The building presently lies empty, and its ultimate future is undecided.

Plate 33: The LSTM in October 1899. Standing is Mr PJ Michelli, Secretary of the SHS (for forty years), and sitting is Dr DC Rees, the Medical Superintendant/Tutor.

Plate 34: The LSTM (left, background), with the Albert Dock Hospital (SHS), soon after its inauguration in 1899.

Plate 35: Interior of the new 'Top Ward' of the Albert Dock Hospital, 1899. This was later named 'Manson Ward'.

Plate 36: Four endowment plaques which were originally on the walls of the 'Top Ward' of the Albert Dock Hospital; most date from the very early days of the establishment of the original LSTM and hospital. They are now at the rebuilt hospital.

Plate 37: The first class at work in the laboratory of the LSTM in 1899. Dr DC Rees is demonstrating the life-cycle of *Plasmodium* sp; also standing is George Warren – laboratory attendant.

Plate 38: Mr (later Sir) James Cantlie (1851–1926): surgeon to the LSTM

Plate 39: Plaque in the main entrance hall of the London School of Hygiene and Tropical Medicine commemorating the role of Sir Patrick Manson in the foundation of the LSTM.

Plate 40: Admission books of the Albert Dock Hospital in the early days of the 20th century; most of these are still extant.

Plate 41: The extension to the LSTM was carried out in 1912 and consisted of laboratories and a student hostel; the covered corridor connecting the School with the Albert Dock Hospital is shown.

Plate 42: Dr Charles Wilberforce Daniels (1862–1927) was the second Superintendent of the LSTM. In 1903 he resigned to become Director of the Institute of Medical Research at Kuala Lumpur. He later became

Director of the LSTM and Physician to the Albert Dock Hospital. When Manson retired, he was appointed Medical Consultant to the Colonial Office. [reproduced by permission of 'The Wellcome Institute Library, London']

Plate 43: (a) Endowment plaque (which remains on display at the Albert Dock Hospital) commemorating the TNT explosion which did a great deal of damage to the hospital and school in 1917. Another plaque (b) commemorates the life of Mrs Maude Ashley - mother of Edwina, Countess Mountbatten of Burma - who died in 1911.

Plate 44: Mr (later Sir) Austen Chamberlain MP who continued to support the LSTM which his father - Mr Joseph Chamberlain - had done so much to initiate.

Plate 45: The box used to convey mosquitoes from Rome to London (a), and (b) its interior - showing one of the wire cages in which some of the mosquitoes survived the journey.

Plate 46: Dr George Carmichael Low (1872–1952) who was to take an important part in the Roman Campagna expedition [reproduced by permission of 'The Wellcome Institute Library, London']. He also played a major role in the development of tropical medicine in London, and in the foundation of *The [Royal] Society of Tropical Medicine and Hygiene*.

Plate 47: Major Ronald Ross pictured in 1908 while Professor of Tropical Medicine at Liverpool.

Plate 48: Plaque on the wall of what was Ross' London home - 18 Cavendish Square, London, W1. This was unveiled in 1985.

Plate 49: The Hospital for Tropical Diseases and LSTM building at 23 Gordon St WC1 (Endsleigh Gardens) at about 1920.

Plate 50: Plaque commemorating Sir Patrick Manson's contributions to the LSTM which was displayed in the clinical theatre at the Endsleigh Gardens building. It was subsequently placed on the wall of the present Albert Dock Hospital.

Plate 51: The staff of the Hospital for Tropical Diseases in 1930; in the middle of the front row: are Sir Leonard Rogers, Dr G C Low, Dr (later Sir) Philip Manson-Bahr, and Dr (later Sir) Neil Hamilton Fairley.

Plate 52: Plaque commemorating the first Director of the LSHTM - Sir Andrew Balfour - in the main entrance hall of the LSHTM.

Plate 53: Professor Robert Thomson Leiper (1881–1969). He joined the staff of the LSTM in 1905, and later became the Founder and first Director of the Institute of Parasitology at Winches Farm, St Albans [reproduced by permission of 'The Wellcome Institute Library, London'].

Plate 54: The seal of the LSHTM, which is described in the accompanying panel.

Plate 55: Foundation stone of the LSHTM.

Plate 56: Mr Neville Chamberlain, who laid the foundation stone of the

LSHTM. He was later the British Prime Minister – who led Britain into World War II - and was succeeded by Mr Winston Churchill in 1940. He died as a result of a gastrointestinal malignancy in 1940.

Plate 57: The London School of Hygiene and Tropical Medicine building under construction in April 1927.

Plate 58: The LSHTM shown in an aerial view in 1990. Gower Street is shown running obliquely from north to south; to the right is Senate House, University of London.

Plate 59: The museum of the new LSHTM showing the Manson collection and an exhibit on malaria and blackwater fever.

Plate 60: An exhibit in the new LSHTM which emphasised the strong hygiene ('sanitation') component in its teaching activities.

Plate 61: The Dreadnought Hospital, Greenwich. 10 beds were made available for Tropical Medicine during the 1939–45 war.

Plate 62: Sir Neil Hamilton Fairley, FRS (1891–1966). Director of Pathology at the LSTM, he was later appointed to the newly established Chair of Clinical Tropical Medicine at the LSHTM [reproduced by permission of 'The Wellcome Institute Library, London'].

Plate 63: 23 Devonshire Street, W1 (left) - the 'home' of Clinical Tropical Medicine from 1946 to 1951.

Plate 64: Foundation stone of the rebuilt workhouse - later to become St Pancras Hospital - in 1890

Plate 65: The Infirmary (now the South Wing of St. Pancras Hospital).

Plate 66: The opening ceremony, which was carried out by the Duchess of Kent on 24 May 1951. She was escorted by Sir Alexander Maxwell, KCMG, Chairman of University College Hospital.

Plate 67: The present Hospital for Tropical Diseases building (a) at its opening (viewed from the south-west) in 1951, and (b) today; the inset shows the current letter-head of the hospital.

Plate 68: St. Pancras Old Church. In the foreground is the Rhodes family tomb; the name of Cecil Rhodes (1853–1902) appears on the marble slab but his remains are in fact interred in the Matopo Hills, Zimbabwe (formerly Southern Rhodesia).

Plate 69: The St Pancras Coroner's Court. In the foreground is the tomb of Sir John Soane, architect of the Bank of England.

Preface

For a century, and more, Britain was pre-eminent in the field of tropical medicine [i.e. the clinical (bed-side) discipline concerned with those diseases more common in warm compared with temperate climes][1-4]; this resulted largely, although not entirely, from her days of Maritime supremacy and Imperial presence in numerous tropical countries. Special expertise was required to manage the exotic diseases encountered in the tropics, some of which were brought back to these shores by the numerous servants of Empire and Raj (often after extended periods of residence in warm climes). Later in the Colonial era, orientation in this field changed, far more emphasis being directed towards prevention - and less frequently management - of the diseases affecting British travellers; greater attention was also paid to the medical problems of indigenous inhabitants of tropical countries (medical education followed later), and more recently members of the minor ethnic groups in this land.

London's 'tropical medicine' began as a *clinical* discipline (with a parasitological input) at the London School of Tropical Medicine (LSTM) which was established in 1899; as well as the care of the 'servants' of Empire, training of medical officers (and the organisation of postgraduate courses for them) was a major activity. When the London School of Hygiene and Tropical Medicine (LSHTM) was founded in 1924 (its new premises were opened in 1929) it became detached from the *clinical* discipline. The *schools* of tropical medicine, in both London and Liverpool, have become progressively far less *clinically* orientated and have reached out increasingly into hygiene, 'sanitation' and preventive medicine in the tropics, and towards public health. The LSHTM is now firmly set on a course designed to transform it into the major public health centre (in research and postgraduate teaching) for the United Kingdom, with only minor emphases on tropical activities. This course was succinctly summarised in 1985 by a former Dean: 'We are concerned with the postgraduate teaching of everything *except the bedside aspects of health* [my italics]. We are interested in vaccines, insecticides, improvement of sanitation, better water supplies, all aspects of the prevention of disease, and promoting community health. We are the only school in Europe which combines all these disciplines'[5]

The last two or three decades have seen changing emphases in the practice of 'tropical medicine'. Techniques and methods of investigation have become far more complex; in research, molecular biology and molecular genetics now dominate the scene. Funding is being targeted to bench research at a highly sophisticated level (e.g. the search for vaccines against parasitic diseases); at the same time, facilities for *clinical* research have diminished. Also more and more clinical problems from the tropics are being dealt with not by the major centres in London and Liverpool, but by communicable (infectious) disease departments throughout the United Kingdom - many of which were threatened with extinction a mere decade or so ago, when it was generally considered that communicable disease in the western world had been conquered! HIV infections (and AIDS) have been especially important in re-kindling the communicable (and tropical) diseases flame – which had been virtually extinguished.

But how did the *clinical* discipline develop during the nineteenth and early twentieth centuries? This is a saga which has never been adequately recorded; I have attempted to address this deficiency. In his presidential address to the Royal Society of Tropical Medicine and Hygiene in 1925, Dr Andrew Balfour (later to become the first Director of the LSHTM) considered, 'there is nothing to compare with the *historical perspective* [my italics] as a means of adjusting our ideas, of clarifying our conceptions, of stimulating our flagging energies', and as a result 'one of the lessons [learned] is very likely to be that of humility [which is] specially true in the case of medicine'[6]. 'We cannot' (he continued) 'but wonder at some of those clinicians of former days who, relying mainly on 'the seeing eye and the understanding heart' grappled successfully with intricate problems and handled disease in a manner which, to this day, commands respect'. It is surely time that the massive contributions of the pioneers of *clinical* tropical medicine were properly acknowledged. It is also noteworthy that in Balfour's view tropical medicine and tropical hygiene were 'of course, inextricably mingled' and that 'preservation of health in hot climates' was (then as now) extremely important; he was therefore wisely commending a balance between *prevention* ('sanitation') and *clinical* medicine, an orientation which we are in danger of overlooking with so much current emphasis on either basic science or public health[7]. This therefore seems an appropriate moment to consider the rise and fall of *clinical* tropical medicine, i.e. while the discipline remains relatively fresh in our minds, and before it is completely obliterated as a separate entity[8]. In this text I have attempted to summarize the development of *clinical* tropical medicine in London from earliest times to the heights which it attained and occupied in those now far-off days of Empire and Raj. The saga contains a great deal of British social (including the formation of the charitable Seamen's Hospital Society in 1821), in addition to a very substantial amount of Colonial (Imperial) history. This account is dominated by the LSTM; the LSHTM will assume second place.

I thank Dr Alex Sakula, former President of the History of Medicine Section of the Royal Society of Medicine who, by inviting me to give a lecture on this subject (to the Section of the History of Medicine of the Royal Society of Medicine)[8] acted as the major catalyst for this work, Mr O R Cross, Miss Mary Gibson and Dr P E C Manson-Bahr for valuable discussion, and Mrs Jayne Ball for typing the entire script from my long-hand. I am grateful to Miss Dawn Lake for help with the index.

This publication is sponsored by the Hospital for Tropical Diseases from their Trustees Funds.

G. C. Cook

1

'Tropical' disease in England before 1900

There is in one sense no such thing as tropical medicine, and in any case many of the most erudite writings of Hippocrates are concerned with maladies which now-a-days are chiefly encountered under tropical or sub-tropical conditions.

Andrew Balfour (1873-1931)[1]

Many communicable diseases which presently fall under the umbrella of 'tropical medicine' were formerly world-wide in their distribution. These include: malaria, leprosy, cholera, dysentery, plague and typhus[2]. The viral infection variola – smallpox – (now extinct) constituted a further example. Tuberculosis and the enteric fevers (typhoid and paratyphoid) are now largely confined to the tropics and subtropics, but nevertheless remain significant problems in many temperate countries. However there are a few diseases which have never gained a foothold in the temperate areas of the globe (since recorded history began), in most cases because the vector or animal reservoir requires a high ambient temperature for survival; leishmaniasis, trypanosomiasis, yellow fever and dengue are examples of protozoan and viral infections, respectively.

Major 'tropical' diseases in England

Malaria (or ague) was commonplace in England up to the present century. The term has been in use in England only since 1887, having been derived from the Italian *mal aria* (bad air)[2]. However, this is a clinical entity which had been clearly documented for many centuries and was undoubtedly known to Hippocrates ('many fell victims to the quotidians'); in fact descriptions date back to 1000 BC[2]. There is reasonably good evidence that many individuals of historical eminence were either seriously debilitated or had their lives cut prematurely short by febrile illnesses which resulted from a *Plasmodium* sp infection[3]; Alexander the Great (323 BC), St Augustine (first Archbishop of Canterbury) (AD 604), King James I, King Charles II, Cardinal Wolsey and Oliver Cromwell

1

provide examples. The disease was known to Chaucer (1340–1400) and later to Shakespeare (1564–1616): 'He is so shak'd of a burning quotidian that it is most lamentable to behold' (Henry V, II; i: 123). This was in fact a major disease entity throughout most of Europe[4]. Clearer descriptions of malaria began with the introduction to Europe of cinchona (Jesuits') bark by Jesuit missionaries, from southern America[3,5]; a clearcut clinical response to specific chemotherapy could then be documented. Cinchona was first introduced into Rome by Spanish priests in 1632 and was included in the *London Pharmacopoeia* (3rd edition) in 1677 as *Cortex peruanus*[3,5]. Its first recorded use in England is in 1656; this is recorded in a Northampton doctor's notebook[5]. Sir Robert Talbor, physician to King Charles II cured the king of a fever with a concoction prepared by leaving macerated powdered bark in port wine for one week; he also added opium to add pain relief to the remedy. Thomas Sydenham (1624–89) (plate 1) (frequently designated the 'English Hippocrates') successfully treated the intermittent fevers in London during the seventeenth century[6]. Although a firm believer in the *miasmatic theory* the Italian physician, G M Lancisi (1654–1720) nevertheless believed that malaria was transmitted, and even suggested that mosquitoes might be relevant[2]; it is of considerable interest that mosquito nets were in use in ancient Rome! However, mosquito transmission of human malaria was not scientifically established until the very late nineteenth century (chapters 4 and 8). In England the disease was formerly endemic in low-lying, ill-drained, swampy areas, eg the Fens of Cambridgeshire, Lincolnshire (and the surrounding counties), the marshes on either side of the Thames estuary in Kent and Essex, the Romsey and Pevensey marshes, and around Bridgwater – near the Bristol Channel. Malaria was prevalent in London as late as 1859; at St Thomas' Hospital 12 to 60 cases per 1000 patients (the numbers obviously fluctuated from year to year) between 1850–60 suffered from malaria[2]. However, this high incidence in London diminished sharply when the Thames Embankment was erected and extensive drainage work was undertaken; by 1864 numbers were greatly reduced. Apart from the occasional case of 'airport malaria' in recent years[3], the last cases acquired in south-east England occurred from troopships at the end of World War II.

Leprosy was also a major problem in northern Europe, including Britain, in the Middle ages[2]; it seems clear for example that Robert the Bruce of Scotland suffered from this bacterial infection[7]. The disease had in the early centuries of the Christian era probably been confined to the East[8], however, cases then appeared along the Mediterranean littoral and thence northwards throughout Europe[9]. Some of the eleventh century Crusaders to the Holy Land undoubtedly returned with the disease, having become infected in the Middle-east. According to one estimate, one person in every 200 in France was at one time suffering from a condition

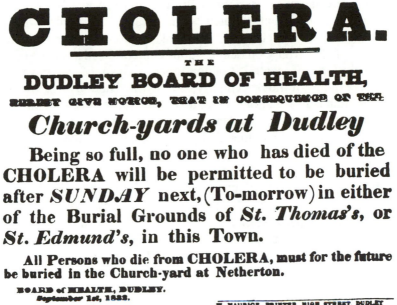

CHOLERA.

THE
DUDLEY BOARD OF HEALTH,
HEREBY GIVE NOTICE, THAT IN CONSEQUENCE OF THE

Church-yards at Dudley

Being so full, no one who has died of the CHOLERA will be permitted to be buried after *SUNDAY* next, (To-morrow) in either of the Burial Grounds of *St. Thomas's*, or *St. Edmund's*, in this Town.

All Persons who die from CHOLERA, must for the future be buried in the Church-yard at Netherton.

BOARD of HEALTH, DUDLEY.
September 1st, 1832.

W. MAURICE, PRINTER, HIGH STREET, DUDLEY

Fig 1.1: Notice dated 1 September 1832 from Dudley, near Birmingham, indicating that the two graveyards were so inundated with the corpses of cholera victims that no further interments could be undertaken in the immediate future.

diagnosed as leprosy[2]. It was from the outset regarded as a contagious disease and the leper was banished from human society. A great deal of work on the prevalence of leprosy in medieval Denmark has been carried out by Møller-Christensen[10]; numerous hospitals dedicated to St Jørgen had their own burial ground and incontrovertible skeletal evidence of this disease[9] has been firmly established.

The Asiatic cholera first reached Britain in October 1831; there were major outbreaks in 1831–2, 1848–9 and 1853–4, and smaller ones in 1868 and 1893[2,11,12]. Fig 1.1 gives an indication of the seriousness of the 1831–2 epidemic, when many thousands of individuals in several of Englands' major cities were smitten by the disease. As late as 1832, it was considered to be a visitation of Divine Providence on sinners. It was not until the close of the 1848–9 epidemic (in London) that the eminent anaesthetist John Snow (1813–58) (plate 2) who had been born in Yorkshire, suggested that material from the excreta of cholera patients could, when accidentally ingested, cause the disease[13,14]. Snow furthermore suggested that cholera was spread by the accidental emptying of sewers, bearing infected excreta, into the drinking water of the community. Most cholera deaths in London had occurred he noted, in a district in which the drinking water was obtained from a point of the

3

Thames where there was serious pollution with sewage. Snow incidentally, suggested that contaminated water could be purified by filtration through sand and gravel, or by allowing it to stand in reservoirs. At the close of the 1854 epidemic, 500 cholera deaths occurred in a very small area of central London over a span of 10 days. As a result of a house-to-house enquiry, Snow (assisted by the Reverend Henry Whitehead[15]) demonstrated that only those who obtained their drinking water from the contaminated Broad Street pump contracted the disease[16]; the legend that following removal of the pump-handle the numbers of new cases rapidly declined is not strictly true. [A plaque commemorating that event now exists in Broadwick St, Soho, beside the 'Dr John Snow' public house]. With hindsight there is no doubt that the outbreak was already subsiding; however, Snow's classical monograph (an expansion of the pamphlet published in 1849)[13] was of enormous importance to epidemiology, and served as a salutary reminder to many generations that contaminated drinking water was the cause of this particular communicable disease. Above all however, this was a clear demonstration that a 'germ-borne disease' could be prevented, long before its cause (or indeed a knowledge of disease germs) was understood.

Dysentery (bloody diarrhoea) was well described in Britain by Sydenham in 1669[6]; it had a seasonal prevalence and was at its peak at the beginning of autumn and 'upon the invasion of the winter . . . totaly ceased'. He considered: 'It is for the most part mortall to old persons, lesse fatall though very dangerous to youth but benigne enough to infants.' Whether this description applied to shigellosis or amoebic colitis (or both) is quite impossible to decipher. The recommended management consisted of the ingestion of large quantities of whey!

Plague is a further 'tropical disease' which was formerly a major problem in temperate countries[2,17]. Whilst in most outbreaks bubos (ie, lymphatic swellings) form the most usual presenting feature (hence bubonic plague), in others a high percentage of cases manifest as a rapidly fatal pneumonia (pneumonic plague*). [When the infection is transmitted to man via the marmoset rather than the rat (see below) the pneumonic form is more common than the bubonic.] The greatest pandemic of plague in history (the Black Death) occurred around 1348; the disease entered Europe in 1346 via the Crimea, and by 1347, Constantinople, Cyprus,

---

* The words of a nursery rhyme which probably originated in the seventeenth century: 'ring-a-ring-o'-roses, a pocket full of posies, atishoo! atishoo! we all fall down', are generally considered to refer to the herbs carried as a protective measure, and the almost inevitable sequel to pneumonic plague, respectively (Opie I, Opie P (eds). *Oxford Dictionary of Nursery Rhymes*. Oxford: Oxford University Press 1951.)

Venice and Sicily had been invaded. By the following year, most of western Europe (including Britain) was smitten, and mortality rates of one third to one half of the population were recorded[18]. Mortality amongst the learned professions was high and the Church in particular suffered severely; also, the economic and agricultural structure of the land was radically changed. Plague became endemic in the UK between 1590 and 1665 and was a major problem in Shakespeare's day[19]: in London, it caused 33,000 deaths in 1603, >35,000 in 1625, >10,000 in 1636, and >9000 between 1644–47. However, in 1665 (the Great Plague)[20], there were as many as >68,000 recorded deaths. Both Samuel Pepys and Daniel Defoe[21] gave excellent accounts of this particular outbreak. Following this there were a few isolated incidents but no further major epidemics in Europe. One example occurred at Marseilles and Toulon in 1720 (where 90 died); however, it had become epidemic in Russia in 1709 (with 150,000 deaths), and persisted in remote parts of Asia. There was a large epidemic in Egypt in 1834. The last great pandemic (which has not yet terminated) began in 1894; in that year it caused 100,000 deaths in Canton, and in the following year 1,300,000 deaths in India. The last recorded cases of plague in England occurred around 1910[22]. Two opposing theories to account for the origin and spread of plague existed from very early times until the latter decades of the nineteenth century: the 'miasmatic' theory (a noxious influence was presumed to be present in the atmosphere, or arose from the earth during plague periods), and the 'contagion' theory (a healthy person developed the disease as a result of a direct contact with a plague sufferer (or via fomites)). By and large, precautions were taken to counteract the latter form of spread, and from the eighteenth century onwards major ports were guarded against the introduction of plague (and other epidemic diseases). It is of interest that as early as 1347–8, patients were forbidden to traffic in articles of food and drink, and from time to time municipal authorities were ordered to put infected patients outside the city gates (as was the case with lepers)[2]. Many plague hospitals and lazarettos were founded at this time. The role of rats (*Rattus rattus* and *R norvegicus*) in transmission was suggested in ancient times, and again in China in 1792 and 1834; in 1894 the plague bacillus *Yersinia pestis* was clearly demonstrated in dead rats. Despite these observations, most authorities doubted a connection! From 1906, however, circumstantial evidence was sufficient to introduce the destruction of rats on ships, the inspection of passengers and crew (when necessary), and to institute quarantine restrictions; these measures (with a single exception – see above) have kept the disease away from the shores of Britain. Firm proof that the rat flea *Xenopsylla cheopis*, and less importantly *Nosopsyllus fasciatus*, transmit the bacillus whilst feeding on a healthy man (or rat) was not forthcoming until 1914.

The major problem regarding an historical evaluation of the group of rickettsial infections collectively known as typhus (usually transmitted by lice[23] and mites) is that early reports did not differentiate them from typhoid or enteric fever (see below). Sir John Pringle (1707–82) (chapter 2) had in fact equated 'jail-fever' (typhus) with hospital fever in an important paper *Experiments upon Septic and Antiseptic Substances, with remarks relating to their use in the Theory of Medicine* published in 1750. There is no doubt that these diseases were extremely common in England in the eighteenth and early nineteenth centuries and were closely associated with poverty[24]. In an unsuccessful attempt to reduce the high prevalence of 'jail-fever' at the old Newgate prison in London, the Reverend Stephen Hales (1677–1761) designed a windmill-type roof-ventilator[2]. In 1789–90, and again in 1794, there were very severe outbreaks of typhus in Manchester[2] and a number of fever wards ('houses of recovery') were constructed at the Manchester Infirmary. A fee of 'one or two shillings' was paid by the physicians to persons giving information on the occurrence of typhus in any house in the district around the Infirmary; furthermore, rewards were also paid to the head of a family if he disinfected his house as well as the patient's clothes after the fever had subsided. In 1838 the prevalence of typhus ('fever') in London became so high that Sir Edwin Chadwick, Secretary of the Poor Law Commission, recommended a special investigation (see below); this began amongst the poor of Wapping and Stepney, Whitechapel and Bethnal Green.

Smallpox was endemic, and periodically epidemic, in England during the seventeenth and eighteenth centuries; Sydenham wrote a graphic account of the disease and its management in 1669[6]. One example was a large outbreak which occurred at Chester in 1774; the prevalence in the 15% of the population which had not already suffered was recorded as 53%, with a death rate of 17% of those actually infected and one of 9% in the entire unprotected population[2]. Since the early eighteenth century, methods of direct inoculation of blood from a patient suffering from a mild attack (certainly not without risk) was widely practised in the East; variolation was introduced to England in 1718 by Lady Mary Wortley Montagu (1689–1762) (wife of the British Ambassador to Turkey) who was taught the technique in Constantinople[25,26]. The eminent English physician Richard Mead (1673–1754) published in 1747 a work which gave the full weight of his considerable authority to the practice of 'inoculation'; use of this procedure spread widely during the next half-century. Some years later the Gloucester general practitioner Edward Jenner (1749–1823) (plate 3) developed the idea which was prevalent in some country districts (milk maids were known to be protected against smallpox), that cowpox infection (which affected the udders of cows) protected *Homo sapiens* from smallpox[2,25]. Jenner vaccinated a boy

(James Phipps) with lymph obtained from cowpox vesicles which had developed on the finger of a dairy-maid, Sarah Nelmes; this event took place on 14 May 1796, and on 1 July of the same year he inoculated the boy with smallpox 'matter' in the accepted way; the boy did *not* develop smallpox[27,28]. In July 1798 Jenner published his important monograph *An inquiry into the Causes and Effects of the Variolae Vaccinae*. Despite varying amounts of opposition in some quarters, the procedure became accepted and was widely practised. In 1802 Parliament awarded Jenner £10,000 for his discovery; an amendment which sought to double this amount was defeated by 3 votes, but in 1807 Jenner was awarded a further £20,000[28]. In 1898 there was an attempt to make smallpox vaccination *compulsory* in Britain, but the Bill failed to get through Parliament (Fig. 1.2). The last known case of this disease was diagnosed on 26 October 1977 in Somalia; a plaque at the London School of Hygiene and Tropical Medicine commemorates this event (Plate 4).

Examples of 'tropical' infections which still exist in temperate climes

John Bunyan (1628–88) was well aware of the consumption (tuberculosis) which so often 'took him down to the grave' (*The Life and Death of Mr Badman*, 1680). This disease has certainly claimed many worthy lives, including those of John Keats, Frédéric Chopin, D H Lawrence, Jane Austen, and R L Stephenson. Richard Morton (1637–98), a young contemporary of Sydenham, published a treatise – *Phthisiologia* in 1689; this work dealt comprehensively with tuberculosis and demonstrated that the formation of 'tubercles' (which he claimed could heal spontaneously) was a necessary component of the pulmonary lesion(s)[2]. The first description of joint tuberculosis ('white swellings') is attributed to Richard Wiseman (1622–76), a British surgeon, in *Severall Chirurgicall Treatises* published in 1676. Giovanni Morgagni (1682–1771) described renal tuberculosis at Bologna, and Richard Bright (1789–1858) laryngeal tuberculosis at Guy's Hospital, London (Morton had almost certainly pre-dated him[2]). Percivall Pott (1714–88), a surgeon at St Bartholomew's Hospital, London, documented vertebral tuberculosis (Pott's disease) in 1779. Although the causative organism had not been identified, this clinico-pathological entity – with its countless and varied manifestations (which remains arguably the most important of all 'tropical' diseases – claiming vast numbers of lives in 'Third-world' countries) was clearly recognised by these and countless subsequent writers[29,30]. In 1825 P C A Louis (1787–1872) published *Recherches anatomico-pathologiques sur la phthisie*; this work which is based upon 123 cases (with post-mortem findings in 50 of them) gave detailed descriptions of the pulmonary form of the disease. In 1826, R T H Laennec (1781–1826) published the second

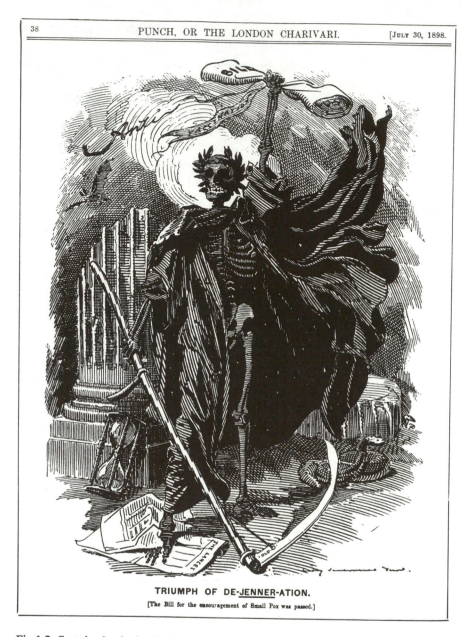

TRIUMPH OF DE-JENNER-ATION.

[The Bill for the encouragement of Small Pox was passed.]

Fig 1.2: Sustained agitation by the anti-vaccinationist lobby (religious as well as political objections were voiced), together with the failure of the British medical profession to fully support smallpox vaccination led to the collapse of proposed *compulsory* vaccination in England. Therefore, under the new Act (and also a later one passed in 1907) parents merely had to state their 'conscientious objections' as a valid reason for not having their child vaccinated. A number of embarrassed British individuals working in India wrote to the correspondence columns of medical journals at home inviting the objectors to come and discover what smallpox was doing to the population there![27] [*Punch* 1898; 30 July: 38].

edition of *Auscultation médiate,* in which he described the development of the tubercle through its various stages. *On The Treatment and Cure of Pulmonary Consumption, on Principles Natural, Rational, and Successful* was published by George Bodington (1799–1882) in 1840. The first institution for the management of pulmonary tuberculosis was established (on open-air lines) at Sutton Coldfield, Warwickshire; although not particularly successful this paved the way for numerous sanatoria, most of which were initially situated on the European continent[2]; these were followed by tuberculosis dispensaries at Edinburgh (1887), Oxfordshire (1910), and Sheffield (1911). Pulmonary tuberculosis became a notifiable disease in England and Wales in 1911. As recently as 1932, 2–13% of samples of raw milk tested in England and Wales contained virulent bovine *Mycobacterium tuberculosis* – especially important in the production of abdominal lesions. An attenuated strain of bovine *M tuberculosis* formed the basis of the Bacille-Calmette-Guérin (BCG) vaccine which was introduced, for use in calves, in 1906. The prevalence of tuberculosis in Britain steadily declined in the first half of the twentieth century; this was hastened by the introduction of streptomycin in 1944, and later by other anti-tuberculosis chemotherapeutic agents[29,30].

In 1750, John Huxham (1692–1768) wrote in his *Essay on Fevers* that the 'small-intestinal lymphoid patches' (which had been described by J C Peyer in 1677) were especially affected in typhoid (enteric) fever[2]. Typhoid (enteric) fever can therefore be identified far back into history; however, a clear distinction from typhus was not made until 1837 (in America) and 1850 (in Britain) by William Gerhard (1809–72) and Sir William Jenner (1815–98), respectively. In 1829 two notable works on typhoid fever were published: a monograph by P F Bretonneau in which he clearly located the disease in small-intestinal Peyer's patches, and Louis' work which was based on 138 cases of the disease (with post-mortem findings in 50 of them)[31]. At Bristol, William Budd (1811–80) hypothesised that typhoid fever was spread by the ingestion of material from an infected patient, and that defective sewers were the most likely source of human infection; this was of course in accord with Snow's work on cholera (see above). However, the work was opposed by the highly influential Charles Murchison (1830–79) – who had served for over two years in the Bengal Army of the East India Company – in his *Treatise on the Continued Fevers of Great Britain* published in 1862 (a second edition came in 1873)[2]; this work also covered typhus and 'remittant fever'. A detailed account has been given of typhoid fever in Britain between 1860 and 1900[32]. Fig 1.3 refers to an outbreak of the disease in 1897. The best documented historical report of a typhoid carrier is that of the cook 'Typhoid Mary', who between 1900 and 1907 certainly infected 26 individuals and probably very many

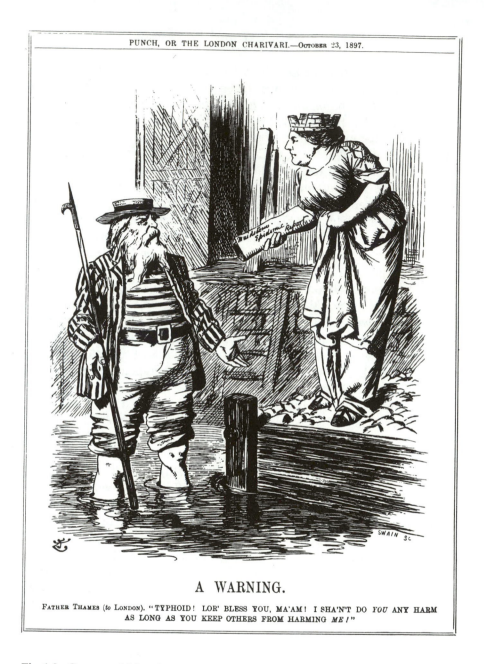

A WARNING.

FATHER THAMES (*to* LONDON). "TYPHOID! LOR' BLESS YOU, MA'AM! I SHA'N'T DO *YOU* ANY HARM
AS LONG AS YOU KEEP OTHERS FROM HARMING *ME!*"

Fig 1.3: Cartoon which refers to an outbreak of typhoid fever at Maidstone, Kent in 1897[31]. The impression is given that this infection is spread predominantly by infected water rather than food; this obviously resulted from an unjustified extrapolation from the work on cholera transmission which was by then well accepted. [*Punch* 1897; 23 October: 187].

10

more[33,34]. Inoculation against typhoid was first carried out on a large scale in British troops during the Boer War, then in India, and during the First World War (1914–18); during these wars the total numbers of cases of typhoid in British troops amounted to 105, and 2.35 per 1000 strength, respectively. Paratyphoid A and B were added to typhoid during the First World War because there was a high prevalence of these diseases on the Eastern Fronts; the resultant inoculum was designated TAB. In England and Wales the annual mortality rates for typhoid declined from 332 per million in 1871–80, to 91 in 1901–10, and 2 in 1941–50[2].

Development of modern sanitation and 'hygiene' in England

Infections which in recent years have come to be regarded as 'Tropical Diseases' were thus commonplace in England until well into the twentieth century, although in several cases a slow decline had begun in the middle of the eighteenth century; this largely reflected the introduction of modern sanitation* and 'hygiene'. Improvements here resulted either from individual effort, or were initiated by the Army and/or Navy[2]; public health in Britain ultimately became a major political, legislative, and administrative matter and *prevention* its watchword. The initial 'alarm' was sounded by the cholera epidemic of 1831–2 (see above) but the dominant figure in the intellectual arousal of the 'public conscience' was undoubtedly Jeremy Bentham (1748–1832). Poor Law reforms heralded the environmental changes which led to improved health for the inhabitants of this country. Sir Edwin Chadwick (1800–90) (plate 5)[35,36] was the prime motivator, assisted by Neil Arnott (who had worked for the East India Company), James Kay (later Sir James Kay-Shuttleworth), and Thomas Southwood Smith (who had worked at the London Fever Hospital); they were subsequently joined by Ashley Cooper (later 7th Earl of Shaftesbury (1801–1885)). Chadwick in particular appreciated the relationship between insanitary housing and excessive sickness, especially that caused by the 'fever' (ie typhus). His *Report on the Sanitary Conditions of the Labouring Population* was published in 1842[37]; the major objective was to prevent disease – still considered to be spread by miasmas (bad smells) – for practical (not necessarily humanitarian) purposes. The main thrust was therefore to instigate external sewerage, to abolish stagnant drains and cesspits, and to improve water supplies[37].

---

* The definition of *Sanitation* (*Shorter Oxford English Dictionary*) is: 'the devising and application of means for the improvement of sanitary conditions' (1848), and *sanitary*: 'of or pertaining to the conditions affecting health, esp. with ref. to cleanliness and precautions against infection, etc; pertaining to or concerned with sanitation' (1842).

Chadwick also paid attention to the plight of children in factories, and the establishment of an efficient Constabulary Force. In 1848 Parliament passed the Public Health Act, and the Nuisances Removal Act. In 1848 also, Liverpool became the first city to appoint a medical officer of health, and Sir John Simon (1816–1904)[37] was shortly afterwards given a similar position in London. Simon's annual reports on the health of the City of London embodied vast quantities of detailed data which were used in the preparation of the great Public Health Act of 1875.

The Victorian contribution to the public health of Britain was therefore enormous, and presents a challenge for the health services of today[37,38]. If the environmental conditions of developing and tropical countries could be raised to those of 'westernised' countries (which took place in the latter days of the nineteenth and early ones of the twentieth centuries), many of the diseases mentioned in this chapter would begin to decline there also. Obviously such measures would exert a lesser impact on those diseases (most of which are viral or protozoan) which require a vector, and can only survive at a relatively high ambient temperature.

2

Disease in the tropics and the British pioneers

. . . Our ancestors have turned a savage wilderness into a glorious empire: and have made the most extensive, and the only honourable conquests, not by destroying, but by promoting the wealth, the number, the happiness of the human race.

Edmund Burke (1729–97)

Long before the formal creation of the specialism *tropical medicine*, numerous British pioneers were making important contributions to medicine in tropical countries[1–3]. Many were quite exceptional and remarkable men. Scotland produced more than its fair share of these medical 'explorers'; the major reason(s) for this seems to be that the educational systems produced far more graduates than was necessary for the country's requirement so that output exceeded demand; also, one should not underestimate a great deal of missionary zeal. These pioneers therefore left these shores and learned and wrote a great deal about the local diseases in several tropical countries; tables 2.1 – 2.3 summarize some of those (with dates of birth and death) who produced valuable contributions (usually monographs) about their experiences with regard to medical practice. The list of individuals mentioned in this chapter[1–3] is by no means definitive but is intended to form a backdrop to the later chapters which trace the development of the discipline *tropical medicine* in London.

The 'English sugar islands' (the Caribbean)

Life expectancy at birth in England during the seventeenth century was around 35 years[4], but in the Caribbean it was considerably less for whites and blacks alike. The Caribbean was indeed a 'white man's grave', but also the black man's too! Negroes imported to the sugar islands (from Africa) died much more rapidly than their infants were born; therefore the slave masters abandoned attempts to keep them long enough to breed a new generation and routinely brought replacements year in and year out[5].

13

By moving to the Caribbean, the colonists escaped some of the worst English 'killers' – eg, plague, smallpox and influenza; tuberculosis and venereal disease(s) were also apparently less common. However, they encountered instead, malaria, yellow fever, dysentery (the 'bloody flux'), 'dropsy', leprosy, yaws, hookworm disease and elephantiasis; some of these diseases, eg yellow fever, had been introduced from Africa by the slave ships[2], and the slaves themselves brought 'new' infections with them, including leprosy, yaws, guinea worm (dracontiasis), elephantiasis, and 'a sleepy disease' (this was not transmitted there – and never has been – because the vector was absent). It is probable that trachoma was also introduced by these slaves. 'Ophthalmia', which was rife amongst them probably consisted of a mix of trachoma, gonococcal, and Koch–Weeks infections. The introduction to the 'new world' of yellow fever from Africa has been well documented: the *Oriflamme* conveyed it to Martinique, and the *Hankey* to Grenada[2]; it was incidentally returned to the west (in fact to Spain) by the *Grand Turc*.

The slave ships employed doctors and paid them so many shillings for every negro who remained alive at the end of the voyage; this provided an obvious inducement to deliver as much as possible of the 'cargo' in a viable state. The average mortality on the voyage in the sixteenth, seventeenth and eighteenth centuries was, however over 30% and occasionally double or even treble this[2]. As a result, there were a great many physicians, surgeons, and apothecaries travelling to and from the 'English islands'[5]. In the seventeenth century, the 'humoral theory' of medicine still held sway; four competing elements: earth, water, air, and fire determined man's physical environment, and these had counterparts in human physiology – the four invisible fluids (humors): – melancholy, phlegm, blood, and choler – which passed through the veins from liver to heart. To remain healthy the four humors had to be kept in a delicate balance.

The most distinguished physician to practice in the Caribbean during the seventeenth century (albeit for only 15 months) was undoubtedly Sir Hans Sloane (table 2.1)[3] (later president of the Royal Society and perhaps better known as the founder of the Chelsea Physic Garden); he had previously lived in the house owned by Sydenham (chapter 1). He clearly had a thorough knowledge of the 'intermittent fevers' for his report: *Of the diseases I observed in Jamaica, and the Method by which I used to Cure them* recorded the management of several hundred cases (both black and white, children and adults, rich and poor); he also wrote on yaws, elephantiasis, and sleeping sickness[1]. Sloane successfully used the Peruvian bark (or Jesuit's powder) for malaria, and laudanum (in conjunction with a bland but nutritious diet) for dysentery; he advocated (and used) 'blood letting' liberally, a not

Table 2.1 British doctors who practised, and also made important literary (as well as other) contributions, in the Caribbean

SLOANE, Sir Hans+	1660 – 1753
HILLARY, William	17(?) – 1763
GRAINGER, James*	1721 – 1766
CHISHOLM, Colin+	17(?) – 1825
WRIGHT, William*+	1735 – 1819
McGRIGOR, Sir James*+	1771 – 1858

[* Born in Scotland; + Fellow of the Royal Society]

entirely appropriate technique for many tropical diseases which frequently produce an associated anaemia.

The Yorkshireman, William Hillary[3,6] lived and practised in Barbadoes from 1752 to 1758. In a monograph he described many of the local diseases; *Observations on the Changes of the Air and the Concomitant Epidemical Diseases, in the Island of Barbados* was published in 1759 (with a second edition in 1766). In this work there is reference to a disease which is considered by some to be tropical sprue (possibly the first description of this disease); however, Hillary's description of this condition is as follows:

> From the best accounts that I can obtain, this malady has been some chance time seen in this island, near these thirty years, though but very seldom; and after I came there in 1747, I did but see one person who had it, in the first four years of my residing here; and three more in the next three years: But within the four last years past, it is become so frequent, that I have seen some scores of patients labouring under it, yet it seems not to be in the least infectious or contagious.

It seems most likely therefore that he had encountered *Giardia lamblia* infection[7]; there can be no doubt that the description referred to an epidemic disease which was probably spread via contaminated water, or possibly food. Hillary also wrote on yellow fever, and was something of a climatologist, carefully correlating some of the prevalent diseases with the prevailing weather conditions[1]. He warned against the dangers of sea-bathing whilst 'overheated'; although an attractive form of exercise, swimming in the Caribbean was not apparently considered a healthy pursuit in the seventeenth century[5].

Dr James Grainger[3] worked at St Kitts from 1759 and contributed: *An Essay on the more common West Indian Diseases, and the remedies which that country itself produces. To which are added some hints on the management of the negroes* which was published in 1764. He wrote about 'Sick Houses' (or estate hospitals), advocated the provision of isolation and venereal wards, described some of the diseases which afflicted negroes, and commented upon the hygiene of slaves; in addition, he distinguished two distinct types of dysentery – possibly for the first time[1]. Grainger was born at Dunse, Berwickshire and educated at Edinburgh University; he subsequently became an Army Surgeon in London, a post which proved not unduly successful and he departed for St Kitts in 1759; he died there of 'fever'. Samuel Johnson described Grainger as one 'who would do any good that was in his power'[1].

Another physician who worked in the West Indies was Colin Chisholm[1,3]; he wrote a monograph on the 'pestilential fever' which was published in 1795: *An Essay on the Malignant Pestilential Fever introduced into the West Indian Islands from Boullam, on the coast of Guinea, as it appeared in 1793 and 1794.*

William Wright[1,3], was born at Crieff in Scotland; he was initially apprenticed to a surgeon at Falkirk, and studied medicine at Edinburgh. Following a voyage to Greenland, he served on the *Intrepid*, a 'plaguey old hulk'[1] in which he contracted typhus. Wright was later involved in several naval engagements, cruised in the Mediterranean, and saw service in the West Indies. After leaving the Navy, he settled in Jamaica where he became a private practitioner, and introduced the use of cold baths for tetanus! He was apparently a botanist of repute and contributed an *Account of the Medicinal Plants growing in Jamaica*. Wright also wrote on many local diseases, including yaws, which he was able to distinguish from syphilis. He wrote two practical guides: *Directions to Officers going to the West Indies*, and *Instructions for a person about to sail for the East Indies and China*; the following quotation comes from the former 'Be sure to draw down the mosquito-net all round, and brush well inside with a large towel to kill such mosquitoes as still be there'[1] – advice which is as acceptable today as it was in the eighteenth century. After leaving Jamaica, Wright returned to England, became a regimental surgeon, was captured by the French and Spaniards, became a prisoner in Spain for some time, returned to England, again sailed for Jamaica (where he again suffered from fever and ague), returned again to England, and later proceeded to Barbadoes, where he had charge of the military hospitals there.

In many ways the most impressive of the early Caribbean pioneers was however, Sir James McGrigor[1,3,8] (Plate 6); he made numerous contributions to medicine in the British Army and to military hygiene[9,10] and it was he who first separated the wounded from those with infectious fevers. It has been said that he was to Wellington what his personal surgeon D J Larrey (1766–1842) was to Napoleon[11], and that he stood up to the former (a mark of moral courage which has been compared with questioning an order from Churchill in 1940!). Despite this, Wellington had considerable respect for McGrigor and considered him 'one of the most industrious, able and successful public servants I have ever met'[11]. Although best known for his unparalleled term of service as Director-General of the Army Medical Department (for 36 years, from 1815–1851), he gained experience in both the East and West Indies, Egypt, and the Peninsula. He wrote: *Medical Sketches of the Expedition to Egypt from India* (1804), and the *Report of Sickness, Mortality and Invaliding in the Army in the West Indies* (1838). He founded the Museum of Natural History and Pathological Anatomy, and the library at Fort Pitt, Chatham, the headquarters of the Army Medical Service before the removal to Netley. In 1789 he had been one of the group of founders of the Aberdeen Medico-Chirurgical Society[12]. McGrigor is today commemorated by a statue in the McGrigor courtyard at the Royal Army Medical College, Millbank[13].

India: early days of the British Raj, and the development of the Indian Medical Service (IMS)

The hazards and depredations of disease in Asia (as elsewhere in the tropics) were viewed in the seventeenth and eighteenth centuries as an established part of a hostile and untamed environment[14]; only through the superior knowledge and skill of European medicine was it considered at all possible to bring them under effective control. Although a few British medical pioneers had reached India by the end of the eighteenth century, it was not until the early nineteenth that their concentration began to expand. The initial objective was to attempt to improve the conditions under which the British soldier worked, and in addition various individual efforts were made to provide comfort and preserve health within the British community[2]; the indigenous people were however allowed to continue as they had done for centuries! Fevers, smallpox[15], plague[16], cholera, and relapsing fever, took a terrible toll – the extent of which will never be known. The enormous amounts of morbidity and mortality produced a sense of fear, if not terror, in the mind of the average European, and this was at a time when in England the example of cholera was producing a great stimulus to sanitary reform, improved housing, refuse disposal, and greater cleanliness in general (chapter 1). Between 1830 and 1846, for example, the proportion of deaths per 100 Europeans serving there which were attributed to four diseases endemic in the Bombay Presidency was: fevers 23.0, dysentery and diarrhoea 32.4, cholera 10.3, and hepatitis and amoebic abscess 9.5[2]. A description of conditions in Bombay (by a municipal commission) as late as 1861 was as follows[2]:

Go into the native town and around you you will see on all sides filth immeasurable and indescribable, and at places almost unfathomable; filthy animals, filthy habits, filthy streets, and with filthy courtyards around the dwellings of the poor; foul and loathsome trades, crowded houses, foul markets, foul meat and food, foul wells, tanks and swamps [the Commissioner's choice of adjectives appears to have been limited!], foul smells at every turn, drains unventilated and sewers choked, and the garbage of an Oriental city. Men, women, and children, the rich and the poor, living with animals of all kinds and vermin, seeing all this and inhaling the deadly atmosphere and dying by the thousand.

However, by 1864, as a result of a new Sanitary Act a health service had been set up, and in 1865 a Town Improvement Act was ratified; by 1868 a significant change in the state of Bombay was recorded[2]:

In three years [the Health Officer] has wrought a marvellous revolution. Except in a few obscure lanes, the city is almost devoid of bad odours. Its area is nearly thrice that of municipal Calcutta and yet every street and house and every road is daily swept as well as watered and the dust is carefully removed. The natural effect has been seen, not merely in the comfort of all classes of the inhabitants, but in the fact that cholera, which used to be endemic in the city . . . has not been known for some time.

At the same time the public health in Rajputana was without doubt, absolutely appalling[2]:

The ways of defiling water and food are innumerable. On the margin of the village tank the dead are burned . . . the buffaloes wallow in the mud, the sacred kine drink, the Brahmans wash their clothes and persons, and the women fill their waterpots. The washing in water inconceivably filthy, merely as a symbolically religious act, the deposit of filth near wells and tanks, the religious obstacles to cleanliness, all contribute to mortal disease. The women are employed for many hours every day in preparing with their hands animal manure as fuel, so it is impossible for the poor to have clean food. Dogs, cows, swine, peafowl, kites and vultures do a large amount of scavenging.

And at Peshawar, once known as the 'graveyard of India'[2]:

No language could be too strong in describing the abomination of the whole existing arrangements . . . Of course the grave and radical defect is the open main channel, exposed to every species of contamination . . . The deeper channel . . . is actually on a lower level than the ordure of the pits . . . the effect on the unhappy dhooly-bearers may be learnt from the records at the station hospital, where in 1870 these poor creatures died

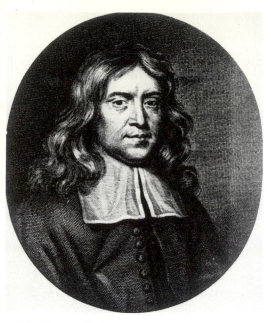

1. Dr Thomas Sydenham

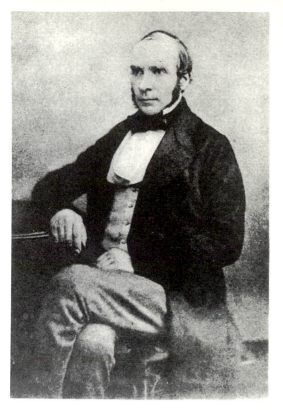

2. Dr John Snow

4. Plaque recording the last case
of smallpox in 1977

John Snow

3. Dr Edward Jenner

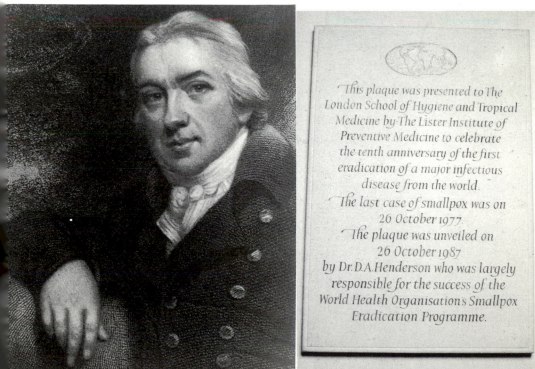

This plaque was presented to The
London School of Hygiene and Tropical
Medicine by The Lister Institute of
Preventive Medicine to celebrate
the tenth anniversary of the first
eradication of a major infectious
disease from the world.
The last case of smallpox was on
26 October 1977.
The plaque was unveiled on
26 October 1987
by Dr. D.A.Henderson who was largely
responsible for the success of the
World Health Organisation's Smallpox
Eradication Programme.

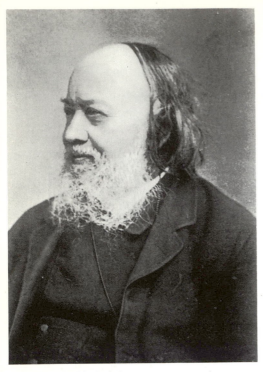

5. Sir Edwin Chadwick

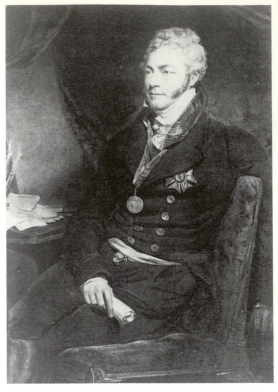

6. Sir James McGrigor

7a & b. Plates in Sir James Annesley's 1828 text

8. Sir Joseph Fayrer

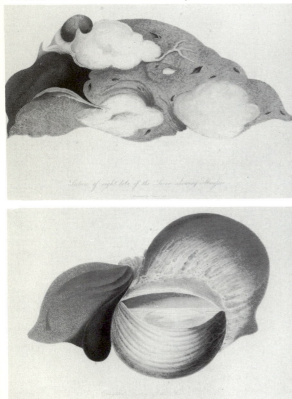

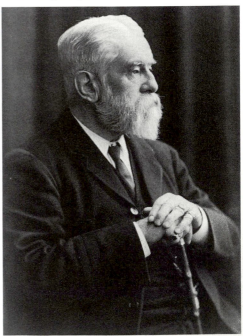

Joseph Fayrer

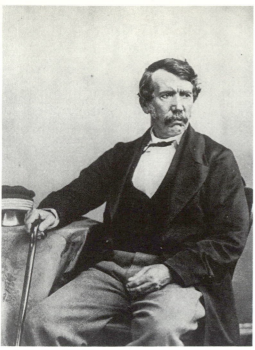

9. Dr David Livingstone

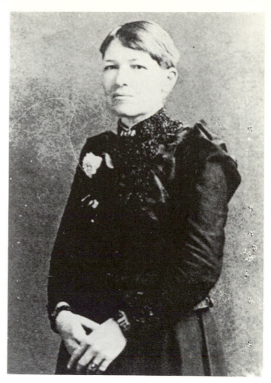

10. Miss Mary Slessor

11. Sir William McGregor

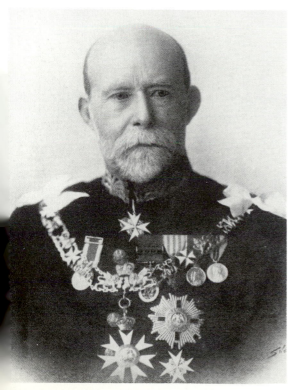

12. Sir John Pringle

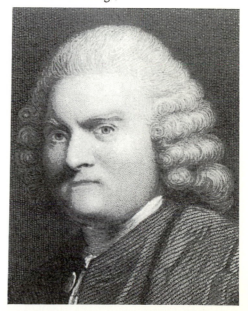

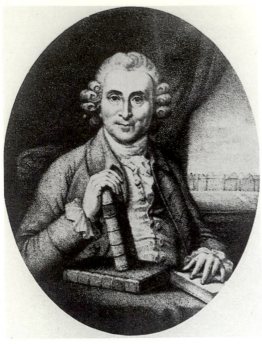

13. Dr James Lind

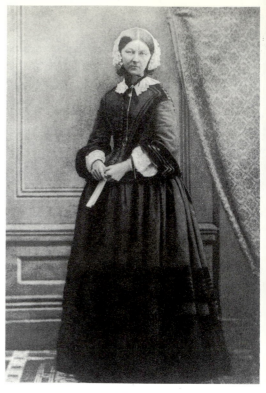

14. Miss Florence Nightingale

15. HMS *Grampus* (25 October 1821 – 30 October 1831)

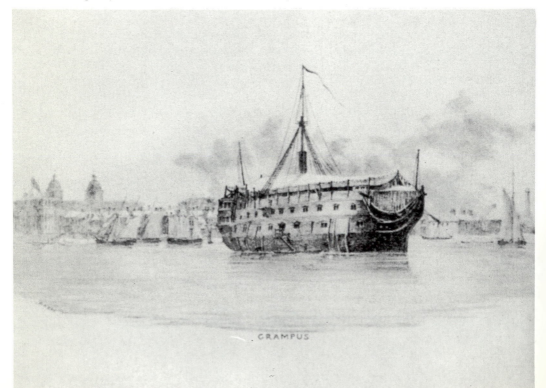

like rotten sheep . . . In conclusion I can only say that I do not see how matters could be worse except in a community which drew no distinction between its cesspools and water-tanks, and used each indiscriminately for all purposes.

Within the great temple of Madura the water tank had been used for hundreds of years as a bathing-place before the people presented offerings to their deity; on average, 200 individuals bathed and washed their clothes daily as a sacred duty (*Report of the Sanitary Commission with the Government of India* (1871)); as late as 1888, a Mr Justice Cunningham wrote:

The tank is often mere sewage. Every shower washes surface filth into it, every dust-storm carries some more; a perpetual series of bathers adds daily to its impurity; clothes and cooking utensils add their modicum of dirt; as the dry season lasts it grows dirtier and dirtier.

A report by the Sanitary Commissioner of Madras in 1875 on the condition of the town of Combum stated[2]:

The chief predisposing causes of the abnormal sickness and mortality of the town were the crowding of every available spot within its limits with corpses, and pollution of its water supply. The exciting cause is malaria arising from a swamp which, owing to partial silting up of an important irrigation channel, has replaced for about two miles the running stream which originally drained efficiently the irrigated lands. More tombs than living persons are visible in the town. The borders of wells and water-channels seem chosen especially for sepulture.

In the wake of efforts in England to reduce the morbidity and mortality from cholera a clean water supply was installed in Calcutta in 1870; this was immediately followed by a significant improvement in the health of the city, and resulted in a marked reduction in the cholera returns[2].

Throughout this period, the future Indian Medical Service (IMS) was developing[17]. From the earliest days of the East India Company, a Marine Medical service existed for the medical requirements of the company's ships and personnel; this company had maintained a hospital at Madras since 1664; in 1676 another had been established at Bombay, and in 1707–8 a further one at Calcutta. In the early days, the conditions of service and pay for the medical officers were exceedingly poor[2]; even the Surgeon–General received only £20–£30 annually for attending daily:

from morning until night, to cure any persons who may be hurt in the service of this Company, and the like in all their ships . . . they shall also

Table 2.2   British doctors who practised, and also made important literary (as well as other) contributions, in India

JOHNSON, James	1777 – 1845
MARTIN, Sir (James) Ranald*+	1793 – 1874
ANNESLEY, Sir James+	1780 – 1847
BALLINGALL, Sir George*	1780 – 1855
WADE, John*	17(?) – 18(?)
TWINING, William	1790 – 1835
MALCOLMSON, John+	1802 – 1844
MOREHEAD, Charles*	1807 – '82
CHEVERS, Norman	1818 – '86
PARKES, Edmund+	1819 – '76
WARING, Edward	1819 – '91
FAYRER, Sir Joseph+	1824 – 1907
CORNISH, William	1827 – '97
CARTER, Henry	1831 – '97
LEWIS, Timothy	1841 – '86
CUNNINGHAM, David*+	1843 – 1914
LAMB, George*	1869 – 1911
BIDIE, George*	1830 – 1913
LUKIS, Sir Charles	1857 – 1917

[* Born in Scotland; + Fellow of the Royal Society]

cut the hayre of the carpenters, saylors, caulkers, labourers and any other workemen in the Companies said yards and ships, once every forty days, in a seemly manner.

The Bengal Medical Service was founded on 20 October 1763, and in January 1764 it became the IMS; the staff were primarily military officers, although there were some in civil employ who were temporarily lent for service duties. In addition, the East India Company (from which the Government of India was transferred to the Crown in 1858) maintained four other medical services.

Regarding medical education in India at this time, Medical Colleges had been set up at Calcutta and Madras in 1835, and the Grant Medical College had been founded at Bombay in 1845. In England, medical education for those intending to serve in India was undertaken at the Army Medical School at Fort Pitt, Chatham (from 1860) and the Royal Victoria Hospital, Netley (from 1863)[9]; the latter institution was also the training school for Royal Navy medical officers until Haslar was opened in 1880[18]. The Royal Army Medical College, Millbank, was not opened until 1907; from then, IMS in addition to Army officers received their education there and also at Aldershot[9].

Table 2.2 summarizes the names of a selection of British doctors who both served in India and made significant literary contributions during this period; this list is by no means definitive, and is intended merely to draw attention to a few of the more important and interesting individuals, and others whose scientific and administrative contributions significantly advanced their various disciplines[1].

Although of Scottish descent James Johnson[1,3] was born in Ireland. In 1798 he was appointed as surgeon's mate in the Navy, cruised in the Mediterranean and was invalided from Egypt. Between 1803 and 1806 he served in India, and also as a naval surgeon for four years in the East. He suffered from amoebic dysentery and liver abscess in the Indian Ocean, and from 'ague' at Walcheren. Johnson apparently advocated calomel (instead of cinchona) for treating the 'remittent fevers' in Bengal, and this according to one writer did a great deal of harm and led to many deaths[1]. His major work was *The Influence of Tropical Climates on European Constitutions* (1812); it ran to numerous editions and had an appendix on Tropical Hygiene. He subsequently took up practice in Portsmouth, and later in London. Sir (James) Ranald Martin[1,3] was born in Skye, studied medicine at St George's Hospital, London and in 1817 became a surgeon at the Bengal Medical Establishment of the East India Company. His *Notes on the Medical Topography of Calcutta* appeared in 1837; this was largely devoted to 'sanitation' (or insanitation!). He later contributed to, and subsequently took over, the editorship of Johnson's book.

Sir James Annesley[1] is best remembered today for a superbly illustrated two-volume quarto work (which contains numerous coloured engravings of post mortem specimens) entitled *Researches into the Causes, Nature and Treatment of the more Prevalent Diseases of India and of Warm Climates generally* published in 1828; this contains a wealth of clinical detail (many case-histories are included); he did not neglect the preventive aspects of medicine in the tropics. Plates 7a and b give examples of some of the illustrations from this work. In addition to this *magnum opus* he wrote a treatise on cholera. Annesley was born in County Down, studied medicine at Trinity College, Dublin and afterwards in London; he sailed to Madras in 1800. Annesley was invalided home from active service, and on his return to India became Garrison Surgeon of Masulipatam; here he studied tropical diseases both in the European and also the 'native'. He later took part in the Java expedition, saw further service in India and gained a very wide clinical experience at Madras. After 37 years of distinguished service he left India due to ill-health. Sir George Ballingall's[1,3] major contribution was his *Observations on the Diseases of European Troops in India*. He differentiated two forms of dysentery on clinical grounds (see above). Ballingall was born in Banffshire, sailed to India in 1806, and later became Regius Professor of Military Surgery at Edinburgh University[1]. Few details of John Wade survive; he studied at Edinburgh, and whilst an Assistant Surgeon in Bengal advocated the formation of local medical libraries. He made three important literary contributions: *Select evidence of a successful method of treating Fever and Dysentery in Bengal* (1791), *Prevention and Treatment of the Disorders of Seamen and Soldiers in Bengal* (1793) and later, *Nature and effect of emetics, purgatives, mercurials and low diet in disorders of Bengal and similar latitudes.*

Many of these early texts were dominated by tropical gastroenterological conditions (involving the small-intestine, colon, and liver); an excellent example is to be found in William Twining's[1,3] *Clinical Illustrations of the more important Diseases of Bengal* published in 1832. Twining was a Nova Scotian who trained at Guy's Hospital, London under Sir Astley Cooper; he served with Wellington in Portugal, was present at Waterloo, and later moved to Ceylon and then India. He became Senior Assistant Physician to the General Hospital in Calcutta, where he died.

John Malcolmson joined the Madras Medical Service in 1823 and became an Assistant-Surgeon of the Madras European Regiment. A prize-winning essay submitted to the Madras Medical Board: *A practical essay on the history and treatment of beri-beri* was published as a book in 1835. He also wrote on liver enlargement and hepatic abscess. After leaving the Medical Service in 1840 he became a partner in a firm – Messrs. Forbes & Co, Madras. Whilst on a geological expedition to Gujarat and Khandesh he contracted hepatitis and died at Dhulia. Yet another Scot, Charles Morehead[1,3] was born and educated in Edinburgh; he later studied medicine in Paris and in 1829 joined the Bombay Medical Service. He became the first Principal of the Grant Medical College (see above) and was widely known as the 'pioneer of medical education in India'[1]. He wrote *Researches upon the Diseases of India* which was published in 1856, and opposed an excessive use of mercury in the management of tropical diseases! Norman Chevers[1] was born at Greenhithe, studied medicine at Guy's Hospital, London and in 1848 obtained a commission in the Bengal Army, from which he retired with the rank of Deputy-Surgeon-General in 1876. Between 1861 to 1876 he was the Principal of the Calcutta Medical College, Professor of Medicine, and First Physician of the College Hospital. He was secretary to the Medical Board in Bengal during the Indian Mutiny (1857–9). He produced: *Commentary of the Diseases of India*, and *Medical Jurisprudence in India*; in addition he was co-editor of the *Indian Annals of Medical Science.*

After graduating from University College Hospital, London, Edmund Parkes[1,3] (he was born at Bloxham, Oxfordshire) sailed to India for a 3-year period from 1842; there he dealt with a great deal of dysentery, hepatitis, and cholera. He wrote about healthy cholera carriers, and advised on the protection and disinfection of water supplies. After retirement from the Army in 1845 he became a noted teacher in clinical medicine at University College, London[1]. However, he was summoned to Turkey during the Crimean War and later gave up clinical medicine to become Professor of Hygiene at the new Army Medical School at Fort Pitt, Chatham (see above). His major literary contribution was a *Manual of Practical hygiene*. He died of tuberculosis. Edward Waring became an authority on the indigenous medicinal plants of India, and wrote: *Bazaar Medicines of India*. His origins were in Shropshire; before going to Madras in 1849 as an Assistant-Surgeon in the Honourable East India Company, he had visited amongst other countries: Sierra Leone, Jamaica, Australia, and the Cape of Good Hope. In Burma he was sent to a lonely out-station where he compiled a *Manual of Practical Therapeutics*. He later moved to Travancore where he collaborated with Parkes (see above) on a text devoted to liver abscess. After returning to England in 1863, he became editor of the *Indian Pharmacopoeia*, and produced *The Tropical Resident at Home*.

One of the greatest and revered names in Indian medicine was that of Sir Joseph Fayrer[1,3,19] (Plate 8). He was born at Plymouth, the son of a naval officer, and received his medical education at Charing Cross Hospital. He entered the Royal Navy, and was posted as Assistant-Surgeon to HMS 'Victory' for service at Haslar Hospital in 1847. Following this he lived on the Continent as private medical attendant to Lord Mount-Edgcumbe. After leaving the Navy in 1847, he obtained a commission as Assistant-Surgeon in the Bengal Medical Service; here he was apprenticed to the Residency-Surgeonship at Lucknow. He was incorrectly reported as being killed in the Mutiny. Fayrer later became Professor of Surgery at Calcutta, and turned his attention to Indian snake bites; he was in fact a pioneer on snake venoms. His greatest work *Thanatophidia of India* was published in 1872; he left India in the same year but returned briefly as medical officer to the Prince of Wales whilst on his Indian tour. He later settled in London. His *Tropical dysentery and chronic diarrhoea* was published in 1881.

William Cornish received his undergraduate training at St George's Hospital, London and in 1854 went to Madras as an Assistant-Surgeon. He later became Sanitary Commissioner for the Presidency. He wrote on dysentery, enteric fever, cholera, and prison dietaries. He made provision for District Civil Surgeons to tour their areas on sanitary duties, introduced changes in famine administration, and revolutionised jail dietaries in Madras. He retired in 1885 after promotion to Surgeon-General. According to Balfour, he 'built for himself a place in the annals of preventive medicine'[1]. Another pioneer – who was both a scientist and an accomplished artist – was Henry Carter. He first set foot in

India in 1858 as an Assistant-Surgeon in the Bombay Medical Service and left with the rank of Deputy-Surgeon-General, IMS in 1888. He discovered the spirochaete of relapsing fever in India; he also studied oriental sore, leprosy, and mycetoma. He unsuccessfully proposed the segregation of lepers (to the Bombay Government) in 1876. Following Laveran's discovery of *Plasmodium* sp in 1880, he demonstrated the existence of three species of the parasite in India. He was also a pioneer in tropical pathology. He died of 'phthisis'.

Balfour considered that Timothy Lewis had been undervalued in previous accounts of the pioneers; his services were it seems not well recognised during his lifetime[1]. Lewis was a Welshman who graduated from University College, London and Aberdeen. He entered the Army Medical Service in 1868 and studied on the Continent before sailing to India. Together with Cunningham (see below) he detected amoebae in cholera stools, and produced the first authentic account of amoebae obtained from the human intestine! He discovered *Filaria sanguinis hominis* (now named *Wuchereria bancrofti* – chapter 4) and correlated its association with chyluria. His monograph *The microscopic organisms found in the blood of man and animals and their relation to disease* was published in 1878; in it he described the spirochaetes of relapsing fever, and the rat trypanosome. He left India (where he held the rank of Surgeon-Major) for England in 1883 and became Assistant Professor of Pathology at Netley. He died three years later of pneumonia. He was described by C Dobell as the 'Godfather of Tropical Medicine'! 'He founded, both in India and at Netley, a school and also a tradition, the fruits of which ultimately became visible to all the world in the researches and discoveries of the officers of the IMS and the Royal Army Medical Corps'[1]. David Cunningham shared many of the scientific triumphs of Lewis. He made the first accurate description of *Entamoeba coli*, *Trichomonas intestinalis*, and *Chilomastix mesnili*; he was also the first person to recognise *Leishmania* sp in 'oriental sore'. He played a part in 'the manufacture of quinine'[1]. A Scot, he graduated at Edinburgh, became Professor of Physiology, and later Professor of Physiology and Pathology, at Calcutta Medical College. However, the climate of Calcutta, and the conditions of work there undermined his health; in1898 he retired to Torquay, Devon as an invalid.

Passing top of the Indian Medical Service list, George Lamb (he had graduated from Glasgow University) then came under the influence of Sir Almoth Wright; following Netley he sailed to India in 1894. After further studies at Netley, and at the Pasteur Institute, Paris he became Assistant to Haffkine at Parel in 1898. He worked on Indian snake venoms and directed researches of the Advisory Committee on plague. George Bidie was born in Banffshire and studied at Edinburgh and

24

Aberdeen Universities; he entered the IMS in 1856 and retired as a Surgeon-General in 1890. He wrote on many topics, including natural history, botany, economic products, and coinage, and in 1867 discovered a preventive against an insect pest which threatened to wipe out the coffee plantations of South India. However, his pioneering work was in three major areas: (i) in 1859–61 he introduced a system of hygiene which (for 8 years) eliminated cholera from a circumscribed area by preventing water pollution by infected 'cholera discharges' (in much the same way that John Snow had done a few years earlier in London (chapter 1)) (ii) he introduced into India the humane treatment for the insane (his measures went beyond those which were currently in operation in Britain)[20], and (iii) in 1886 he instituted (throughout the Presidency of Madras) the systematic medical inspection of schools.

The last of the Indian pioneers to enter into this account is Sir Charles Lukis. He qualified in medicine from St Bartholomew's Hospital, London, entered the IMS in 1880 and subsequently became Director-General. As well as his outstanding scientific ability, he was 'a wise and far-seeing administrator'[1]; he did much to advance hygiene in India. He was largely instrumental in developing research opportunities and was described as a 'foster parent' to the Calcutta School of Tropical Medicine (chapter 8). According to Balfour, he 'wielded an excellent pen'[1].

Early contributions to medicine in Africa

A superb contemporary account of the living conditions, morbidity and mortality encountered by the indigenous population of Sierra Leone which was published in 1803[21] was written by Thomas Winterbottom[3]; his name is most widely linked with cervical lymphadenopathy in *Trypanosoma gambiense* (sleeping sickness) infection (Winterbottom's sign). Another account of the problems facing Nigeria's indigenous population in the nineteenth century has also been provided[22]. British pioneers in Africa were far fewer numerically than those in either India or the Caribbean. Conditions were more hazardous than elsewhere, the range of unknown diseases being far greater[21,22]; British colonisation therefore came later. Yellow fever was a particular threat to the European (fig 2.1)[2,23,24]. Whereas in the Caribbean and India, the colonialists had introduced new diseases (eg sexually transmitted diseases)[14], it seems unlikely that they contributed significantly to Africa's problems. British pioneers went to Africa for largely different reasons. They were not there solely to protect the health of British soldiers, and the servants of the Raj. In some cases, missionary zeal had a great deal to do with their sojourn. Table 2.3 lists the names of a few remarkable individuals.

Without doubt David Livingstone (Plate 9) remains the best known of

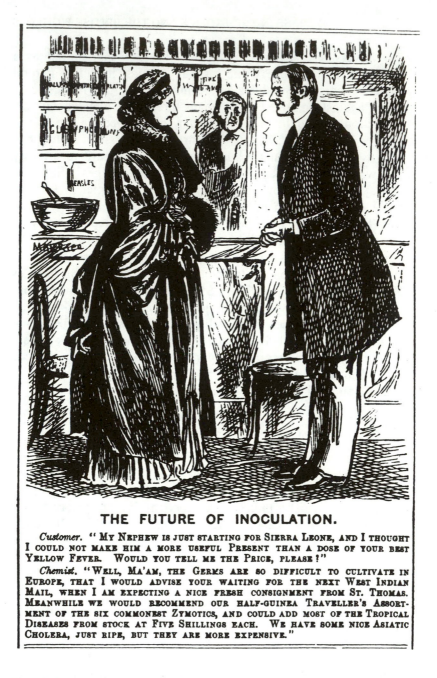

THE FUTURE OF INOCULATION.

Customer. " MY NEPHEW IS JUST STARTING FOR SIERRA LEONE, AND I THOUGHT I COULD NOT MAKE HIM A MORE USEFUL PRESENT THAN A DOSE OF YOUR BEST YELLOW FEVER. WOULD YOU TELL ME THE PRICE, PLEASE !"

Chemist. "WELL, MA'AM, THE GERMS ARE SO DIFFICULT TO CULTIVATE IN EUROPE, THAT I WOULD ADVISE YOUR WAITING FOR THE NEXT WEST INDIAN MAIL, WHEN I AM EXPECTING A NICE FRESH CONSIGNMENT FROM ST. THOMAS. MEANWHILE WE WOULD RECOMMEND OUR HALF-GUINEA TRAVELLER'S ASSORTMENT OF THE SIX COMMONEST ZYMOTICS, AND COULD ADD MOST OF THE TROPICAL DISEASES FROM STOCK AT FIVE SHILLINGS EACH. WE HAVE SOME NICE ASIATIC CHOLERA, JUST RIPE, BUT THEY ARE MORE EXPENSIVE."

Fig 2.1: Prospects for vaccination in the nineteenth century [*Punch* 1881; 19 November: 230]: it was still some 50 years before a satisfactory vaccine against yellow fever was to be introduced.

Table 2.3 Some early British contributors to medicine and/or public health in Africa

LIVINGSTONE, David*+	1813 - '73
BOYLE, James	18(?) - 18(?)
KINGSLEY, Mary	1862 - 1900
SLESSOR, Mary*	1848 - 1915
McGREGOR, Sir William*	1846 - 1919

[* Born in Scotland; + Fellow of the Royal Society]

the early missionary doctors in Africa[3,25,26]. In his presidential address to the Royal Society of Tropical Medicine and Hygiene in 1925, Balfour considered:

> There is no need to tell [his] story, which now-a-days has found its way into the film world and provides an infinitely better subject than half the trash which thrills a decadent public.

Livingstone was born at Blantyre, Scotland and educated at Glasgow University; he personally financed his early education whilst working at a cotton factory. After entering the service of the London Missionary Society (LMS), he studied medicine in London, and embarked as a missionary for the Cape of Good Hope. Livingstone made journeys 'into the interior' in 1841, 1842 and 1843; he 'discovered' Lake Ngami in 1849, and the Zambesi in 1851. After further travels he visited England in 1856, and was awarded a DCL by Oxford University. His connections with the LMS were severed in 1857. After further travels in Africa, he again visited England in 1864, and published *The Zambesi and its Tributaries*. Back in Africa, he reached Ujiji, where he was rescued in 1871 by H M Stanley. He subsequently made further expeditions in order to discover the source of the Nile and died at a village in Ilala (now in Zambia). His body which was conveyed to England by his servants was subsequently buried in Westminster Abbey, in 1874. Arnold considers, rather unsympathetically, that he offered a way to rescue Africa from its suffering state, 'civilise it', and prepare it for the blessings of Christianity[14]. Be that as it may, Balfour considered, probably correctly, that Livingstone tends to be categorised as a missionary or explorer rather than as a physician and pioneer in tropical medicine[1]; his account of the tsetse fly *Glossina morsitans* was accurate, as was his description of *nagana* (animal trypanosomiasis): 'throughout his writings there is evidence of the trained scientific observer. . . . He opened up tropical Africa, not only to the missionary, the trader, the soldier, and the administrator, but to the scientific enquirer, and, more especially, the

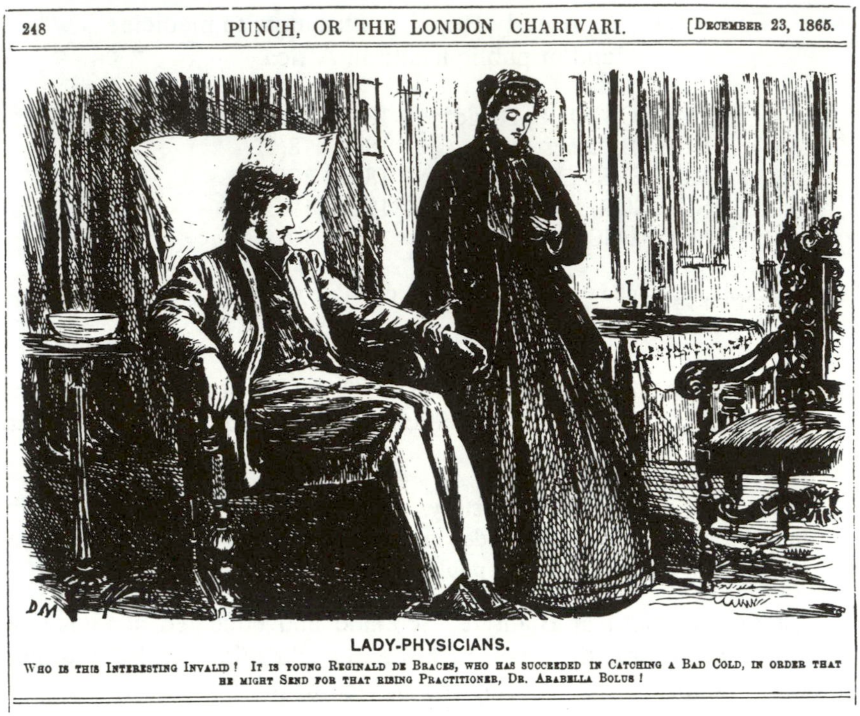

248 PUNCH, OR THE LONDON CHARIVARI. [December 23, 1865.
DM
LADY-PHYSICIANS.
Who is this Interesting Invalid! It is young Reginald de Braces, who has succeeded in Catching a Bad Cold, in order that he might Send for that rising Practitioner, Dr. Arabella Bolus!

Fig 2.2: Cartoon referring to the first women medical practitioners in England. [*Punch* 1865; 23 December: 248].

tropical diseases expert. . . . He did more than anyone to bring the Dark Continent into the limelight, and for that reason alone deserves a place amongst our pioneers.'

James Boyle worked in Sierra Leone (following a period in India), and published a monograph (with a rather long title) on the topography, causes, symptoms and treatment of the fevers he encountered there; this was published in 1831[1]: *A practical medico-historical account of the western coast of Africa: embracing a topographical description of its shores, rivers, and settlements, with their seasons and comparative healthiness; together with the causes, symptoms, and treatment, of the fevers of western Africa; and a similar account respecting the other diseases which prevail there.*

There were no women amongst the early pioneer doctors; this is not surprising because medical graduation in Britain did not begin until 1865; Elizabeth Garrett Anderson was the first woman to obtain an English diploma – the LMSA[27]. Fig 2.2 refers to this historical event. However, two outstanding non-medical women made substantial contributions in west Africa. Mary Kingsley[3,28,29] was fully aware of the extent to which the unhealthiness of the West Coast hampered progress; she did much 'to dispel the apathy with which [Britain's] West Coast Colonies were regarded, and drew attention to the absolute necessity of taking steps to lessen their morbidity and mortality[1]'. Her book *Travels in West Africa* was published in 1897. She died of enteric fever at the relatively early age of 38 years[3]. But her contributions to preventive medicine had a profound effect in the early days of the Liverpool School of Tropical Medicine (chapter 7) and her reputation persists there today. Mary Slessor (Plate 10) was a Christian missionary. This truly amazing woman began life as a poor factory girl in Scotland, and pursued her life throughout with genuine missionary zeal. She lived and worked in Calabar, eastern Nigeria for 39 years where she dissuaded the indigenous population from many local superstitions and deadly practices, attempted to prevent infanticide, and introduced various humane techniques. She was a pioneer in health education and was known locally as Ma Akamba (the 'Great Mother'); Sir Frederick (later Lord) Lugard (the great colonial administrator) wrote of her death as 'a great loss to Nigeria'[1].

In many respects the greatest and most remarkable of the early African pioneers was Sir William McGregor[1,3,30] (Plate 11). As well as being a medical scientist, he was another great Colonial Administrator. He was born at Fowie, Aberdeenshire, the son of a farm labourer. He read medicine at Anderson College, Glasgow, and graduated at Aberdeen University. After house appointments he sailed in 1873 to the Seychelles as Assistant Government Medical Officer; following this he moved to Mauritius, and a year later became Chief Medical Officer in Fiji. At this point in his career he turned to administration and became in turn High Commissioner and Consul-General for the Western Pacific, Administrator (and later Lieutenant-Governor) of British New Guinea, Governor of Lagos, Governor of Newfoundland, and finally Governor of Queensland; he retired in 1914. MacGregor was a teetotaller and did not smoke. Every night he read from his Greek Testament; he was also skilled in French and Italian and 'knew something of many 'barbarous tongues''[1]. In addition he was a mathematician, surveyor, lapidary, and a master of many arts. His particular medical contribution was to advance the cause of 'tropical medicine' (especially hygiene) in the colonies in which he served; from a very early stage he recognised the necessity for the provision of facilities for training the *natives* in medicine[1]; in this he took the lead in Fiji. Sir Ronald Ross who formed a rather special relationship with him later (chapter 8) wrote of him: 'he recognised the superlative value of sanitation in the development of a colony and was, I think, the only high British official who ever grasped the real importance of the general anti-malaria schemes which I proposed in 1899'.

Table 2.4   Some other British medical personnel who made important contributions to the diseases of warm climates

PRINGLE, Sir John*+	1707 - '83
LIND, James*	1716 - '94
NIGHTINGALE, Florence	1820 - 1910
DAVIDSON, Andrew*	1833 - 1918
MANSON, Sir Patrick*+	1844 - 1922
ROSS, Sir Ronald+	1857 - 1932

[* Born in Scotland; + Fellow of the Royal Society]

Other early contributors to tropical medicine

By no means all early contributions were made by doctors actually working in the tropics. Jenner's contribution to smallpox control[15], and Snow's with regard to cholera[2] are examples which have been cited in chapter 1; neither of these pioneers ever left the shores of England but their contributions were of monumental importance to medicine in the tropics. Similarly, Sir Christopher Wren, FRS (1632–1723)[3] – better known for his architectural contributions – should be given due credit for demonstrating the value of intravenous rehydration in a series of animal experiments; prior to the recent introduction of oral rehydration regimens this formed an essential technique in the management of cholera and other acute tropical diarrhoeas. In India in 1838, the accepted (but somewhat impractical) method used for rehydration was 'to inject saline . . . into the vein from its having been discovered by chemical tests that the serum of blood in cholera patients is deficient in some of its natural saline ingredients'[1].

Table 2.4 summarizes some other individuals who made substantial contributions to medicine in the tropics. Two great men who served in the Army and Navy respectively – Pringle and Lind – provided major literary contributions. In Balfour's words: 'In our island story war has usually meant service abroad, frequently in hot climates'[1]. Sir John Pringle[1,3,9] (Plate 12) was born at Stobs, Roxburghshire, and educated at Edinburgh and Leyden. He was a Professor in 'non-medical subjects' at Edinburgh University and practised as a physician in that city; he moved to Flanders with the Earl of Stair, and later became Physician-General to His Majesty's Forces in the Low Countries (and Physician to the Royal Hospitals there). Later he served in Scotland with the Duke of Cumberland but afterwards returned to the Army, on the continent. Pringle eventually settled in London where he became President of the Royal Society. He was apparently a great leader; he was 'opposed to indifference, ignorance, and barbarity', and had (according to Balfour) to 'grope his way in the dark and trust largely to the results of his personal observations in the field'[1]. Pringle's *magnum opus Observations on the Diseases of the Army* ran to seven editions; it is one of the classics of medicine and contains numerous clinical descriptions of tropical diseases, including malaria, dysentery, typhus, and influenza. 'He traced a connection between foul straw, filthy privies and dysentery, discoursed on climatology, pleaded for ventilation and cleanliness, and did not forget to deal with . . . a most important branch of army hygiene . . . the rationing and diet of the soldier'[1]. At a clinical level, he apparently favoured bleeding before the 'exhibition of bark [cinchona]' in the management of malaria; in Balfour's view 'anyone who has passed through the furnace of a severe attack of acute malaria, with throbbing temples, congested face, and splitting headache must, I think, have felt that a little 'tapping of his claret' might have brought relief'[1]. James Lind[1,2,3,31,32] (Plate 13) was the founder of naval hygiene; he had one important advantage over Pringle, ie, he actually served in the tropics; moreover, he had many sailors with tropical diseases under his care whilst he was a physician to the Royal Naval Hospital, Haslar. Balfour considered that he did for the Navy what Pringle had done for the Army. Lind joined the Naval Medical Service at the age of 23 and spent most of the next 10 years on the Guinea Coast or the West Indies; in 1758 he was appointed Physician at Haslar. His major literary contributions were on tropical hygiene, and scurvy. His *Treatise on the Scurvy* was published in 1753, and the *Most Effectual Means of Preserving the Health of Seamen* in 1757. These monographs were followed by a third book: *An Essay on Diseases incidental to Europeans in Hot Climates, with the Method of preventing their fatal Consequences*, which was published in 1768[2].

Florence Nightingale (Plate 14)[1,3,9,33,34] revolutionised army nursing (and indeed nursing in general); she campaigned against insanitary conditions – in which 'cholera, enteric fever, and dysentery ran rife' – and made ceaseless efforts to improve the hygienic state of the British soldier both at home and abroad. She wrote: *Observations on the Sanitary Conditions of the British Army in India* in 1863. She considered that her work was not only a noble task; it was nothing less than 'creating India anew'. Arnold[14] considers that she 'saw the creation of a public health department for India as part of a mission to bring a higher civilisation into India'. Much of her best known work was carried out in the Crimea and at Scutari, Turkey.

Andrew Davidson was without doubt the best known physician in tropical diseases in England before Patrick Manson set up in London following his years in South-east Asia (chapter 4). He was born at Kinneff, Kincardineshire, graduated at Edinburgh University, and in 1862 sailed to

Madagascar as Resident Medical Officer to the Royal Court; he produced a book on the diseases of Madagascar, established the first hospital there, and produced text-books in Malagassy for the indigenous medical students. In 1877 he moved to Mauritius; here, he carried out investigations into rinderpest, malaria and leprosy. After leaving the Colonial Service, he became Medical Adviser to the Crown for the Colonial Office in Scotland, and was appointed lecturer in Tropical Diseases at Edinburgh University. He wrote: *Geographical Pathology*, and *Hygiene and Diseases of Warm Climates*; the latter was superceded by Manson's great textbook published in 1898 (chapter 4). Balfour considered it 'conceivable that the work of Davidson paved the way in some measure for the establishment of Schools of Tropical Medicine in this country'[1].

Two major pioneers – who are automatically associated with the London and Liverpool Schools of Tropical Medicine respectively – were Sir Patrick Manson (chapter 4) and Sir Ronald Ross (chapter 8); their lives will be related later. However, as Balfour has aptly emphasised, a vast amount of observation and writing had preceded them, and as this chapter shows, understanding of the diseases of the tropics by British doctors and scientists had slowly evolved over several centuries; indeed some of the most important diseases were of course known to Hippocrates. By including scientific personnel amongst his crew, the voyages of James Cook, FRS (1728–79) had ensured that a practical knowledge of newly discovered parts of the world could match the progress in England[35]. Numerous achievements in medical progress during the nineteenth century were dependent on the existence of the British Empire[14]; this was the great catalyst for many pioneering achievements. By the closing years of the century, medicine had become a means of demonstrating the superior political, technical and military powers of the West (the 'innate superiority of the European'). It was perhaps a celebration of Imperialism itself[14]!

3

The Seamen's Hospital Society

The Foster Mother of Tropical Medicine in London
Philip Manson-Bahr (1881–1966)

When the Napoleonic wars ended in the early nineteenth century, England was on the threshold of a lengthy period of peace and prosperity. Seamen left their ships to return to their families, find alternative jobs, or to join other ships. However, the Industrial Revolution was in full swing and whole families had moved to find work in growing industrial areas; as a result, many seamen were unable to trace their families and homes[1]. The cramped and unsatisfactory conditions under which seamen worked on board ship around this time have been well described[2]. Now, mariners were no longer desperately needed, and even if they were to find a ship they were paid a mere fraction of their war-time wage. Therefore, a social problem of substantial magnitude surrounded the lot of mariners who had experienced disease or injury in the long struggles against the French; many were both without work and were also homeless; they could be found wandering, friendless, around the streets of London. They faced an untimely death resulting from physical handicap, chronic disease (syphilis was then a major illness), and poverty; no provision had hitherto been made for the relief of their suffering.

In the realisation that the nation had a responsibility for these men who had served her so well, and defeated Napoleon, a group of philanthropists – which included William Wilberforce (1759–1833) and Zachary Macaulay (1768–1835) – conceived, in 1816, a plan to establish a hospital which would be devoted to the care of these seamen[1]. [Wilberforce is of course best remembered for his role in the anti-slavery campaign[3].] A Marine Charity was formed in the winter (which was apparently a particularly severe one) of 1817–18; the general public contributed to the fund which had been launched to provide temporary relief for these distressed mariners. A plan was formulated to establish a hospital solely for merchant seamen; they were to be treated during their illness, and assisted in finding employment on other ships after discharge from medical care. On 8 March 1821 the first meeting of the Committee of Management of the Seamen's Hospital took place

33

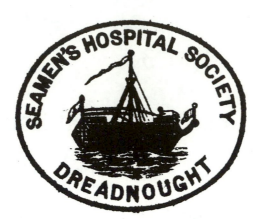

Fig 3.1   The seal of the SHS – which remains in use as the 'letterhead' today.

at the 'City of London Tavern'; this date has since been observed as Founder's Day. It was also in fact a very significant day for the future development of *tropical medicine* in London, for many of these seamen brought with them infections (and other diseases) from the tropics and subtropics. It is not surprising therefore that the resultant Seamen's Hospital Society (SHS) has been called the 'Foster Mother of Tropical Medicine'[4]. Fig 3.1 shows the seal of the SHS. The first minute book of the SHS reads[5]:

> At a Meeting at the City of London Tavern, This Day (the 8th of March 1821) for the purpose of establishing, by public Voluntary Subscriptions, a Floating Hospital, for the Assistance and Relief of Sick and Helpless Seamen, under the Patronage of His Majesty.
> The Right Reverend the Lord Bishop of Chester in the Chair.
> The Reports of the Committee for the Relief of distressed Seamen was read; on which it was Moved by William Wilberforce Esq, MP and Seconded by The Earl of Rocksavage . . .

Amongst others present at that meeting were: Lord Ellenborough; Rear Admiral Sir Edward Codrington; Thomas Wilson Esq, MP; Will[m] Taylor Money Esq, MP; The Honble Sir George Grey, Bart; Rear Admiral Spranger; the Right Honble The Earl of Darnley; the Honble Capt[n] Waldegrave RN; Tho[s] Rowcroft Esq, and Sir George Keith.

The meeting agreed: a 'Provisional Committee for framing Rules and Regulations for the government of the said Hospital, with authority to add to their numbers, who shall fix a day for a General Meeting of Subscribers, for the election of a Committee, for the promotion and management of the Interests and Concerns of the Charity.'

This consisted of: John W Buckle Esq; Aaron Chapman Esq, Captain C C Owen, RN; Sir John Will[m] Lubbock, Bart; John Deacon Esq, and George Lyall Esq. William Williams Esq, MP, was elected treasurer.

This committee laid before a General Meeting on 11th April 1821 the 'Rules and Regulations for the Government of the Society prepared by them'.

From the outset, Royal Patronage was forthcoming; in 1821 His Majesty King George IV (1762–1830) accepted an invitation, and by 1833 the Vice Patrons included: His Imperial Majesty The Emperor of all the Russias, and Their Majesties the King of Prussia, the King of Denmark, and the King of the Belgians. The minutes of an early meeting also contain the following observations[1]:

> sailors in general are bred up to their occupation from early youth and retain few of the habits of persons employed on shore. Their great failing and principal occasion of all their misfortunes is an almost total absence of foresight and consideration for the morrow. They appear to have no conception of the possible approach of misery until it is too late to escape it and when at length they become subject to its visitation they are appalled and sink beneath its weight. If informed of or directed to hospitals, asylums, or other places of relief ashore which do not bear the name 'Seamen's' they are unwilling to approach them and will submit to be driven to such receptacles only by extreme misery. A sailor, rather than repair to an hospital on shore will strip almost the last rag off his back for the means of obtaining a cure; it is well known to every person acquainted with the habits of these peculiar beings that they will at any time prefer to remain on board their ships, even approaching death, rather than consent to be taken to an hospital on shore, although with the prospect of returning health.

Following the first meeting, the Admiralty agreed to loan a disused 48-gun ship (a stores ship) for use as a floating hospital. During the period in which the *Grampus* (Plate 15) (the first of the hospital-ships) was fitting out the Charity agreed to render assistance to any sick seaman who requested it; for this they used a house in Wapping which was loaned by the London Dock Company. On 11 May 1821, a temporary hospital was opened at the Farm House at Stepney Green; a Medical Officer attended three days each week, and seriously ill patients were transferred to the (now Royal) London Hospital. 171 patients were apparently 'relieved' at this establishment[1]. Ten patients remained there when the transfer to *Grampus* took place. Now converted for use as a hospital ship (repairs and alterations had been carried out at Deptford

Yard and took many months to complete), HMS *Grampus* was moored off Greenwich in the most central and suitable position in the Port of London; this site was considered the most convenient one on the Thames for taking sick men from their ships as they passed upstream. On 19 October 1821 the ship, victualled by Seamen's Hospital funds (the bedding and linen having been provided by the Royal Naval Hospital, Haslar) was ready to receive patients; they boarded her on 25 October. The lower decks were used as wards, whilst the top deck was fitted with canvas shelters for convalescent patients. There was accommodation for 181 patients and the two low-ceilinged wards were lighted by whale-oil burning lamps. Surgical operations were undertaken on the lower decks and were sometimes carried out by candle-light. Rowing boats were provided to convey patients, staff and visitors to and from the shore. In 1821, the staff consisted of a Superintendent (Lieutenant Somerville), Surgeon (Mr Arnott), Steward and Clerk, Boatswain and Carpenter, 2 Boatswain's Mates, 3 Nurses, a Cook and a Washerwoman. In addition, Dr Halliday (Domestic Physician to HRH the Duke of Clarence), Dr Mackintosh, Dr G E Jones (Visiting Physician), and Mr Vance (Surgeon to Greenwich Hospital) offered their services free. A Chaplain, The Reverend David Jones, went aboard each day. Rations consisted of 14oz bread daily, ½ lb butter weekly, 6oz cheese weekly, meat on 3 days each week (½ lb when dressed with vegetables), gruel for breakfast, and 2 pints of beer daily. During 1821, 413 patients were admitted of whom only 3 died[1]; only 14 however seem to have been cured *and* discharged to their own homes. Subsequent numbers of admissions, with outcome, can be found in Appendix 1. In 1831 the nursing staff (all male) was increased from six to nine in number, and they were joined by 'a man for night-duty, who shall undertake the work of barber'.

As a general rule, patients requiring hospital care at that time had to be 'sponsored' by a member of the Board of Governors of a general hospital; this stipulation was however not applied on the *Grampus*. Any sick or injured seaman was immediately received on presenting himself alongside, and *without* a letter of recommendation. His apparent condition, together with the fact that he voluntarily sought medical assistance were considered adequate grounds for his being taken aboard. No limit was placed upon the length of stay aboard ship. Patients at most hospitals were usually discharged to their homes for convalescence where relations were expected to care for them. This was not possible for most seamen and they were able to remain on board for convalescence until they had completely recovered and were fit to resume work. During this period every effort was made by (i) the seaman, and (ii) the members of the

Committee (who had connections with shipping) to obtain satisfactory employment.*

By 27 September 1822, the work of the Seamen's Hospital had impressed the Board of Admiralty to such a degree that the Lords Commissioners issued a warrant whereby the *Grampus* was authorised to fly the *Jack and Pendant of the Sovereign's Ships*; this was, and remains to this day a jealously guarded prerogative of the Royal Navy[1]:

> Special Warrant issued by My Lords Commissioners of the Admiralty authorising the *Grampus* to wear the Jack and Pendant of the Sovereign's Ships.
>
> 5th October, 1822
Admiral of the United Kingdom
of Great Britain and Ireland etc.
>
> Whereas we think that the *Grampus* used as a Seamen's Hospital in the River Thames shall be allowed to wear an Union Jack and Pendant while she is so employed, or until further orders. We do hereby authorize you to hoist an Union Jack and Pendant on board the *Grampus* and to wear the same whilst she is so employed as above mentioned or until further orders, accordingly, and for your wearing the said Jack and Pendant this shall be your Warrant.
>
> Given under our hands and the Seal and
of the Office of Admiralty,
the 27th day of September, 1822.
(signed) J. Osborn
G. Cockburn
>
> To the Superintendent of the *Grampus* used as a Seamen's Hospital in the River Thames
>
> By command of their Lordships
(signed) John Barrow

By 1824, 3369 patients had been treated; the figure totalled 1481 in 1825 alone.

The second report of the Charity (issued in 1823) confirmed the value of the service(s) provided on board *Grampus*[1]:

> The Committee would observe that upon its first establishment, the complaints of many of the objects admitted were so far advanced as to place them almost beyond the reach of medical skill; whereas the greater number of cases in the past year have been in a much earlier state of

---

* Since 1821, a mariner has continued to be able to seek medical advice at any of the SHS hospitals without the formality of a doctor's letter. To this day the SHS sponsors two wards at St Thomas' Hospital, London.

sickness which can only be attributed to the more general knowledge of the Charity, and the facility with which seamen of all nations are received on board the *Grampus*.

However, life on *Grampus* was clearly not without medical 'politics'. The following anonymous note appeared for example in *The Lancet* for 1828[6]:

A Subscriber suggests, that great caution should be exercised in electing a surgeon to the Hospital Ship 'Grampus', as the late surgeon sent his 'lithotomy cases' to the London and other Hospitals.

This brought forth the following rather irate reply[7]:

To the Editor of The Lancet.

Sir, – I am authorised to request the favour of your inserting the following fact, in answer to an anonymous, false, and malignant statement, which appeared in THE LANCET of the 11th inst., reflecting upon the surgical practice of the Grampus Hospital Ship: the only case of stone in the bladder, received on board the Grampus, was under treatment in the last summer, and removed by the express desire of the parents of the patient (contrary to the wish of the surgeon), to St. Thomas's Hospital, for the purpose of undergoing the operation; he has since left St. Thomas's Hospital, without the operation having been performed, constantly refusing his consent to undergo the same, both on board the Grampus, and at St. Thomas's Hospital. I am, Sir,

R. HARLEY, Secretary [SHS].
19 Bishopsgate Within, Oct. 22, 1828.

In 1832 a very significant event occurred: a member of Lloyds of London – Mr John Lydekker, died from cholera and left in his Will four vessels of his fleet, which had returned from the Far East, together with their cargoes, for the benefit of the Seamen's Hospital[1].

London July 23rd, 1832

. . . all the residue of my property after paying the aforesaid legacies I give and bequeath to the Trustees of the Seamen's Hospital Ship for the Sick and Diseased Seamen in the River Thames.

John Lydekker

The proceeds amounted to the vast sum of £55,000 which gave the Charity much needed financial stability. Details of subsequent donations, receipts, and expenditure during the hospital-ship days can be found in Appendix

1. On 6 May 1833 the Charity formally took the title of the *Seamen's Hospital Society* (incorporated by an Act of Parliament), and the terms of reference were: 'for the charitable relief of sick and distressed Seamen of all Nations in the Port of London and for providing them with medical and surgical aid, lodging, support and clothing until convalescence and until employment can be again found for them in their meritorious Calling[1]'.

However, the year before Lydekker's beneficence, the *Grampus* had been replaced by a larger ship. The 98-gun vessel HMS *Dreadnought* (Plate 16) which had flown the flag of Vice-Admiral Collingwood (between May and October 1805), and had been commanded by Captain Conn (a distant cousin of Nelson) at the Battle of Trafalgar was taken over in 1831; she had in fact captured the Spanish vessel *San Juan Nepomuceno*. Before her removal to Greenwich, she had been used as a hospital-ship at Milford Haven by the Royal Navy. The conversion cost £2393 18s 7d, and the accommodation was 250 patients and 150 convalescents; this ship was brought into service on 31 October 1831 (and remained in use until January 1857). Cholera became a problem at this time, and the hospital-ships were maintained as isolation hospitals by the Central Board of Health (CBH)[1]. In 1832, the cholera situation on the Thames was so serious that HMS *Dover* was fitted up as a Hospital-ship for the reception of 200 seamen, to join the *Dreadnought* and the *Iphigenia* at Greenwich. By 1835 the CBH decided not to maintain the *Dover* any longer, but because cholera was then so prevalent, the SHS took over the ship in 1835 and kept it at its own expense. Later, the SHS also took over other ships including HMS *Devonshire* (see below) and the *Belle Isle* – to deal with subsequent cholera outbreaks[1]. A contemporary account of the *Dreadnought* in 1850 is as follows[1]:

Having taken a boat from the pier at Greenwich, I soon reached the landing stage of the Dreadnought. No special order of admission being required, I mounted the gangway and was at once conducted aft by the quartermaster on duty. The neat and orderly appearance of the spar deck was noted. 'All accommodation above the main deck was occupied for general purposes such as the accommodation of officers and for recreation by convalescent patients. Down on the first deck were the Nurses' quarters, hammocks slung for convalescent patients and 'about amidship on the starboard side, is a very complete little chapel. Service is performed here by the Chaplain twice a day . . .' The medical officers' cabins were also on this deck. Below was the hospital proper 'Here in a ward extending fore and aft be some forty or fifty sick sailors from all quarters of the globe [Plate 17].' This was the surgical ward, the medical cases being housed in the middle deck, and on the lowest deck minor surgical cases. 'From this deck (being level with the landing stage) are hoisted through the hatchways all severe cases of accident, many of which arrive from the ship-building yards situated on both banks'. It may be mentioned that all severe casualties are received here, whether the sufferer be a sailor or not.

In 1837 the University of Edinburgh recognised the *Dreadnought* for medical student training in surgery and anatomy[1]; the students also had the opportunity to learn about *tropical* diseases from which many of the seamen suffered. In 1843, one of the assistant surgeons, Mr George Busk*, documented a previously unknown trematode (fluke) in the duodenum of an Indian seaman (a lascar); the organism was documented by G Budd in 1845[8], named *Distoma buski* by Lankester in 1857[9], and subsequently *Fasciolopsis buski*; it was described in detail by T Spencer Cobbold (1828–86) – the foremost parasitologist of his day in 1859.

In July 1840, the ship had sprung a leak and was removed to dry dock (repairs were carried out in 4 days[1]); during this time the patients were removed to Guy's and King's College Hospitals.

In July 1849, the ship was again 'docked and examined, in order that a better provision may be made for ventilating her lower deck'[13]; during this time the patients were transferred to the *Iphigenia*, the late Marine Society's receiving ship. The 1853 anniversary dinner of the SHS was recorded in *The Lancet*[14]:

> The anniversary dinner of the Seamen's Hospital Society, for sick and diseased seamen of all nations in the port of London, was held on Wednesday evening at the London Tavern, Bishopsgate-street, under the presidency of the First Lord of the Admiralty, Sir James Graham, Bart., supported by a company very influential in the mercantile world, most of whom have for many years given their cordial patronage to an institution into which sick seamen of every nation on presenting themselves are immediately received, without the necessity of any recommendatory letters, their own apparent condition being sufficient to obtain their admission. There were about 150 gentlemen present, amongst whom were the members for Greenwich, the deputy master of the Trinity House, Sir James Lushington, John Labouchere, Esq., Richard Green, Esq., &c.

---

* Busk was born at St Petersburgh in 1807, qualified in medicine in 1830, and became Assistant Surgeon on the *Grampus* in 1832; he subsequently became a surgeon in 1839, visiting surgeon in 1854, and subsequently consulting surgeon until his death in 1886. He was to go on to great distinction both as a surgeon and scientist[10]. He was elected President of the Royal College of Surgeons in 1871, and also a Fellow of the Royal Society. He was also Vice-President of the Linnean Society, and a prominent member of several other learned societies. Some of his most interesting scientific contributions incidentally, relate to early descriptions of Neanderthal man[11,12].

The evening passed off with much cordiality of feeling, and the right hon. baronet in the chair promised that if invited next year, whether at the Admiralty or not, he would attend the festival.

Later that year, the *Dreadnought* was joined by a *Cholera ship*; however, on this occasion 'the cholera' was not a vast problem, at least on the Thames[15]:

On Tuesday a quarterly general court of the governors of this charity was held at the offices, 74, King William-street, City. It was announced that the Government had been applied to with respect to 'a cholera ship,' for the purpose of receiving cases of cholera occurring amongst the sailors on the river. To this judicious request the Government has acceded; and her Majesty's ship the *Devonshire* has been granted for that purpose. It is moored near the *Dreadnought*, off Greenwich, and patients are received at all hours of the day and night. As yet there have been but 20 cases, as we are informed, on the river, and the prevalence of the disease is decreasing rather than otherwise, so far as the Thames is concerned. The *Devonshire*, the 'Cholera ship,' has accommodation for two hundred. There are ample provisions in the way of nurses, physicians, &c. It will be remembered that the same course was adopted by this charity when the cholera last visited our shores. On that occasion the ship *Iphigenia* was granted for that purpose, and 250 cases were treated therein. The agents of the society are now also engaged in distributing a medicine found useful and adapted to sailors, gratuitously, at the sailors' homes, Thames church-ship, and other places, that all may have recourse to it when the preliminary symptoms appear. The following notice, too, has been, and is being, profusely scattered up and down the river:–

To Captains of Ships, and Seamen generally. - The committee of the 'Seamen's Hospital Society,' knowing the vital importance of the earliest possible medical treatment, whereby, under the blessing of Almighty God, the progress of the cholera may be arrested, earnestly exhort all captains to send every seaman, on the first symptoms of diarrhoea appearing, on board the Hospital ship, lying near the *Dreadnought*, off Greenwich, which is set apart solely for immediate attention to such cases, and where admission is freely given at any hour.

"By order of the committee,
(signed) "S. KEMBALL COOK", Sec.

This is issued by way of cautioning captains not to detain their men, as is too frequently done, until they are almost beyond the reach of medical skill. In the *Dreadnought*, which is the general hospital of this society, seamen of every grade and nation, whatever their ailment, are unhesitatingly received without the vexatious delay of recommendatory letters. Large numbers are taken from ships entering the Thames after long voyages, and in all cases when medicine can no longer avail, a conveyance is provided for them to their homes, with every comfort needful for the journey . . .

In 1857, 'Dreadnought' was replaced by the third hospital ship, HMS *Caledonia* (Plate 18). *Caledonia* was larger than the *Dreadnought*; she was a 120-gun ship, and had been the flag-ship of Lord Exmouth[1]. Extensive alterations were required and these were carried out in the Woolwich Dockyard under the supervision of the Admiralty at a cost to the SHS of £15,000. The work was completed by 26 January 1857, after which time she was also moored at Greenwich. However, the name of the former vessel was by then so familiar to seamen of all nationalities, and had such a special meaning for them, that the new ship was renamed HMS *Dreadnought*, permission having been granted by the Admiralty. In February 1857, an anonymous writer in *The Lancet* described the demise of the first *Dreadnought*[16]:

> The old *Dreadnought*, so long moored in the Thames at Greenwich, and employed as a hospital ship, is about to give place to another vessel similarly fitted and appointed. The tough old ship, that has 'braved a thousand storms, the battle, and the breeze,' is condemned to demolition, and will be shortly towed away to some nautical knacker's yard, and there broken up. The well-known title will be transferred to the new vessel. Erstwhile its name was the *Caledonia* – selected, perchance, in tender remembrance of the lines of Scott –
>
>   "Oh! Caledonia, stern and wild,
>   Meet nurse for a poetic child," –
>
> though the patients now to be nursed are of somewhat tougher sort and coarser grain. The new *Dreadnought* – 'le roi est mort, vive le roi!' – is already fitted and moored alongside the old ship, than which it is both larger and more convenient. Particular attention has been paid to ventilation, and it contains five decks, which are thus arranged: – The upper or weather deck is appointed for the committee-room and commander's apartments; the main deck comprises a mess-room for the medical and other officers, and the chapel; the surgery and dispensary occupy the gun deck; and on the lower gun decks are disposed the nurses' bedrooms and pathological museum. The orlop or lower deck only is appropriated to patients, an allowance that seems somewhat meagre.

However, this report contained some inaccuracies which were pointed out in a subsequent letter to the Editor[17]:

> SIR,– My attention has been called to the following statement in your paper of the 7th inst., relative to the fitting up of the *Dreadnought* (late *Caledonia*) for this Society's Hospital, in lieu of the present *Dreadnought*: – 'The upper or weather deck is appointed for the committee-room and commander's apartments; the main deck comprises a mess-room for the medical and other officers, and the chapel; the surgery and dispensary occupy the gun deck; and on the lower gun decks are disposed the

nurses' bedrooms and pathological museum. The orlop or lower deck only is appropriated to patients, an allowance that seems somewhat meagre.'

The fact being entirely at variance with such statement, I venture to request that you will give the same publicity to my report, *that every deck is devoted to the use of the patients.*

The Weather Deck will be used by the convalescents for the enjoyment of air and exercise. Seats are there provided for them, and they will be protected by proper awnings when needful.

The Main Deck is screened off on the starboard side as a chapel for Divine worship, and the larboard side, where seventy hammocks can be hung, is appropriated to the sleeping accommodation of those removed from the sick wards as convalescents.

The Middle Deck is set apart for the surgical patients, and (with the beds six feet apart) contains space for seventy beds.

The Lower Deck is allotted to the medical cases, and, allowing the same space, it holds eighty beds.

The Orlop Deck is devoted to venereal cases, and in the same way it admits sixty-five beds.

In the Hold are the furnaces, boiler, &c., for warming the decks, and for hot-water baths, space for 100 tons of coals, besides coke and various store-rooms.

The committee reserve no accommodation exclusively to themselves, as the superintendent is permitted to use the apartment in which they meet.

The officers' and attendants' cabins, the various offices, provision and store rooms, surgery, dispensary, operating-room, baths, lavatories, &c. &c., are placed at the fore and after part of the various decks, as most convenient for the purposes of the hospital.

Such are also the arrangements which have always prevailed on board the present Hospital Ship, although from the larger size of the late *Caledonia* increased advantages are afforded.

The committee are very anxious that the public generally should visit the new hospital, in order to satisfy themselves with the arrangements made for the health, comfort, and convenience of the patients.

I am, Sir, your obedient servant,

KEMBALL COOK, Secretary.
King William-street, E.C., Feb. 1857.

Shortly afterwards the following note appeared[18]:–

THE OLD 'DREADNOUGHT'. – On Tuesday last commenced the sale of this old vessel, which has been used for so many years as a floating hospital off Greenwich. Eighty-five lots of timber, &c., fetched £370. It is computed that her copper will fetch £2000.

The medical staff of the *new Dreadnought* consisted of: two physicians: Dr Barnes and Dr S H Ward; two surgeons: Mr Busk and Mr Tudor; an Assistant Surgeon Mr Croft; and a physician's assistant Mr Corner[19]. Mr

John Tudor recorded 15 operations which were carried out on the ship, but by way of introduction gave details of the hygienic standards on board[20]:

> It may, I presume, be confidently asserted as a general rule, that the mortality following surgical operations does not depend so much upon the operation itself, or the particular mode in which it is performed, as upon the circumstances under which the patient is afterwards treated. The sanitary arrangements of hospitals, both civil and military, have at all periods occupied the serious attention, not only of the profession, but also of that section of the public whose philanthropy leads them to devote their time and means to the prosecution and support of a subject of such vital importance; and upon this topic I beg to offer a few remarks . . .
>
> Upon these grounds, I beg to submit a list of operations performed on board the hospital ship *Dreadnought*, during the year 1857–58. Out of fifteen cases of importance, it will be observed that only one death occurred, and that was of a negro, who had mortification in consequence of a frost-bite of the foot and lower part of the leg. This man, from the first, was of a desponding temperament, and sank from pyaemia a week after the operation. As several of the above cases have already been published, they require but brief notice here.
>
> The ventilation afforded on the surgeons' deck of the *Dreadnought* I hold to be particularly favourable for the treatment of surgical cases, as the admission of air through the port windows – seventeen in number on each side – can be regulated with the greatest facility, according to the state of the weather, and the condition and requirements of the hospital atmosphere. The planking of the deck above is open down its centre, through the length nearly of the whole ship, and to about eight feet in breadth, the space thus included being enclosed in a continuous glass shaft, terminating in five skylights twelve feet square, with lateral sliding doors, on the uppermost or weather-deck. It will be observed that, with the lateral currents from below, a ready outlet, with sufficient draught to ensure a free and continuous passage of fresh air, the force of which can be increased at will by raising or lowering the port windows, is thus secured; and in the early morning, and after the dressing of the patients has been attended to, the entire deck can, as it were, be 'flushed' of its impurities; and I must here remark that these impurities are capable of being greatly diminished by observing the following precautions: – All dressings, where there is any offensive discharge, are invariably saturated with some disinfectant fluid – either the chlorides of zinc, or soda, or Condy's solution, but I am more inclined to favour the former. It appears to me very desirable also, in such cases, to annihilate offensive emanations before they are diffused, by freely disinfecting the dressings as they are removed. I also make a practice of using the chlorine baths to offensive sores, or in case a stump shows a tendency to a foul condition, either from decomposed blood or sloughing cellular tissue: the parts are freely and frequently washed with

the same fluids, by means of a large syringe. In some cases, I find it advantageous to suspend upon strings around a patient's bed rags wetted with one or other of the same solutions.

Another very important consideration is the cleanliness of the wards, more especially the prevention of the collection of flue, the neglect of which is, I am persuaded, more productive of mischief, in retaining infectious material, than almost anything else. This is avoided by carefully sweeping with hand-brooms at least three or four times daily – a duty which is performed by the convalescent patients. I see no objection to the deck being washed with soap and warm water once or twice a week, except the weather be damp and cold, and especially if erysipelas prevails. The ship being heated on both sides with hot-water pipes, of four inches in diameter, the drying process is much facilitated, which greatly diminishes the risk. Again, to prevent contagion being carried by the hands, another constant source of evil, I wash after touching every sore, and this practice I inculcate upon my dressers and nurses.

The number of beds which I have upon one deck for the reception of surgical cases, immediately under my own treatment, is fifty-six, arranged in two rows on either side of the ship, which admits of about six or seven feet between each bed, so that there is no crowding. The height is not more than seven feet between decks, but as the length is 180 feet, and the breadth about forty-four feet, each patient obtains, as nearly as possible, 1000 cubic feet of space.

The general and immediate treatment which I adopt in operations consists in –

First. The most liberal and nutritious diet which a patient can take, and stimulants to any extent which I may consider requisite; at the same time carefully watching the effect, protecting the digestion, and sedulously regulating the secretions in general. I believe it to be a mistake sometimes committed, to change, unnecessarily, the diet immediately after, and for several days following, an operation – a period, according to my judgment, when the patient, from the effect of the shock, is most dependent upon our support, and when, à fortiori, the sustaining powers should be most carefully maintained. And I must here do the managing committee of this hospital the justice to remark, that they implicitly rely upon the judgment of their medical officers. I was surprised to find the high rate of mortality following surgical operations in the Paris hospitals; and from inquiries made on the spot, I am inclined to believe that this might be greatly diminished, by the adoption of a more liberal dietary, and substituting good, sound stimulants in place of the present miserably thin wine given to the patients.

Secondly. I pay great attention to the cleanliness and dressing of the patients, and prefer the dry application, which consists of cotton wadding, unless suppuration becomes profuse or offensive. In the latter case, I invariably substitute lint and 'moist cotton;' the latter, which is common cotton wadding steeped in water until thoroughly wetted, when it can be separated into layers, and cut to any size, forming a very convenient

45

Table 3.1

Summary of the diagnoses relating to 1000 consecutive medical admissions to the 'Dreadnought' hospital ship in 1860, under a single physician[21].

General Disease

Fever - typhoid, 60; typhus, 1; relapsing 2; febricula, 46	109
Ague, 94; hemicrania, 1; ague cachexia, 7	102
Anaemia and debility	40
Rheumatism - acute, 53; chronic and slight, 44	97
Exanthemata - measles, 5; scarlatina, 11	16
Erysipelas	11
Skin diseases	14
Periostitis	3
Anasarca	8
Cholera	1
Opium-eating, effects of	1
Scurvy	96
	498

Thoracic Viscera

Heart and large vessels	23
Asthma	3
Bronchitis - acute, 24; chronic and slight, 42	66
Emphysema	3
Haemoptysis	6
Laryngitis (subacute and chronic)	5
Pleuritis	5
Pleurodynia	1
Pneumonia and pleuro-pneumonia	41
Phthisis	77
	230

Abdominal Viscera

Oesophagus, schirrus of	1
Constipation	1
Colic	5
Diarrhoea	47
Dysentery	56
Dyspepsia	5
Epiploitis	1
Peritonitis	6
Stomach, derangement and disease of	7
Tonsillitis	15
Worms	4
Spleen, disease of	7
Liver, disease of, including cirrhosis and abscess	23
Kidneys, disease of	17
	197

Brain and Nervous System

Cerebral congestion	5
Delirium tremens	19
Epilepsy	10
Insanity	2
Neuralgia	2
Paralysis	24
Spinal debility	1
Sciatica	11
Tetanus	1
	75

and cleanly dressing, and adapted to take up almost any quantity of disinfectant fluid

Lastly. Strict attention is observed in the provision of clean bed-linen, and part of this, as a rule, is changed daily; and in cases where a patient is confined to bed for a long time, I am in the habit of having him changed from one bed to another twice or thrice a week, which, with proper care, can be effected without risk or discomfort . . .

In conclusion, I would remark that the less the medical staff is interfered with, and the more they are trusted and encouraged by the governing authorities of any hospital, so much the better will it be for the patients committed to their charge, and for the credit and reputation of the institution. Indeed, I am persuaded of this, that in any hospital, whether civil or military, the greatest success will follow in the train of that wisdom which confides the most in and meddles the least with those men who devote so great a portion of their time and experience, with much zealous care and anxiety, to the relief of suffering and disease in every shape and form . . .

The following year, Dr Stephen Ward produced a 'breakdown' of the diagnoses of 1000 consecutive cases admitted under his personal care to the *Dreadnought* (table 3.1)[21];

It will, he wrote: 'correct the notion entertained, not only by the public, but by many medical men, that the *Dreadnought* is little better than a 'refuge' for patients suffering under scurvy and chronic dysentery. While it constitutes a peculiar field for the study of organic and blood diseases contracted in tropical climates, and of the behaviour under and relative liability to disease of different races, it also, as will be seen by reference to the subjoined table, affords ample materials for the study of the acute and chronic diseases to be met with in other metropolitan hospitals.

References to reports of some specific diseases can be found in Appendix 2. Some of the practical problems encountered in using the ships as hospitals have been summarized by Manson-Bahr[4]:

Each ship in turn was moored in the most easily accessible and convenient berth that could be found in the Thames, off Greenwich. Soon, however, it became evident that the position of the *Dreadnought* became injuriously affected by the gradually increasing congestion on the river banks on each side. Moreover the din and disturbance proceeding on both sides from the ship-building yards and the incessant clamour which arose both by day and night interfered with the nursing and treatment of patients. Other difficulties were 'obstruction to navigation, the shallowness of the water, and lack of ready access to the shore.' 'So defective was the ventilation system that it led to the spread of infectious diseases among the patients. The opening of portholes produced an icy draught which impinged upon the cots and beds, and in foggy or windy weather they had to be closed so that the conditions within became intolerable. . . . Lack of adequate lighting in the winter months interfered with operations, which had to be undertaken by candlelight.'

By 1865, the committee of the SHS had resolved that 'the use of the hospital-ship *Dreadnought* shall be discontinued, and that a suitable site, with a river frontage, and accessible by boats, shall be procured'[22]. In March 1865, the SHS wrote to Her Majesty's Treasury with a view to obtaining a grant of £20,000 from the unclaimed wages and effects of deceased seamen; this request was refused[1]. Application was then made to the Lords of the Admiralty for the Greenwich Hospital (see below) (which was at that time almost empty) to be made available to the Society; it was considered that because Merchant Seamen had been compelled for many years to pay contributions to the Greenwich Hospital, and from which they had received no benefits, this was a reasonable request. As a result of a deputation to the Prime Minister, the Earl of Derby, on 4 March 1867 agreement to use a part of the Greenwich Hospital was granted[1]. After protracted negotiations with the Lords of the Admiralty, the First Lord suggested on 8 November 1869, that the Society should make formal application to use the Infirmary; this was sent on 15 November 1869. These years seem however to have been ones of considerable uncertainty[23]:

The *Dreadnought* is now empty, and undergoing extensive repairs, the Society having for the time reduced their number of patients, and transferred them, with the medical staff, to the *Belleisle*, which ship did good service in the Thames during the epidemic of cholera two years ago. The *Belleisle* will accommodate about ninety patients, and is a very fair specimen of navy hulks used for the reception of the sick and wounded in time of war. It would, however, be a subject of great regret if the repairs now proceeding on board the *Dreadnought* are likely to lead to a renewal of her lease of existence as an hospital ship. Several years have now elapsed since the Committee of the Society, acting upon the advice of their medical officers, determined to close the floating establishment as soon as a home on shore could be found. It needs no sophistry, and but a very slight acquaintance with the laws of hygiene, to show that this determination, though tardy, was wise, and all those interested in the welfare of our mercantile marine were glad to hear of the projected change, albeit at the sacrifice of the largest floating hospital extant. But to what extent have the Committee of the Society advanced since the shore scheme was broached? They have expended a large sum in the purchase of a site close to the water's edge, and they have petitioned Parliament for money or for a certain vacant wing of Greenwich Hospital, hitherto without success. They cannot build without money, and it is currently reported that no subscriptions will be obtained from shipowners as long as the wards of Greenwich Hospital remain as now, a reproach and a disgrace to the Board of Admiralty. There is now no doubt that the Society should have accepted the quarter originally offered by the Government, and have trusted to their own perseverance and the influence of public opinion for the eventual result; but, under present circumstances, it will be to the advantage of the Society's patients, and the Society itself, that, when the naval medical school is established at Greenwich Hospital, our sick sailors should be received within the walls of that institution for the purpose of affording clinical instruction to the medical officers of the Royal Navy. Such an arrangement, as we have before intimated, would tend greatly to the advantage of that class who form the special clients of this very useful Society.

On 22 January 1870, the Lordships of the Admiralty agreed to lease the Infirmary together with the adjoining Somerset Ward to the Society for 99-years at a nominal rent of one shilling per annum[1]. By March 1870 it was abundantly clear that the ship would definitely be vacated[24]:

The authorities of the Seamen's Hospital Society are actively engaged in preparing for removal, and it is probable that the *Dreadnought* Hospital Ship will be vacated during the ensuing month. Rumours exist that the old vessel is to be utilised as a training or reformatory ship, but we trust that the Admiralty, under the advice of their Medical Director-General, will see the wisdom of not granting her to any Society for such a purpose. It is well known to the professional staff of the *Dreadnought*, both past and present, that, after a ship had been inhabited by the clients of the Society for a certain number of years, wounds did badly, and hospital gangrene prevailed. On this, as well as on other accounts, the 'habitat' of the Society has been changed no less than three times, H.M. *Grampus*, *Dreadnought*, and *Caledonia* having been successively lent by the Admiralty. Any utilisation of this ship (which has now been used as an hospital for thirteen years) for the purposes indicated above is, therefore, strongly to be deprecated.

On 13 April 1870, the patients were moved from the ship to the newly acquired buildings (Plate 19); this removal was apparently accomplished within a 2-hour period[4].

The Cardiff venture

In 1867, *The Lancet* recorded a similar enterprise at Cardiff; a hospital-ship was set up there, also. But, here also, reservations were raised concerning the use of a ship as a hospital[25]:

A SEAMEN'S HOSPITAL SOCIETY has been recently formed at the port of Cardiff, and now has its head-quarters on board the *Hamadryad*, a frigate that was granted by the Government last year, and has received patients within its walls since the beginning of November. From the half-yearly report, compiled by Mr. F. Vavasour, Sandford, the surgeon superintendent, and lately issued, we find that 254 patients have passed through the books of the ship, 102 being classed as medical, and 152 as surgical cases. Among the former are found eleven cases of scurvy. The nationality of patients shows about in the same proportion as that of the seamen admitted into the *Dreadnought*, except that the *Hamadryad* appears to have received a comparatively large number of Austrians. The wisdom of putting sick seamen for treatment on board any ship (and particularly one constantly in dock) is very questionable, but it is satisfactory to know that the rise and progress of establishments such as that represented by the *Hamadryad* indicate an increasing interest in the welfare of merchant seamen.

By 1870, activities at Cardiff seem to have been in full swing, albeit on a far smaller scale than at Greenwich[26]:

The annual meeting of this institution (which is established on board her Majesty's ship *Hamadryad*) took place a few days ago. The Report shows that 1214 cases, including out-patients, have been treated during the past year, at a total cost of £1426. The sanitary state of the ship appears to have been remarkably good, for it was announced by Dr. H.M. Dixon, the resident medical superintendent, that thirty cases only had ended fatally, and that the mortality from fever was but 1 in 38. This result is very satisfactory, though we cannot on that account allow that a ship is by any means a good habitation for the sick. We are glad to record that the Committee acknowledged the services of their medical officer by a cordial and unanimous vote of thanks, a kind of compliment not always paid to the stipendary staff of our public hospitals.

However, this report contained an important error![27]:

To the Editor of THE LANCET

Sir, – Will you allow me to correct an inaccuracy in your report of this hospital in your impression of March 19th. The number of deaths during the year 1869 was only 12 (not 30, as stated in THE LANCET) out of 1214 cases treated by me; and of this number, 6 were cases which died within a few hours after admission. – Yours faithfully,

HALLAM M. DIXON, Medical Superintendent.
H.M.S. *Hamadryad*, Cardiff, March 24th 1870.

A new role for HMS 'Dreadnought'

It was decided, after removal of the patients to the Greenwich Hospital Infirmary, that the *Dreadnought* would continue to play a role in the health-care of seamen; the vessel was in fact to be converted into a convalescent smallpox hospital[28]:

> At the meeting of the Metropolitan Asylums Board* on Saturday, it was resolved to accept the offer of the Admiralty, and to fit up the *Dreadnought* as a Convalescent Small-pox Hospital. We took occasion some six weeks since to refer to a suggestion that was made as to the propriety of utilising the ship as a temporary receptacle for small-pox cases, and pointed out at that time the advantages that would arise on the score of isolation,and the close proximity of the ship to those districts most in need of hospital accommodation. The scheme was propounded about two months ago, but the authorities at Gwydyr House cast cold water upon it, asserting, according the *The Times*, that 'the ship could not give the space required for this epidemic,' though it does not appear that they had ascertained the cubical capacity of the vessel, or that they made any statement whatever as to the number that she was calculated to accommodate. It was, indeed, hastily and unreasonably presumed at the head-quarters of the Poor-law Board that because the old ship had been very properly vacated by the Seamen's Hospital Society as unsuitable for the purposes of a permanent establishment for the sick, she was ill-adapted for the purposes of a temporary hospital during the prevalence of epidemics. We believe that the *Dreadnought* is worth keeping afloat (if cheeseparing proclivities will permit) for this very purpose for some years to come, and hence congratulate the General Purposes Committee of the Metropolitan Asylums Board on their success with the Lords of the Admiralty in obtaining a loan of the ship. The Seamen's Hospital Society having paid dearly for their fittings in 1856, cleared everything away last year, and have left a clean sweep fore and aft. There are four entire decks, varying from 150 ft. to 200 ft. in length, and two, or at all events three, only of these should be occupied by patients. No need exists for any warming apparatus during the next seven months, by which time we may fairly hope that the epidemic will have ceased. Cooling arrangements can be easily constructed under the forecastle, there is abundance of room for nurses and servants' quarters under the poop, and a very large deck space exists for air and exercise. The Committee declare their ability to have the ship ready for the reception of patients a few days from this date, and we shall look forward with interest to the

---

* The *Metropolitan Asylums Board*[29] had been set up in 1867 to provide and maintain hospitals and institutions in London for many branches of medicine, including infectious diseases. Although most of its hospitals were land-based, the majority of smallpox cases were looked after on one of the small-pox boats anchored at Long Reach – 15 miles below London Bridge[29,30].

accomplishment of a scheme that we have consistently and persistently advocated.

The 'Dreadnought' was thus ready to join the other Thames Hospital-ships[30] which were used for small-pox cases, and it was not long before the ship was ready to carry out this entirely new service under the aegis of the Metropolitan Asylums Board[31]:

> The arrangements for the reception of small-pox convalescents on board the *Dreadnought* hospital-ship are fast approaching completion. Cabins have been erected under the poop deck for the accommodation of a medical officer, ward master, steward, watchman &c., and the kitchen range, wash-house, laundry and other offices are built up under the forecastle. The steward's pantry, bread-room, &c., are on the forward part of the main deck, which deck will be used as a dining-room, and will give ample sitting accommodation for at least 200 persons. The middle, lower, and orlop decks are left entirely clear, with the exception of bath-rooms that have been built up forward, and which certainly tend in some measure to mar ventilation. A pipe will be laid along the bed of the river, and communicating as before with the Kent Waterworks, and closets are being erected very much in the same places and on the same principles as those in use when the Seamen's Hospital Society were in possession. We venture to predict that the ship, in this new phase of her existence, will serve a very useful purpose, and the hulk that has been obtained by the Asylums Board should be moored off, or a little below, Woolwich, on the north side of the river. The old *Belleisle* has been lent more than once to the Seamen's Hospital Society, and appeared to serve their purposes very well indeed during the last epidemic of cholera. She would hold at least 100 convalescent patients, and is (or was up to a very recent date) fitted with kitchen-range, water-tanks, &c., on a very large scale. It is a matter of great regret that the authorities of the Seamen's Hospital were unable to anticipate events by twelve months, inasmuch as they might have disposed of their fittings to the Metropolitan Asylums Board, as well as much valuable material that was sold by auction for an absurdly small sum of money. We believe that the *Dreadnought* will be ready for the reception of patients on Monday next.

And, according to *The Lancet*[32], things were working out reasonably well:

> The system of draughting convalescent patients from the small-pox hospitals opened under the auspices of the Metropolitan Asylums Board to the *Dreadnought* hospital-ship off Greenwich, appears to answer particularly well. The inmates now number over 200, but we think the resolution arrived at, to increase the number to 250, a very injudicious determination. There is a fair cubic allowance of air for the patients now accommodated,

all proper deductions being made for the many peculiarities inci-
dent to a floating hospital. We recommend the Metropolitan Asylums
Board to 'let well alone.' The old *Dreadnought* thus far has done
the work allotted to her in connexion with this epidemic exceedingly well, but the addition of another 50 inmates may foul the
nest, so as to make a lazarette of the worst kind out of what is
now a very complete isolated hospital for small-pox convalescents.

But this new role for the *Dreadnought* lasted only a short time[33]:

The 'Dreadnought' Committee of the Metropolitan Asylums Board have
arranged to close the vessel finally for the reception of small-pox
convalescents on the 14th prox [September 1871]. The ship was fitted
up very simply and very quickly in the spring of the year, and was
formally opened on the 8th of May, under the medical superintendence
of Mr. Thomas S. Horsford. A total of 1021 cases have been taken on
board; three deaths only have occurred, and the discharges have averaged
about 50 per week. The general health of the inmates has been excellent.
All the patients have convalesced rapidly, and there can be no doubt
that this floating hospital has in her old age been utilised to very good
purpose. A process of disinfection is being carried out, which consists in
whitewashing the sides and beams, scrubbing the decks with a solution of
chloride of lime, and burning sulphur on all the decks. The Metropolitan
Asylums Board at their last meeting passed a cordial vote of thanks to Mr.
Horsford, who has performed the administrative as well as the medical
duties connected with this hospital with great skill and assiduity. It is the
present intention of the Board to keep the *Dreadnought* for any epidemic
emergency that may arise; and the local authorities of the port of London,
who are now organising a system of surveillance of the shipping, have
obtained possession of the vessel in order to utilise her as a receiving
ship for any cases of cholera that may now or next year occur on board
the vessels in the pool or in the docks.

It was not long (September 1871) before 'the Asiatic cholera' raised its
ugly head again – this time in the Port of London – and yet another new
role for *Dreadnought* was recorded in *The Lancet*[34]:

The Medical Department of the Privy Council appear at last to have
stirred up the local authorities bordering the Thames to some purpose.
A deputation waited on the President of the Local Government Board
on Wednesday, to lay before him certain difficulties under which
the authorities laboured in endeavouring to carry out efficiently the
recommendations of the Privy Council. It was also urged that the
Government should take the matter into their own hands, and not
make the local authorities responsible for that which must benefit the
entire population of the metropolis. Mr Stansfeld discussed the matter

very fully with the deputation, and said that the subject should receive his prompt and earnest attention. Two meetings of the sub-committee appointed by the local authorities have recently been held, at which three important resolutions were proposed and adopted: (1) To place a floating hospital at Gravesend for the reception of cases of cholera; (2) to obtain permission from the Metropolitan Asylums Board to send cases of cholera to the *Dreadnought* hospital-ship; (3) to appoint a medical adviser and superintendent, to conduct an inspection of the shipping lying in the river and the docks, and to inaugurate and carry out such hygienic arrangements as may be required. The Mayor of Gravesend and Dr. Letheby have made arrangements with the Government for the conveyance of the *Rhin*, now lying in the Medway, to moorings at Gravesend when required, and it is stated that she can be sent round in about twelve hours. The Committee, in accordance with their resolution, have obtained leave from the Metropolitan Asylums Board to make use of the *Dreadnought* if required. There are still two districts (those of Rotherhithe and West Ham) the authorities of which object to unity of action, so that these districts will be compelled to provide for their own sick at their own cost. We hope to record next week that the port of London is at all events as well protected against the advance of cholera as the outposts, and hence that, practically, the piecemeal system of sanitary *surveillance*, against which we have so long protested, has ceased to exist.

A proposed decision to sell the smallpox/cholera hospital-ship seems to have aroused little enthusiasm[35]:

The Hackney Vestry have advertised the sale of the temporary hospital for small-pox. We cannot but regard this proceeding as very ill-timed. The question of hospital provision for cholera is still under consideration, and it may be that the vestry will require a similar structure next year. It would therefore have been wiser to delay taking action in the matter until the question of hospital accommodation shall be put on a satisfactory footing. Moreover, the sale of boards and windowpanes salivated with the infection of small-pox is, to say the least, imprudent, if not positively dangerous. Disinfecting processes are at present by no means so certain that they should be relied upon implicitly, whilst a year's exposure to the influence of the atmosphere would certainly reduce the danger to a minimum. On all grounds, we think it would be wise and economical to retain all the temporary small-pox hospitals for at least another year.

On 30 November 1872, the *Dreadnought* parted from her moorings at Greenwich Reach and a famous landmark which had been familiar to countless Merchant Seamen disappeared; this event also marked the end of the first era in the history of the SHS[1].

The land-based hospital

Although the new land-based facilities at Greenwich had certain advantages, there were nevertheless some drawbacks as this *Lancet* reporter outlined[36]:

> ... The Royal infirmary is lavishly furnished with all requisites for hospital administration. There is a splendid kitchen, bathrooms that may almost be called luxuries, a dispensary and adjoining store-rooms that can hardly be surpassed in point of convenience in any British hospital, and an abundance of officers' quarters. The gas and water arrangements are equally complete. But the wards are very small, and, unless some structural changes are made, efficiency will be purchased at the cost of a very large nursing staff. Meanwhile there can be no doubt that our sick seamen will have a far more comfortable resting-place in the port of London than heretofore; and if energy and industry be displayed by the officers of the institution, this hospital should take and maintain a very advanced position in the large list of metropolitan charities; for it must be remembered that, though located at Greenwich, the institution is essentially connected with, and derives its status from, the city and port of London. The Committee of the Society have appointed Mr. S. Kemball Cook, their very able and energetic secretary, to be house-governor; but no change has occurred in the medical staff. The patients of the Seamen's Hospital Society were transferred from the *Dreadnought* to the Royal Infirmary, Greenwich, on Wednesday last, and the new home for our sick seamen of the mercantile marine is now fairly established.

The hospital could accommodate 300 patients in 88 wards – the majority of which contained 3 beds[4]; there was no doubt therefore that conditions for the patients were infinitely better than they had been on the three successive ships.

Plate 20 shows the Greenwich Hospital as it appeared in the eighteenth century. It was founded in 1694 by William and Mary; they had envisaged it as the naval equivalent of the Chelsea hospital, which had been built by King Charles II to house Army pensioners. The first pensioners arrived there in 1705, but the building – designed by Sir Christopher Wren and several contemporary architects – was not completed until 1745. The infirmary, which was situated to the south-west of the Hospital (fig 3.2), was opened in 1767. In 1805 the Hospital was the setting of an extremely important national event: after his death at Trafalgar, Lord Nelson's body lay in state in the painted hall before being taken ceremoniously (amongst a large flotilla of ships) to Westminster and thence to St Paul's Cathedral. By 1814, 2710 pensioners were housed there; however, during the peaceful years following Waterloo the numbers declined dramatically, and in 1869 the Hospital closed. This left the Infirmary, together with the Somerset ward

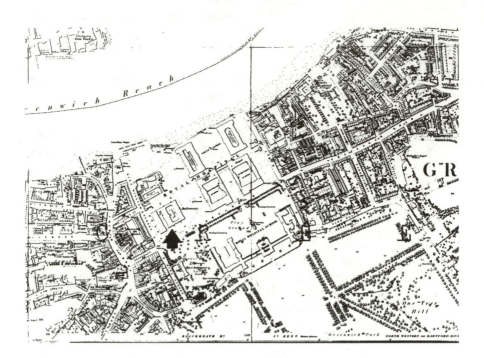

Fig 3.2 Ordnance survey map of 1867 (25 inches = 1 mile) showing The Royal Hospital Greenwich and its Infirmary – arrowed [reproduced by permission of the Guildhall Library, City of London].

(which was also situated to the south-west of the Hospital) unused, and it was these buildings which were to become the new *Dreadnought* Hospital. Plate 21 shows the Greenwich Hospital in 1841 (with the *Dreadnought* pictured in the foreground). In 1873 the Greenwich Hospital became the Royal Naval College; this had previously been housed at Portsmouth.

Once ashore, the SHS medical and nursing staff expanded; the *Dreadnought* now had a Matron and female nursing staff. However, significant administrative problems arose[37]:

> It is very remarkable that, while the great hospitals of the Royal Navy have for the last three years been most satisfactorily worked, under the sole authority of a medical officer in place of the formerly existing captain-superintendent, the Seamen's Hospital at Greenwich should be making progress in exactly the opposite direction, a layman being appointed to supervise the medical men. When the old *Dreadnought* was in use the senior medical officer was the superintendent, and has continued until recently to exercise the same functions. Now, however, when comfortable quarters on shore are added, the Secretary of the Society, who formerly resided in London, has persuaded the old naval officers who rule the institution, and who are no doubt glad to avenge the wrongs of their fellows in the matter of naval hospitals, to appoint

56

him house governor, and to him the medical officers are to be responsible, even (in the case of the juniors) to the extent of asking leave of absence. We are not surprised to hear that such an arrangement has been protested against by the entire medical staff, and that Dr. Swan, one of the house-surgeons, has preferred to vacate his office rather than submit. The whole matter is so preposterous that we feel certain that some alteration must be made if the hospital is not to be deprived of all its officers, for no professional man will submit to such treatment from a lay committee.

This was followed up in a further report[38]:

... [The] resolution, 'that in the absence of the House Committee [composed of old naval officers with some few civilians, but entirely wanting the medical element] the house-governor alone shall be responsible for any departure from the printed instructions laid down for the guidance of the officers of the institution,' it will be seen, placed the entire establishment under the control of the lay governor as soon as the necessity for any deviation from the ordinary routine should arise. In order, however, to understand the resolution more clearly, the whole of the medical staff met, and referred it back to its authors for explanation and confirmation; but no reply was received. Surely the House Committee, as a body of gentlemen, cannot have counted the cost of this decision when applied to their medical officers, whose social position, independent of their high professional standing, forbids them to ask any layman for deviations in the working of the hospital which they alone can comprehend or properly estimate ... We understand that the stipend of the house-governor exceeds that of the whole medical staff, and we respectfully direct the attention of all interested in the Seamen's Hospital to this fact ...

In September 1873, *The Lancet* devoted an entire leading article to the administration and finances of the Seamen's Hospital[39]:

Some twelve months have elapsed since we took occasion to direct the attention of our readers to the administration of the Seamen's Hospital, and to point out several items of faulty or defective organisation. Time has passed on, and changes and events have occurred in this as in all other institutions. But the changes have taken place in the staff, not in the administration; and the events cannot be said to be a source of congratulation to the Managing Committee. For within a space of rather more than eighteen months four medical officers have been dismissed from duty – a fact, as we take it, unprecedented in any hospital in the United Kingdom. A special Committee has been held, convened by the chairman in the absence of the secretary, at which no minutes were taken, and of course none were forthcoming when required. ... The sum of the matter is this – that the Managing Committee of the Seamen's Hospital, unlike most other hospital committees, have not yet discovered the wisdom of consulting the senior members of their medical staff; and until this is

57

done, and done constantly, its members will never get beyond a 'fringe' of knowledge as to the actual internal administration of their hospital.

Following other unfavourable reports[40,41], the matter seems to have been resolved satisfactorily – at least in the eyes of *The Lancet*'s correspondent[42]:

> The Committee of the Seamen's Hospital have commenced a new career of usefulness, and, as we hope, of prosperity. They have given the professional administration of their hospital into the hands of their chief professional officer, they have abolished the obnoxious title of house-governor, and have relegated the secretary to his proper post – that of regulating and improving the financial aspects of this very admirable institution.

[A potentially disastrous fire broke out in 1874[43]:

> The basement of the west wing of the Seamen's Hospital caught fire on Wednesday morning, at about 2 o'clock. Mr. Johnson Smith, the surgeon, and Mr. Duncan and Mr. Tom Pink, the assistant medical officers, were on the spot immediately; and through the exertions of the hospital steward and the fire brigade of the Royal Naval College, the fire was speedily extinguished, though for some time it seriously threatened the safety of the entire building. The cause of the fire is unknown.]

Despite persisting financial problems, the land-based *Dreadnought* Hospital was by 1875 firmly established, and was dealing with the largest number of patients since the *Grampus* was opened more than 50 years before[44]:

> The annual meeting of this Society was held on Wednesday, the 3rd instant, under the presidency of Captain the Hon. F. Maude, R.N. From the report read by Mr. H.C. [later Sir Henry] Burdett, the Secretary, it appears that a total of 2067 patients were admitted during the past year, the largest number received in one year since the hospital was established fifty-four years ago. The total income amounted to £8209, as compared with £9936 in 1873, this marked difference being due, however, chiefly to the small number of legacies received during the past year. The expenditure amounted ot £11,227, as compared with £8968; but this comparative increase is due to the increased cost of coals and provisions, and to repairs and maintenance of the building, which latter, under a special agreement with the Admiralty, constitutes a heavy item of cost every alternate year; and the building is now saddled with a separate assessment, which will entail an additional expenditure of more than £300 annually.
>
> It will thus be seen that, in spite of recent judicious reductions in the working expenses, this institution is in by no means a flourishing state as to funds, although during 1874 more practical good has been done by its

means than in any previous year. We cannot urge too strongly the claims of this hospital on the general as well as the mercantile community. 'How to man our merchant fleets' is now the topic of the day, and a Bill to aid, among other things, this now difficult object has just been introduced into the House of Commons by the Government. But it is poor policy to establish scholarships and train boys for the sea if we are not prepared to lend them a helping hand when they come home to us again debilitated by disease or disabled by storm and shipwreck. We counsel the authorities of this very useful Society to make a special appeal to the public without delay. THE LANCET of the 9th ultimo, in an article on the Marine Hospital Service of the United States, showed that we might take a leaf out of the book of our transatlantic neighbours. But as regards the old *Dreadnought* Hospital, this can hardly be necessary, for it has hitherto had, and we believe always will have, the sympathy and support of all who realise the true source of England's power and prosperity.

But the Charity continued to be underfunded[45]:

The authorities of the Seamen's Hospital have forwarded to us an appeal which has been addressed to the charitable public, but which does not appear to have met with much sympathy or attention from the daily journals. We have always advocated the claims of this hospital to a due share of support, and have pointed out very often and very emphatically that the Society, though housed in Admiralty buildings, receives no financial aid from the Government, and is by no means, as some suppose, a foster-child of the Admiralty. It has worked and won its way with the public up to the present time most successfully, and as we have very lately indicated, the present agitation about ships and seamen should give an impetus to *Dreadnought* subscriptions. Our contemporary the *Pall Mall Gazette* has on several occasions said a good word for this institution, and we are sure that *The Times* and other daily journals are equally glad to lend a helping hand to this hospital, which has been a temporary home as well as an infirmary for sick seamen arriving in the port of London during the last half century

and in May 1876[46]:

. . . The Committee of Governors desire to draw public attention to the fact that since patients were removed from the old *Dreadnought* to the building on shore very few sums have been bequeathed to the Society, and they fear that this diminution in such an important source of revenue is due to an impression that the hospital is now wholly or partially supported by Government. They therefore desire to state that no money is received from such a quarter towards the annual income, but that the Committee are mainly dependent on voluntary contributions. We trust this explanation will be effectual in securing increased support for a most deserving institution.

In seconding the adoption of the annual hospital report for 1878[47]:

> . . . Mr. Macgregor (Rob Roy) . . . dwelt on the fact that the removal of such a well-known object as the old hospital-ship *Dreadnought* would account much for the diminished support of the charity, as the public were not reminded every time they passed up and down the river of the excellent work that was being carried on by the Seamen's Hospital Society. Mr. Macgregor expressed a hope that some means might be devised by which this lost interest might be regained. It is to be desired that some day the liberality of the public will enable the committee to procure a river-side frontage on which to erect a building which will not only serve to attract the notice of the public, but will be more convenient and suitable for hospital purposes than the building at present occupied, which is dwarfed into insignificance by the grandeur of the buildings forming the Naval School, and the small wards of which add greatly to the cost of management . . .

The Lancet continued its very considerable interest in the Seamen's Hospital but became increasingly critical of the quality of the facilities provided in the 'new' accommodation; suggestions for improved services to the sailor are outlined[48]:

> The policy of the managers of the Seamen's Hospital Society is already beginning to bear fruit, and the with-holding of a grant by the Common Council of the City of London shows that at length public criticism is being brought to bear on the conduct of the institution. It appears that the Seamen's Hospital Society holds an invested capital of £112,000, besides the use of the hospital premises rent-free from Government. The hospital is situated in Greenwich, on the side of the river opposite to the docks, and therefore inconveniently places for the reception of sick sailors, who on their arrival in port have to be transported some way round or across the river before they are able to enjoy the rest and comfort which ought to be waiting for them close at hand. To maintain a hospital for sick sailors at a spot where no sick sailors land, is as absurd as it would be to place a casualty Hospital like St. Bartholomew's, for instance, on the top of Highgate-hill. The committee have partly seen this, and have so far condescended to stretch the assistance at their command, as to establish a dispensary where out-patients can obtain medicine without coming an afternoon's journey for it. But this dispensary does not touch the evil of having to transport sailors suffering from acute disease across the river. No wonder that increasing numbers of sailors seized with sudden and severe illness apply for admission at the hospitals on the side of the river on which the docks are situated. Moreover, it is difficult to see why the committee cling so fondly to their present building, seeing it is anything but fitted for a general hospital. Owing to the smallness of the wards, the expense of management and the difficulties of nursing must be in excess of what would be the case in wards of better construction, whilst there can be

no doubt of their being less wholesome. The committee of the Seamen's Hospital love to pose as the friends of 'poor Jack'; but really if they had his interests at heart they would provide him with a hospital better suited for his accommodation, and also place that accommodation near him, so that he might at once find refuge instead of having to seek for it in his hour of need. With a hospital building rent-free, accumulated funds of £112,000, and an obstinate adherence to a position which cannot be of the least value to the sick sailor, we do not think the Committee can make a very serious claim on private charity.

Also with regard to funding, the following notice in *The Lancet* for 1880 is pertinent[49]:

A striking feature in the report of the last year's proceedings of this valuable charity, which has been lately published, shows how grateful the seamen themselves are for the benefits which they and their comrades have received from the present medical staff and their predecessors on board of the old *Dreadnought*. One-tenth of the annual cost of the institution – i.e., a sum of £1200 – has been contributed by the seamen themselves out of their scanty earnings in answer to a hope that collections on board ships would be made in aid of so deserving a charity. The wages of seamen during the past year have been so low, and the number of those unemployed so great, that the response is gratifying in the extreme. In no hospital in London, and probably in none in the provinces, has the class which derives medical attendance and aid therefrom done so much towards maintaining the institution whose object is their welfare and succour. 'Poor Jack,' in one way at least, sets a worthy example to the working-classes on shore, whose wages, as a rule, far exceed his.

Patients continued to be admitted (as they had been during the days of the hospital-ships) with a wide range of diagnoses. The continuing importance of scurvy was stressed[50,51,52]; 'enteric fever (with a mortality rate of about 11%), scarlatina, granular ophthalmia, and parasitic diseases of the skin' were important causes for admission, whilst there was 'a progressive falling off in those applying on account of venereal disease'. The following comments on tuberculosis are of interest[52]:

. . . Phthisis, as usual, figures prominently in the mortality list, and the writer quotes Dr. A.C. Hamlin, of the United States Marine Hospital Service, who considers the prevalence of this disease among sailors to be due to 'constant dampness, foul air, great variations of heat and cold in the sleeping quarters, and improper food.' The report before us records, moreover, a remarkable fact – viz, that among English and American sailors, as well as among foreigners who serve in British ships, the proportion of cases of this disease is very low – in the case of British subjects only 3.2 per cent. But among sailors 'from France and the south of Europe, who seldom serve but in vessels belonging to their own ports, the proportion is very high; with the Greeks and Spaniards, for instance, being 11.7 per cent . . .

The 1879 annual report[53] noted:

. . . The most noteworthy feature in the annals of this hospital for the year 1878 is the decided and progressive decrease in the number of cases of pyaemia. Mr. Smith says: In 1875 the number of deaths from this cause had fallen from 10 to 7; in 1876 there were 6 deaths, in 1877 4 deaths, and in the past year 2 deaths only. Since 1875 there has been but one death from erysipelas. Whilst from 1871 to 1874 inclusive there were 43 fatal cases of pyaemia and erysipelas, and the proportion of these to the total number of deaths from all causes was about 10.5 per cent., from 1875 to 1878 the deaths from the above causes were 20 in number, and the proportion to all the deaths during this period not higher than 4.5 per cent. He attributes this very good result to the antiseptic treatment (Lister's) adopted since 1874, and instances some cases that occurred under the hands of his colleague, Mr. Davies Colley, who has treated venous varicosity in the lower limbs by excising portions of the dilated veins, as well as one interesting operation performed by Mr. Amphlett (as acting surgeon) for the reunion of widely separated portions of fractured patella. We take it that in the later days of the old *Dreadnought* such operations in the surgical and lowest deck of that ship would most assuredly have, so to speak, 'gone wrong' in a pyaemic, gangrenous, or some other mal-hygienic sense. It is proper, however, to record that this sanitary condition of the wards has been, or should be, very much enhanced by sundry improvements in the drainage arrangements that have been made in this Admiralty property by the committee of a charitable institution, at a total cost of nearly £300, £120 having, according to the report of Mr. Burdett, been spent last year, and some £150 in 1875 . . .

A further insight into the disease pattern encountered at the Seamen's Hospital is provided in 1891[54]:

Statistics of Medical Cases admitted into the Seamen's Hospital, 1880–89. – Dr. JOHN CURNOW and Mr. W. JOHNSON SMITH gave an account of the total number of medical cases admitted during the decade, which were 7718. They gave (1) the number and percentage of common diseases, such as rheumatism, cardiac valvular disease, pleurisy, pneumonia, phthisis, and chronic albuminuria; and (2) of the rarer diseases from which sailors in the mercantile marine suffer in greater proportion than residents in this country, such as enteric fever, ague, aneurysms, dysentery, and abscess of the liver. The authors specially called attention to the large number of cases of phthisis (nearly one-seventh of the whole), and believe that with better food and improved ventilation of the sleeping rooms, this could be materially decreased; to the proportion of cases of aneurysm to cardiac valvular diseases, which is as 1 to 3, an enormous excess in proportion to that found among the ordinary population, and which they attribute to syphilis as a factor in the causation as well as to the mere strain of work. Chronic rheumatism, as might have been anticipated from the constant exposure to wet and cold, and from a poor diet, figures very largely. Pneumonia, they stated, is very variable in its incidence, and is always very severe. A very large number of cases die within forty-eight hours after admission, and hence the percentage of deaths is much higher than in ordinary hospitals (37 per cent). Chronic albuminuria is less common than would be supposed from the sailor's habits, but here the long periods of enforced sobriety must be taken into consideration. Enteric fever is still very common, and, like dysentery, is due to the water-supply being infected. In every case, on inquiry being made, it was found that the water had been taken into the ship, or that the patient had drunk water from a source of doubtful purity. The proportion of deaths from both enteric fever and dysentery is very small, especially in later years. The cases of enteric fever are all adults, and often exceptionally severe. The number of cases of abscess of the liver was only nineteen, but of these twelve were fatal. In every case there was either coexistent dysentery or a previous history of that disease. In the present year 1891, one case of chyluria, with filariae in the blood, died in the hospital.

The SHS expands its services

In 1877, the 'Dreadnought School for Nurses' – one of the earliest training schools run on the lines prescribed by Florence Nightingale (chapter 2) – was founded. The SHS later considered that a branch hospital was necessary to provide care for the seamen who entered the Royal Victoria and Albert Docks (sailors from all over the globe were flooding into this vicinity); the latter had been opened in 1880. The foundation stone of this new building was laid on 15 July 1889 (Plate 22). This event was recorded in the *Illustrated London News*[55]:

> Prince George of Wales, attended by Captain Stephenson, R.N., on July 15 performed the ceremony of laying the foundation-stone of a new branch hospital at the Royal Victoria and Albert Docks, in connection with the Seamen's Hospital Society . . .
>
> The accommodation for in-patients at the Greenwich Hospital, with its 225 beds, has for some time past been found inadequate to the needs of the great number of seafaring men in a long stretch of the river far below London, and especially below Blackwall, in the neighbourhood of the Albert and Victoria Docks. There are over 80,000 sailors passing in and out of the Docks every year, and a large population is growing up about Canning Town and in the immediate vicinity of the Docks. Many accidents occur, in which the men injured have to be conveyed a long

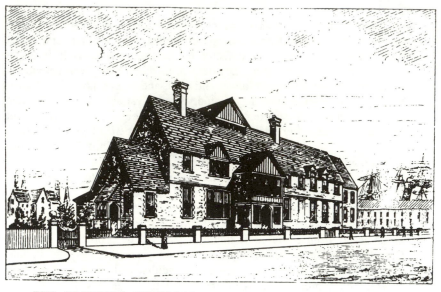

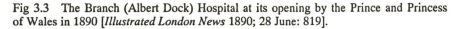

THE SEAMEN'S HOSPITAL, VICTORIA AND ALBERT DOCKS,
OPENED BY THE PRINCE AND PRINCESS OF WALES.

Fig 3.3 The Branch (Albert Dock) Hospital at its opening by the Prince and Princess of Wales in 1890 [*Illustrated London News* 1890; 28 June: 819].

distance, often causing both danger and suffering. The Committee of the Society therefore resolved to establish a branch or auxiliary Hospital on a site close to the Victoria and Albert Docks, and nearly three miles from any other hospital. This branch will contain fourteen beds, and will have a large out-patient department. Arrangements will be made for conveying, by ambulance, convalescent and slighter cases to the Hospital at Greenwich. It is estimated that the cost of the new building will be about £5000, and that it will cost £1000 per annum to maintain. We recommend this object to public support in the shape of increased subscriptions to the funds of the Seamen's Hospital Society.

On 24 June 1890 the hospital was officially opened by their Royal Highnesses, the Prince and Princess of Wales. This event had previously been announced in *The Lancet*[56]:

On the 24th inst., the Prince and Princess of Wales will proceed down the river, by special steamer from the Westminster stairs, to the site of the new branch hospital of this Society, at the Royal Victoria and Albert Docks. The opening ceremony will take place in a commodious shed at the docks, and their Royal Highnesses will subsequently inspect the building. The sanction of the Princess will be asked for a ward to be designated the Alexandra.

The new hospital (fig 3.3) immediately became an outstanding success[57]:

64

Sir Thomas Sutherland presided at the seventieth annual court, held on Tuesday. The report submitted stated that the first branch hospital adjacent to the docks, opened in June last, had been almost constantly full since its opening. The cost of the building and furnishing amounted to £6798, which had to be provided out of capital. During the year the number of patients at the hospital at Greenwich had been in excess of any previous year in the existence of the Society. The dispensaries [see below] also had done good work. Excluding the legacies, the revenue showed an increase of £200. The yearly expenditure of the Society was £13,000, while the reliable income was less than £4000.

This institution was later to form the direct link between the SHS and the discipline of *clinical tropical medicine* which was to emerge later (chapter 7).

Two dispensaries were also established – one at Gravesend and the other in East India Dock Road; they were used as 'clearing stations' for seamen arriving at outlying berths of the Port of London and remained open until 1921 and 1930, respectively. The opening of the latter was recorded in *The Lancet*[58]:

> At a general Court of Governors of this Society held last week, it was reported that the Society had opened a dispensary at 51, East India Dock-road, in consequence of the increasing number of sailors who now congregate in the district. The work of the institution is zealously carried on. The number of patients at the Dreadnought Hospital, Greenwich, and at the branch hospital, Royal Victoria and Albert Docks, had been in excess of any former period, while the patients at the dispensaries were above the average.

The Society's staff-list which was published in September 1892 is of interest in that the name of Dr Patrick Manson (chapter 4) appears for the first time[59]:

> SEAMEN'S HOSPITAL SOCIETY, Dreadnought Hospital, Greenwich, S.E. (235 beds). – Royal Victoria and Albert Dock Hospital, E. (18 beds). Dispensaries: East India Dock-road, E., and Gravesend. This institution is established for the relief of seamen of all nations. Casualties are received at all hours. Apartments are provided in the house of the Principal Medical Officer for students. Honorary Consulting Physicians: Dr. Robert Barnes, FRCP, and Sir Richard Quain, Bart., FRCP. Visiting Physicians: Dr. John Curnow, FRCP, and Dr. John Anderson, CIE, MRCP. Visiting Physician to the Royal Victoria and Albert Dock Hospital: Dr. Patrick Manson, LLD., MRCP. Honorary Consulting Surgeon: Mr. J.N. Davies-Colley, FRCS. Visiting Surgeon: Mr. G. Robertson Turner, FRCS. Principal Medical Officer:

Mr. W. Johnson Smith, FRCS. Ophthalmic Surgeon: Mr. D.S. Gunn, FRCS. House Physician: Dr. M. Spencer, MRCP. House Surgeon: Mr. Arthur Jervis, MB, BS, MRCS. Branch Hospital: – House Surgeon: Dr. C.H. Preston, LRCP. Junior House Surgeon: Dr. Frank L. Wod, Ch.B. Gravesend Dispensary: – Surgeon: Mr. O.R. Richmond. Secretary: Mr. P. Micelli [*sic*].

An interesting change of title of the honorary medical staff, which on the face of it seems of little consequence was announced in 1897[60]:

To the Editors of THE LANCET.

SIRS, – The attention of my committee has been drawn to a letter that appeared in your paper on the subject of the titles of the honorary medical staff of this society, and I am directed to send you the following copy of a minute which was passed on April 10th, 1896:–

'That in future the title of all honorary medical officers' appointed to the branch hospital be Visiting Physician or Surgeon (as the case may be) of the Seamen's Hospital attached to the Branch Hospital: and that in future appointments to the Hospital at Greenwich the title of Visiting Physician or Surgeon (as the case may be) of the Seamen's Hospital attached to the Dreadnought Hospital.'

I am, Sirs, yours faithfully,

P. MICHELLI, Secretary.

Greenwich, Dec. 8th, 1897.

** The letter to which our correspondent refers is probably one which appeared in our issue of Oct. 30th, 1897, under the heading 'Beri-beri and Erroneous Diagnoses.' – ED. L.

More will be heard of this and subsequent correspondence in chapter 6. As will become clear in later chapters, the SHS continued to play a crucial role not only in the care of seamen generally, but in the newly developing discipline – *tropical* (or *colonial*) *medicine*. An 'Upper Deck' for convalescing sailors was presented to the SHS in 1918; Mrs L G Angas had donated her house at Cudham, Kent – and this became the Angas Convalescent Home[1]. The 'King George's Sanatorium for Sailors' was established at Bramshott Place, Liphook, Hampshire in 1921; this was made possible by a fund collected by the first Earl of Inchcape. The 'Passmore Edwards Hospital' at the Tilbury Docks was handed over to the SHS in 1924 (this became the Tilbury Hospital); a 'pavilion' was devoted to Lascar seamen. In order to provide hospital treatment for seamen in a foreign port, a lease of the Queen Alexandra Memorial Hospital, Marseilles, was taken out in 1928; owing to numerous problems – not least the economic climate in Europe around 1932 – this project ran into serious difficulties. The 'Devonport Pathological Laboratory' and 'Devonport Nurses Home' were built in 1929 and officially opened on 15 July 1929 by the Duke of York (later King George VI) (1895–1952) –

President of the SHS – and the Duchess of York. A hostel – 'Nairne House' – was opened directly opposite the *Dreadnought* Hospital in 1951 to provide accommodation for visitors of seamen in the hospital.

The Albert Dock Hospital which was to form the focal point for London's tropical medicine between 1899 and 1920[61], was rebuilt in 1937–38*, and together with the *Dreadnought* Hospital and its various branches remained part of the SHS until they were all taken over by the Ministry of Health under the National Health Service Act, on 5 July 1948. Since 1958, the Society (with the approval of the Charity Commissioners) has been able to extend financial help to any seaman's immediate dependent(s) who is in difficulty because of his illness or death[1]. In 1962, with the co-operation of Trinity House, the 'Dreadnought Nursing Wing' was built at the Trinity Homes, Walmer, Kent. This institution takes care of those officers of the British Mercantile Marine and their dependents who are temporarily prevented by age or illness from looking after themselves at home.

The SHS continues to this day! The administrative headquarters are situated at 29 King William Walk, Greenwich, SE10 9HX; since 1986 the Society has had charge of two wards at St Thomas' Hospital, London, which continue to be devoted to the care of Seamen: 'Any seafarer who works on a ferry, a dredger, a tug boat or supply boat, coastal tanker, water tender or any other specialist craft is entitled to take advantage of the facilities available at the Dreadnought Unit'.

---

* This hospital was to play a major role in dealing with injuries acquired during the bombing of the docks in 1940. At present, it is used in part as a psychogeriatric unit and in part for the mentally handicapped, but its future is undecided.

4

Emergence of Dr Patrick Manson on the London medical scene

Early years in Scotland

Patrick Manson was born of Orcadian stock on 3 October 1844 at Oldmeldrum, some 18 miles north of Aberdeen; the family had long been settled in Aberdeenshire[1-4]. Plate 23 shows his birthplace. His father, John Manson was manager of the local branch of the British Linen Bank, and was also laird of Fingask (an estate which bordered on the town). His mother was Elizabeth Blaikie (a distant cousin of David Livingstone)[4]. He was the second son in a family of nine children (5 sons and 4 daughters). During his childhood he apparently took a more than average interest in natural history, and somewhat later he took to fishing and shooting. In 1857 the family moved to Aberdeen where he attended the Gymnasium school, and subsequently the West End Academy. When aged 15, on account of an interest in carpentry and mechanics he was apprenticed to Blaikie Brothers, ironmasters, in Aberdeen. However, whilst there he developed a 'curvature of the spine' with paresis of the right arm – which necessitated cessation of work and a period of prolonged rest[2]. In 1860 Manson entered the University of Aberdeen to read medicine; he also studied at Edinburgh University during the summer sessions. He qualified in medicine before he was 20, and being too young to graduate he travelled to London to visit some of the medical schools, hospitals and museums. In October 1865, Manson graduated MB, CM and was shortly afterwards appointed Assistant Medical Officer to the Durham Lunatic Asylum, a post which he occupied for a period of 7 months only. Researches on cerebral vasculature, which resulted from a series of post-mortem dissections[2], gained him the MD (Aberdeen) degree in July 1866.

The China Years

An event which was to prove of enormous significance to the development of the future discipline of *tropical medicine* came late in 1866 when

Manson applied for, and was appointed to, the Chinese Imperial Maritime Customs; his elder brother was at this time already working at Shanghai. He lived in Takao, Formosa (now Taiwan) for 5 years, where his duties were to 'inspect the ships calling at the port, and to treat their crews, and also to keep up the meteorological record'[2]; he also developed a private practice (both European and Chinese), and attended a native missionary hospital daily. At that time the European community consisted of 16 individuals, most of whom were engaged in the tea trade. His leisure interests were riding, gardening, bathing and fishing in the lagoon. By the end of his third year there (1869) he was able to repay his father the entire cost of his medical education – £700[2], a filial duty which was frequently carried out in those far off days! The reason(s) he left Formosa is not entirely clear, but it is known that he had become involved with the Japanese political service – whilst assisting China in the purchase of ponies during a Chino-Japanese dispute.

In 1871 he moved to Amoy, a large port (in fact a Treaty-Port) in the Bay of Hiu Tau on the Chinese mainland; here he remained for most of the next 13 years, before leaving for Hong Kong in December 1883. Amoy, which is 1° north of the Tropic of Cancer, had a 'large' European population of 150 who lived, as did Manson, at Koolongsu. As Medical Officer to the Imperial Maritime Customs, he had medical charge of the shipping, and also a hospital for European seamen; he also devoted some of his time to the Baptist Missionary Society's hospital and a Dispensary for the Chinese. Manson, who was a Scottish Presbyterian apparently became involved in a conflict with the missionaries; they felt that he was attempting to turn their hospital into a medical school, instead of 'forging it into an instrument for the spreading of the Christian Gospel'[4]. What was of prime importance to them was 'the winning of souls' and not the advancement of the art and science of healing! Following this he spent most of his time at the Seamen's Hospital in the native quarter. A glimpse of Manson's life-style at Amoy has been recorded retrospectively[5]; 'his appearance of health and vigour [were] more suggestive of a British hunting-squire than of a student on the eve of a discovery that has wrought so much for the benefit of mankind.' He seems to have spent a great deal of time using his rather primitive microscope, and looking after his Chinese patients at the private hospital. He also undertook a good deal of surgery – including many lithotomies. It was here that he invented an apparatus for draining liver abscesses[6]. Leprosy, typhoid, cholera, smallpox, tinea imbricata, malaria and beri-beri were other diseases in which he took a considerable interest[2,4]; he wrote about some of these in a series of contributions in the *Medical Reports of the Imperial Customs* (see below). Some of his other pursuits into clinical investigation have been summarized by Manson-Bahr and Alcock[2]; one of these was 'malabsorption in the tropics', for which Manson first used the Dutch term *sprouw* (then in use in Java, Dutch East Indies) to describe what came to be known as 'tropical sprue'[3,7,8]. Between 1873 and '75 he was joined by his brother David, also a doctor; he unfortunately died of sunstroke in 1878 whilst playing cricket at Foochow[5]. It has been pointed out by his biographers that Manson was intellectually isolated at Amoy[2]; there were no libraries, museums, scientific meetings, or critical colleagues. Nor had he emerged from an academic milieu in Scotland. Rather later (on 27 November 1877) he wrote to (T) Spencer Cobbold (1828–86), the foremost British parasitologist of the day:

> I live in an out of the world place, away from libraries, out of the run of what is going on, so I do not know very well the value of my work, or if it has been done before, or better[4].

and on 20 June 1879:

> . . . Men, like myself, in general practice, are but poor and very slow investigators, crippled as we are with the necessity of making our daily bread[9].

This was therefore a pretty sterile environment in which to undertake clinical research.

Elephantiasis (often with scrotal involvement) was common amongst his Chinese patients, and he subjected some of them to successful surgery; his interest in lymphatic filariasis, which ultimately led to the seminal discoveries for which he is best remembered in a research context resulted indirectly from observations on these cases[1,9].

At the end of 1874, Manson sailed from Amoy for a period of leave in Scotland and England. He attended the Moorfields Eye hospital. He also spent much time at the British (Museum) Library at Bloomsbury (currently being used by Karl Marx while writing *Das Kapital*[4]) where he delved into the extant literature on the cause(s) of elephantiasis and chyluria. During this leave he met T R Lewis (1841–86) (Chapter 2). While working at Calcutta in 1870–72 Lewis had demonstrated the nematode 'embryo' *Filaria sanguinis hominis* in both urine and peripheral blood of a patient who was suffering from chyluria. [Incidentally, this organism had actually been visualised before this, in hydrocele fluid, by the French surgeon J N Demarquay (1814–75) while working in Havana in 1863[2].] In August 1877, Lewis demonstrated the male and female *adult* nematodes in an elephantoid scrotum; peripheral blood contained the 'embryos' (microfilariae). In the meantime J Bancroft had demonstrated, in 1876, microfilariae in the peripheral blood of patients suffering from chyluria at Brisbane, Australia; these were subsequently examined by Cobbold – who recognised them as 'embryos'; the *adults* were visualised by Bancroft on 21 December 1876 in a 'lymphatic abscess' of the arm[10] and after confirmation of its identity, it was named (also by Cobbold) *Filaria bancrofti*[10,11]. Cobbold also confirmed that Lewis' *Filaria sanguinis hominis* and *Filaria bancrofti* represented the same species[11]. Before he returned to Amoy, Manson had apparently constructed a working hypothesis based on what was known about the dog filarial nematode *Filaria immitis*[2,12]: he surmised that *Filaria bancrofti* was attached to the wall, or neighbourhood, of an artery, vein, or lymphatic vessel – probably the latter; this would account for the various clinical manifestations of the disease (including 'lymph scrotum') with which he was by now very familiar.

On the day before Manson left England to return to Amoy (21 December 1875), he married the 17-year old Miss Henrietta Isabella Thurburn – second daughter of Captain J P Thurburn RN who was commanding the training ship *Arethusa* – at St George's Church, Campden Hill[2]. Plate 24 shows Manson at about this time. Back in Amoy in 1876 (aided by a far more powerful microscope – manufactured by Nachet Fils of Paris[2,4]) Manson resumed work on the life-cycle of *Filaria bancrofti*. By late 1877* he had examined 670 'natives' in Amoy, and found that one in every 10.8 was infected; this ratio increased from 1:17.5 in 10–20 year old individuals to 1:3 in those >70 years; furthermore, the presence of infection correlated roughly with the presence of clinical manifestations, although the majority of those who were infected remained asymptomatic[14]. The microfilariae were sheathed, but when cooled down (by contact with ice) the sheath ruptured and they swam around freely[4]. This suggested to Manson that part of the life-cycle took place *outside* the human body. He focused on the mosquito (*Culex fatigans*) as the most likely insect vector (he surmised that it had the correct nocturnal feeding habits); he apparently dismissed fleas, bugs, lice and sandflies as being unlikely candidates.

An early piece of clinical investigation was to feed mosquitoes upon his servant Hin Lo, whose blood he had already demonstrated contained a high concentration of 'embryos'. This piece of clinical research was carried out in a square wooden frame (10 x 6.5 feet) which was covered with fine mosquito-gauze; after Hin Lo had settled down on a bench

---

* In June 1877, Manson began a detailed diary; he continued this until 1897 – after settling in London[13]. His rather square hand-writing is not easily decipherable. Two other diaries are also extant: a Formosa diary (1866–68), and one for 1875 which consists largely of abstracts of published papers. These are housed in the library of the London School of Hygiene and Tropical Medicine, Keppel Street, London, WC1E 7HT.

for the night the door was left open for 30 minutes in order to attract mosquitoes inside (with a light); at this point the door was closed, and the following morning the engorged mosquitoes (female *C fatigans*) were caught beneath an inverted wine glass, transferred to phials, and subsequently dissected by Manson[4,14]. He immediately demonstrated a high concentration of 'embryos' in the stomachs of the mosquitoes[2,14]. He wrote as follows:

> I shall not easily forget the first mosquito I dissected. I tore off its abdomen and succeeded in expressing the blood the stomach contained . . . And now I saw a curious thing. The little sack or bag containing the filaria, which hitherto had muzzled it and prevented it from penetrating the wall of the blood-vessels in the human body, was broken through and discarded[1].

and later:

> I ultimately succeeded in tracing the filaria through the stomach-wall into the abdominal cavity, and then into the thoracic muscles of the mosquito. I ascertained that during this passage the little parasite increased enormously in size. It developed a mouth, an alimentary canal and other organs . . . Manifestly it was on the road to a new human host[1].

These observations were communicated by Cobbold to the Linnean Society of London (of which he was President) on 7 March 1878[1,3,4,15]. The next line of research was to demonstrate the development of the 'embryos' within the mosquito; the whole series of events was later communicated by Manson to the Linnean Society in 1884[16] [these results were later summarised by G C Low[17].] He did not however establish the mosquito–man portion of the cycle (chapter 8); his hunch was that man became infected via water which was 'contaminated' by mosquitos. Another major interest concerned the nocturnal periodicity of the 'embryos' (and the possible explanation for this); they could not be demonstrated in peripheral blood during the daylight hours[18,19]. This regular periodicity in peripheral blood was plotted by Manson after performing serial microfilaria counts on two 21-year old volunteers – Li Kha and Tiong Seng who both came from a highly endemic area for filariasis three days' journey to the north of Amoy. He later demonstrated, in 1881, that the rhythm of periodicity changed when night was turned into day, making it likely that sleeping and waking were the crucial factors. The fact that the 'embryos' actually migrate to the lungs during the day was not demonstrated until 19 February 1897 – also by Manson, who was at that time working in London[20]. A West Indian patient with bancroftian filariasis (*Filaria bancrofti*) committed suicide at 8.30 one morning by swallowing a large amount of prussic acid; on examining the lung histology (obtained at post-mortem) Manson demonstrated a very high concentration of microfilariae, thus clinching their whereabouts during the day-light hours[4].

Attempts at the elucidation of the life-cycle of another parasite (*Distoma ringeri*) were also made during this period[21]. A Portuguese patient who was infected with this helminth died in Formosa in 1878 and Manson asked Dr B S Ringer to carry out a post-mortem examination[3]; the lungs contained eggs of the parasite – which had been named by Cobbold, in London, *Distoma ringeri*. On 24 April 1880, a Chinese mandarin consulted Manson on account of a cough and haemoptysis ('endemic haemoptysis')[4]; his sputum produced 'embryos' (miracidia) in fresh water. In a search for an intermediate host he persuaded R R Hungerford (in Hong Kong) to send him some fresh-water snails – *Melania libertina*[3]; it transpired that the geographical distribution of endemic haemoptysis correlated with that of this snail species. [The complete life-cycle of the parasite – *Paragonimus westermani* – was worked out in 1916, by the Japanese, K Nakagawa]. While at Amoy, Manson also took an interest in other filarial parasites[22]: *Filaria immitis* and *Filaria sanguinolenta* (in dogs), *Filaria corvi-torquati* (Chinese white-necked crow), *Filaria picae-mediae* (magpie), *Filaria papillosa* (horse), and *Filaria mansoni* (*Oxyspiura mansoni*) (domestic fowl). He also made observations on trichinellosis (trichinosis), and *Bothriocephalus* (*Diphyllobothrium*) *mansoni*[4].

Other writing was devoted to hepatitis, and liver abscess (which was to figure prominently in his forthcoming text book published in 1898 – see below) and its surgical treatment[23]. [A complete bibliography of Manson's published work can be found in reference 2].

Manson-Bahr and Alcock[2] have attempted to put Manson's observations on filariasis into context: '[he] was the first to discover by laborious experiment in a new field that the intermediation of a particular bloodsucking insect as a 'nurse' is a *necessity* in the propagation of a specific disease of man – a discovery that threw floods of light into the fields of biology and pathology in a definite direction.' This discovery undoubtedly paved the way for the elucidation of the man-mosquito cycle of *Plasmodium* sp, the malaria parasite (see below). [Looked at in retrospect, the series of observations which culminated in the conclusion that a blood-sucking arthropod serves as a mandatory intermediary in the transmission of a human parasite, signalled the birth of medical entomology[9] and hence *tropical medicine*; however Manson had not conclusively demonstrated mosquito-transmission of this infection[9].]

During his time in southeast Asia he enjoyed good health according to his biographers, apart from attacks of gout which incidentally plagued him for the rest of his life.

In late 1882 Manson returned to Littlewood, Aberdeenshire to devote some time to shooting and fishing. However in the early summer of 1883 he returned to Amoy.

Removal to Hong Kong

In December 1883 Manson and his family – his elder son had been born in 1877 and his first daughter in 1879 (there were ultimately 2 sons and 3 daughters) – left for Hong Kong. There he settled into private practice. The primary objective of this removal was apparently to raise his financial status in order to support his growing family[2]; but his principal biographers consider that 'it was [however] as a zealous missionary of the medical persuasion that Manson revealed his strength in Hong Kong.' He worked at his office at Queen's Road for 10–12 hours daily and operated at the Civil and Memorial Hospitals. On 3 September 1886 he gave his inaugural speech as President of the local Medical Society[2]. [In 1886, the University of Aberdeen conferred the LLD degree on Manson.] He was particularly interested in the poor Europeans and Eurasians of Hong Kong. He also played a leading role in importing a herd of European cows, and in the establishment of a Dairy Farm to supply 'pure' cow's milk for children and the sick[2].

Manson's major contribution in Hong Kong was however in the field of medical education. He established a school of medicine within the Alice Memorial Hospital which formed the basis for the present Medical School of Hong Kong (which was absorbed into the University of Hong Kong in 1911); in the autumn of 1886 he became Chairman of the Hospital Committee, and by August 1887 had been elected Dean of the proposed College of Medicine for the Chinese. At a public inauguration ceremony on 1 October 1887, he made a stirring Inaugural Address (a formidable performance of five thousand words) in this capacity[2]. In 1886 he was joined by the surgeon Mr (later Sir) James Cantlie (1851–1926)[24,25] who took over a good deal of Manson's surgical practice. Cantlie was to have an important future in 'tropical medicine' and his name will reappear in chapters 7 and 8. By 1889 however (he had then served in south-east Asia for 23 years) Manson considered that, having accumulated a great deal of wealth, he was in a position to retire.

Back in Scotland he rented the sporting Lodge of the Castle of Kildrummy on Donside, and during the 1889–90 winter apparently lived the life of a country gentleman; however by the spring-summer of 1890, the Chinese dollar had depreciated sharply, and in fact soon plummeted to such depths that he felt obliged (for financial reasons) to enter practice in London[2,4].

Setting up in London: a 'new career'

At the age of 46, Manson (Plate 25 shows him at about this time) started what was in effect a new career. He moved into 21 Queen Anne St, W1 (his home for 23 years) – a 5-storey Georgian house; practice did not come easily but perseverance apparently paid off. He built up a library and small laboratory. In 1890 he was admitted to the Membership of the Royal College of Physicians (by examination) – he was elected FRCP in 1895 – and in May 1892 was elected Physician to the SHS; here he had charge of a ward of 15 beds at the Albert Dock Hospital (chapters 3 and 6–8), and apparently visited the Dreadnought Hospital, Greenwich at frequent intervals. Further details of the duties associated with this appointment will emerge in chapter 6. In December 1893 Manson is claimed to have demonstrated *Plasmodium* sp in a peripheral blood film at University College, London[2]. While in China and also London, Manson had carefully followed the malaria saga from Alphonse Laveran's (1845–1922) first visualisation of *Plasmodium* sp in Algeria in 1880. He formed an hypothesis that the mosquito acted as the insect vector as it did with *Filaria sanguinis hominis* (*W bancrofti*) infection; this detailed 'mosquito-malaria theory' had been very clearly worked out, and was published in the *British Medical Journal* in 1894[26]. [It has been suggested incidentally that Laveran had preceded Manson in developing this theory[27]]. In the light of this working hypothesis Ronald Ross embarked on his investigations in India[1,3]; in 1900 Ross recorded his thoughts on Manson's hypothesis[28]:

> It is perhaps impossible for any one, except one who has spent years in revolving this subject, to understand the full value and force of this remarkable induction . . . It is true that he endeavoured to predict the history of the parasites a little too far, and that he was in error (as will presently appear) regarding the immediate nature of the motile filaments; but the centre of his theory was invaluable. I have no hesitation in saying that it was Manson's theory, and no other, which actually solved the problem; and, to be frank, I am equally certain that but for Manson's theory the problem would have remained unsolved at the present day.

Whether or not he was the first to formulate the hypothesis, however, he was largely instrumental in guiding Ross throughout his researches in a series of letters (many of which have survived)[2–4,29].

Manson also kept up a lively interest in various other parasitoses during his London days. He was largely responsible for working out the life-cycle of *Dracunculus medinensis*, which involves the water-flea *Cyclops*[4,22]. He also forecast the life-cycle of *Loa loa*[3] – this was later established by his pupil R T Leiper in 1912 – and he took an interest in *Filaria perstans* (*Mansonella perstans*[4,22]) which he initially considered to be the cause of African sleeping-sickness. Much of this research was carried out on specimens sent to him from various tropical countries, most of them in Africa; he corresponded liberally with numerous collaborators during this period.

African trypanosomiasis was, and continued to be, of very considerable interest to Manson for some years to come. A very detailed clinico-parasitological study of a case was reported by him in 1903 (with C W Daniels)[30]. Although trypanosomes were visualised in horse blood in *nagana* by Lt-Colonel (later Sir) David Bruce in 1896, the human parasite was not identified until 1901 (chapter 8). This infection was considered by Manson to be a very important tropical disease which led to serious disability of large numbers of Africans; indeed, it was 'the exemplar' of a tropical disease[31].

By 1894, Manson had embarked on a series of public lectures on tropical diseases at the Livingstone College at Leytonstone (to missionaries proceeding on tropical service), Charing Cross Hospital, and St George's Hospital. The courses seem to have had their origin during a conversation between him and Sir Isambard Owen, Dean of St George's Medical School, towards the end of 1894; Manson had pointed out the backward state of knowledge of tropical medicine in the English medical schools. Two later addresses have survived[32,33]. The former was delivered at St George's Hospital on 1 October 1897 and the latter at the then newly opened London School of Tropical Medicine in 1899 (chapter 7). An advertisement for one series of lectures appeared in *The Lancet* in May 1897[34]:

> A course of lectures on Diseases of Tropical Climates will be delivered by Dr. Patrick Manson in the medical school of St. George's Hospital on Tuesday, May 18th, and every succeeding Friday and Tuesday till July 23rd, at 5pm. The course is intended for medical men intending to practise in the tropics or in Eastern Asia, and as far as practicable will be illustrated by living specimens and by demonstrations of parasitic organisms associated with these diseases. The fee for the course will be three guineas, and application should be made to Dr. Isambard Owen, Dean of the Medical School, St. George's Hospital, S.W., from whom cards of admission may be obtained.

Manson had by this time been appointed Lecturer in Tropical Diseases at St George's, and before recounting several cases from his personal experience, had this to say[32]:

> Ere many years are over, [the systematic teaching of tropical medicine]

will be universal in our medical schools. Those who can read the signs of the times and who are best able to judge regard this as inevitable. Why? Because our country is the centre of a great and growing tropical empire; and, second, because tropical disease in many respects is widely different from the diseases of temperate climates, which, practically, are the only diseases about which at present the student receives instruction. ... Candidates for medical degrees know very well that they will not be asked any questions about tropical disease by their examiners, and so they have not demanded instruction on this subject. And the reason why questions are rarely put on tropical medicine is that the leaders of the profession, those who man our hospitals, who fill the teaching chairs, who examine for degrees, who grant licences to practise, who make the regulations for the education of the youth of the profession are, in almost every instance, men who have never practised in warm countries, and who themselves have never felt the necessity for a wider and more practical knowledge of the diseases peculiar to these climates. Not having themselves felt the want, they have been slow to acknowledge that such a want exists, and slower still to apply the remedy. ... The course of instruction in general medicine usually received in this country is utterly inadequate to qualify for tropical practice. I say so emphatically, basing my assertion on my own experience, my own mistakes, and what I have seen and still daily see of the mistakes of others ...

and he concluded this lecture:

It seems to me ... urgently necessary (1) that a course of lectures on the hygiene and diseases of warm climates should be instituted in each medical school; (2) that a certificate of qualification in these subjects be granted by the licensing bodies after examination to those who have attended this course of lectures; and (3) that the Government should encourage the study of tropical pathology by giving a preference to those possessed of this certificate if equally proficient in other subjects, and that appointments made from home of medical officers for tropical and sub-tropical colonies should be restricted to men holding this qualification. If these suggestions are acted on, not only would vast benefits accrue to the natives of warm climates and to those Europeans who have to reside among them, but an enormous impetus would be given to tropical pathology and therapeutics, and, doubtless, indirectly to medical science in general.

It is astonishing how true most of these remarks remain today. Manson gave the Goulstonian lectures to the Royal College of Physicians in 1896 on the 'Life-History of the Malaria Germ outside the Human Body' (*Lancet* 1896; i: 695–698, 751–754, and 831–833). Looked at in retrospect, it was these various lectures which did more than anything else to launch the new discipline – *tropical medicine* (chapter 5).

Another major achievement during his early years in London was the publication of his classical 624 page monograph: *Tropical Diseases: a manual of the diseases of warm climates* (1898) — 10s 6d. Although many of the pioneers of medicine in the tropics (chapter 2) had produced monographs which recorded disease in their particular locality, Manson's text was the first to bring together those 'exotic' diseases (largely parasitic in origin) which exist in most of the tropical regions of the world. *The Lancet* considered it 'a good book, conceived and written in a scientific spirit and well up to date, and — not to omit in these utilitarian days a practical view of its merits — it strikes us as sound and judicious in regard to the general dietetic and therapeutical treatment of the maladies which it describes[35]'. The *British Medical Journal*'s anonymous reviewer felt that: 'It will be useful not only to those who intend to practise in the tropics, but to those whose lines are cast in our seaports or on our ocean steamboats.' . . . 'The book is especially opportune at a time when so much attention is being directed to the necessity for the study of tropical diseases[36]'. The text was translated into French and Spanish and during Manson's life time went to 6 editions; the 20th edition is currently in preparation.

Various aspects of Manson's physical appearance, personality, and philosophy of life have been succinctly recorded by his son-in-law Sir Philip Manson-Bahr (formerly Dr P H Bahr)[2–4]. Alcock[1] considered that in calculating Manson's place in the history of medicine,

> . . . we must also include the personal element; and the telling fact in this regard is that Manson's work was done amid all the traffic of a general medical practice, and far from any academic suggestion or influence; it was in the highest sense original — almost entirely the product of his own inspiration.

and Manson-Bahr[3] speaking in 1944, at the centenary of Manson's birth considered:

> . . . to the ordinary man, he embodied the personification of a great and well beloved physician and was best remembered as a sane, sympathetic and eminently practical doctor by his patients in Amoy, Hong Kong or London — wherever his footsteps led him.

Later life and honours

In 1904, Manson narrowly missed election to the Regius Chair of Medicine at Oxford; his name, with that of the successful candidate (Sir William Osler), had been forwarded to the Prime Minister[37]. The crowning glory of Manson's career was undoubtedly the founding (with powerful support from the Secretary of State for the Colonies — Joseph Chamberlain) of the London School of Tropical Medicine. Much of this story is related in chapters 5–7. He also played a very important role in the early days of the LSTM (chapter 8). Plate 26 shows a commemorative plaque at the original 'home' of the School – the Albert Dock Hospital. When he retired in July 1912 (from the post of Medical Adviser to the Colonial Office and also from consulting practice) he travelled to Ceylon (November 1912 – March 1913) and later South Africa and Southern Rhodesia (now Zimbabwe). In 1914 he moved to County Galway, Ireland where he indulged in some of his favourite pastimes, including fishing and gardening.

It is perhaps pertinent at this point to outline a few of the remarkable list of honours which were later to be conferred on Manson. He was appointed CMG and elected to the Fellowship of the Royal Society in 1900. From 1900 – 1902 he was President of the Epidemiological Society. In 1903 he was appointed KCMG, and in 1904 received an honorary DSc from the University of Oxford. He was elected first President of the newly established Society of Tropical Medicine & Hygiene in 1907. In 1912 he was appointed GCMG. Numerous other honours from many national and international Societies, Colleges, etc followed[2]. Cambridge University conferred the LLD degree in 1921.

Manson died in London on 9 April 1922 having suffered from myocardial ischaemia for nearly a year; a memorial service was held at St Paul's Cathedral on 12 April[38], and he was buried at the Manson family grave at Allendale Cemetery, Aberdeen. Amongst the many obituary notices were those in *The Times*[39], *The Lancet*[40], the *British Medical Journal*[41] and the *Transactions of the Royal Society of Tropical Medicine and Hygiene*[1]. *The Lancet* described him as 'the distinguished physician and parasitologist'. *The Times* considered that 'As the pioneer and founder of tropical medicine [he . . .] was one of the builders of the British Empire'. A blue plaque was later placed on the wall of the London house to which Manson moved, briefly, after he left Queen Anne Street; this was unveiled in 1985 (Plate 27).

5

The Manson-Chamberlain collaboration

> Learn to think imperially
> *Joseph Chamberlain (1904)*

The Right Honourable Joseph Chamberlain*, Secretary of State for the Colonies from 1895 to 1903, and a 'Statesman of vision', became either by chance or was positively made aware of, Manson's enthusiasm for the establishment of a new discipline – *tropical medicine* (chapter 4). Plate 28 shows Joseph Chamberlain accompanied by his first wife whilst Colonial Secretary, and Fig 5.1 is a cartoon drawn shortly after he was appointed to this position. Chamberlain was a great favourite with contemporary cartoonists; fig 5.2 shows him in his orchid house, and fig 5.3 with the Prime Minister, the Marquess of Salisbury.

Some months after Manson had begun his plans for a series of lectures at St George's Hospital, Chamberlain had written to the Dean of that school (Sir Isambard Owen) requesting notices of these addresses in order that they could be distributed to the Colonial Surgeons who were on leave in the British Isles[1]. This overt enthusiasm from such an extremely influential politician must have been very gratifying for Manson, since he had found little support from his professional colleagues for his idea to start a School of Tropical Medicine; these men had little or no interest even in the recent discoveries in tropical medicine (including Laveran's visualisation of the *Plasmodium* sp)[2]. Furthermore, as we shall see in chapter 6, some of them were to do their best to prevent the developments which Manson envisaged. Clearly with Empire and Raj

---

* Joseph Chamberlain PC, LLD, DCL, FRS (1836–1914) was Member of Parliament for West Birmingham, having previously been Mayor of that city. He held office under W E Gladstone, and later Lord Salisbury. Chamberlain held strongly patriotic and nationalist opinions on foreign affairs, combined with extreme radical views on internal matters. In a speech at Liverpool in 1903 he 'proclaimed himself a convinced imperialist'.

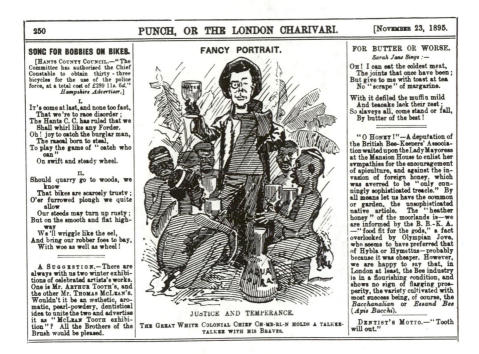

Fig 5.1 Cartoon of Joseph Chamberlain soon after his appointment as Secretary of State for the Colonies. [*Punch* 1895; 23 November: 250].

at its height, a facility for training Colonial Medical Officers in the 'exotic' diseases in (and from) the tropics was not only an attractive idea, but of paramount importance to future Colonial development and expansion. The abysmal lack of training in tropical medicine at this time was apparent from the following correspondence in the *British Medical Journal* for 23 July 1898[3]; this actually concerned Medical Officers in the Royal Navy:

> The President of the Council of the British Medical Association, in accordance with the resolution adopted at the last meeting of the Council, has addressed the following letter to the First Lord of the Admiralty respecting the desirability of making provision for instruction in tropical diseases for the officers of the Medical Service of the Royal Navy.
>
> British Medical Association,
> 429, Strand, W.C.,
> July 11th, 1898
>
> To the Right Honourable G.J. Goschen, M.P.,
> First Lord of the Admiralty.
>
> SIR, – It has been a surprise to the medical profession to learn, as it

81

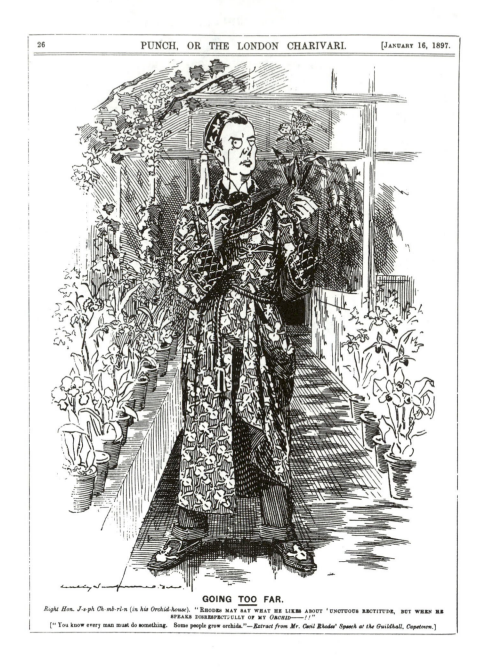

GOING TOO FAR.

Right Hon. J-s-ph Ch-mb-rl-n (in his Orchid-house). "RHODES MAY SAY WHAT HE LIKES ABOUT 'UNCTUOUS RECTITUDE, BUT WHEN HE SPEAKS DISRESPECTFULLY OF MY ORCHID——!!"

[" You know every man must do something. Some people grow orchids."—*Extract from Mr. Cecil Rhodes' Speech at the Guildhall, Capetown.*]

Fig 5.2 Joseph Chamberlain pictured as an orchid enthusiast. [*Punch* 1897; 16 January: 26].

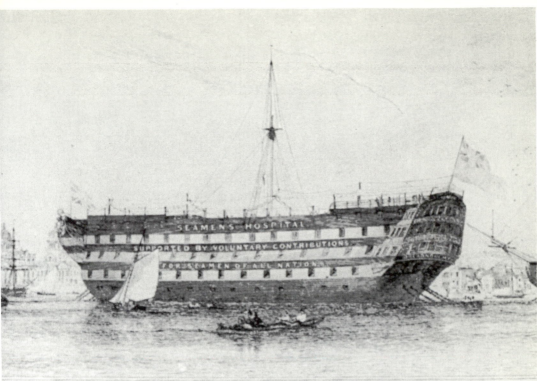

THE DREADNOUGHT, 104 GUNS, UNTIL RECENTLY LYING OFF GREENWICH.

16. HMS *Dreadnought* (31 October 1831 - 25 January 1857)

17. Ward in the *Dreadnought* hospital-ship

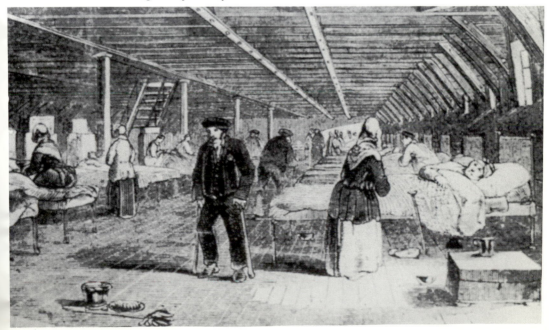

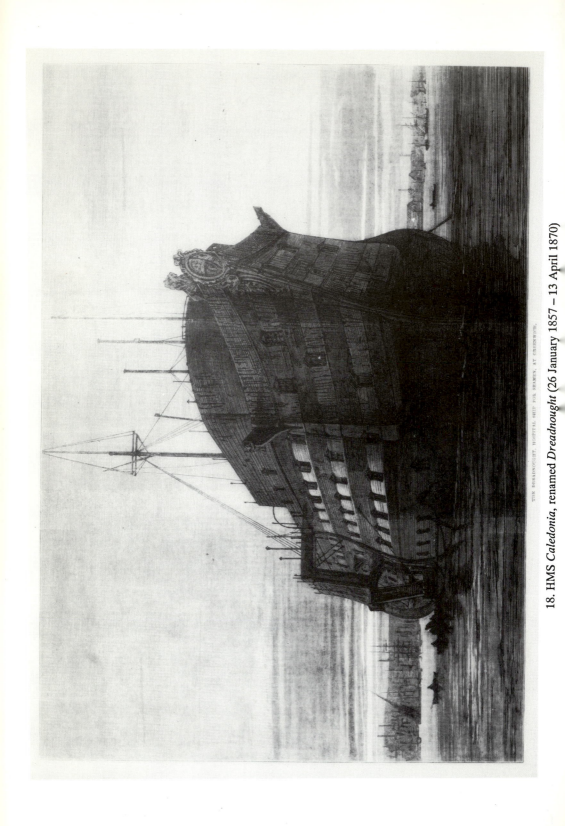

THE DREADNOUGHT, HOSPITAL SHIP FOR SEAMEN, AT GREENWICH.

18. HMS *Caledonia*, renamed *Dreadnought* (26 January 1857 – 13 April 1870)

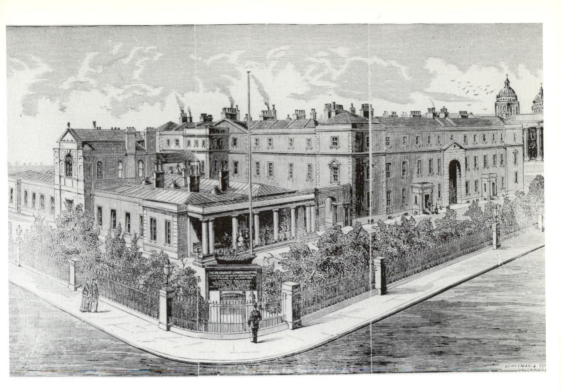

19. The *Dreadnought* Hospital, Greenwich, 1870

20. The Greenwich Hospital in a painting of 1771

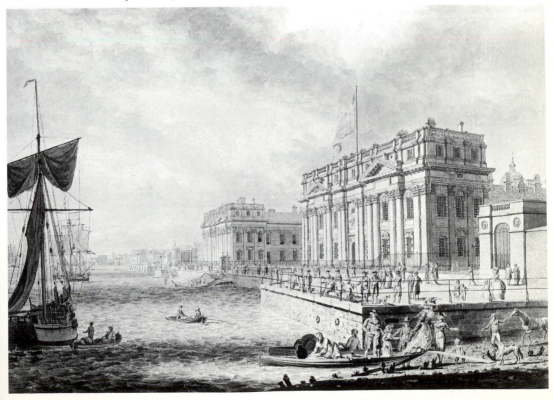

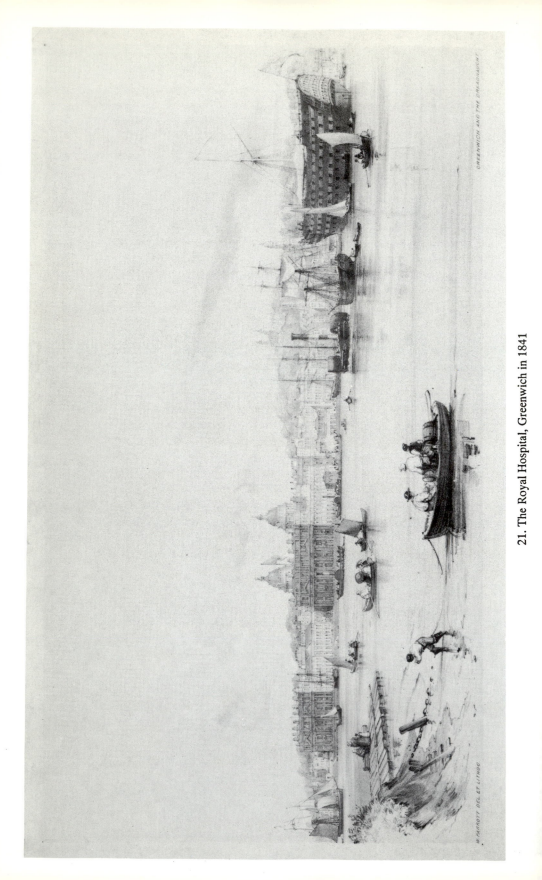

21. The Royal Hospital, Greenwich in 1841

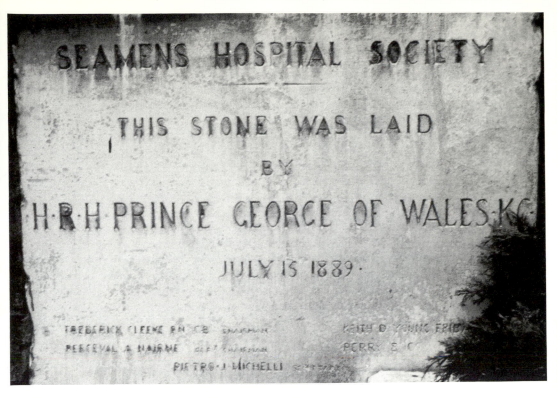

22. The Foundation Stone of the Albert Dock Hospital - 15 July 1889

23. Cromlet Hill, Oldmeldrum, Aberdeenshire - Manson's birthplace - and (inset)
    plaque commemorating Manson

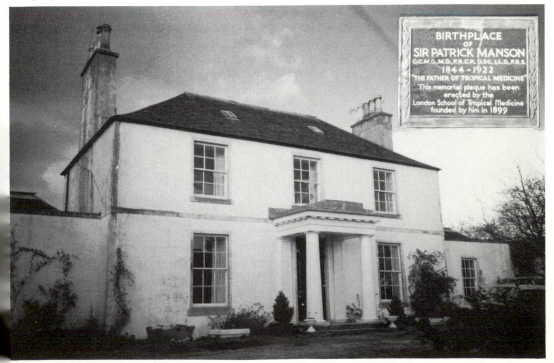

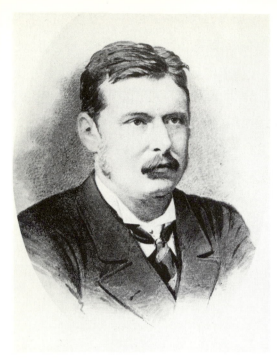

24. Dr Patrick Manson in 1876 - age 31

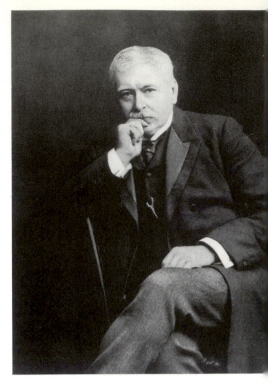

25. Dr Patrick Manson - about 1890

26. Wall plaque commemorating Sir Patrick Manson

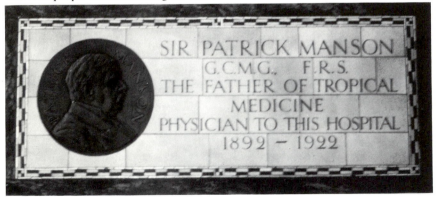

27. Blue plaque at 50, Welbeck Street, W1

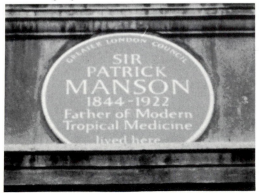

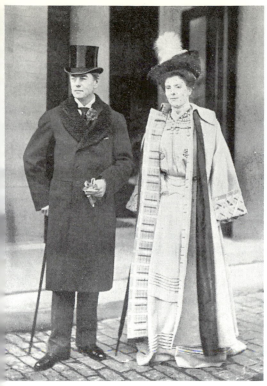

28. The Right Honourable Joseph Chamberlain
with Mrs Chamberlain

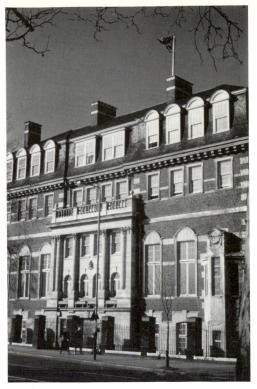

30. The Royal Army Medical College, Millbank

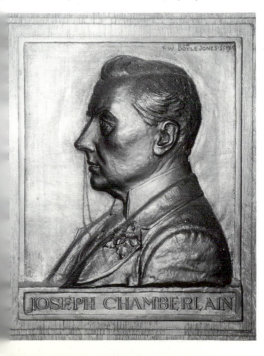

31a. Mr Joseph Chamberlain MP - plaque at HTD

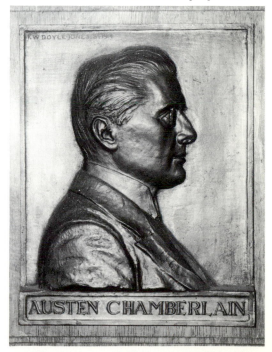

31b. Sir Austen Chamberlain MP - plaque at HTD

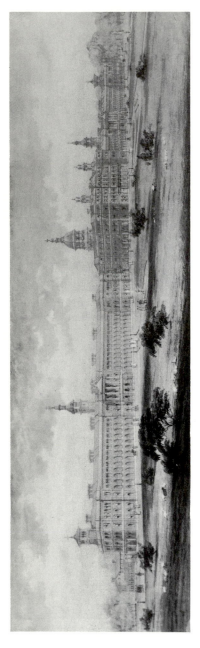

29a. The Royal Victoria Hospital, Netley

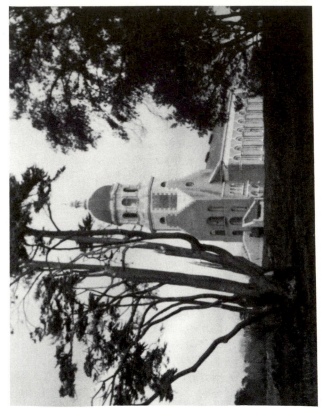

29b. The sole remaining part (the chapel) of the Royal Victoria Hospital in 1991

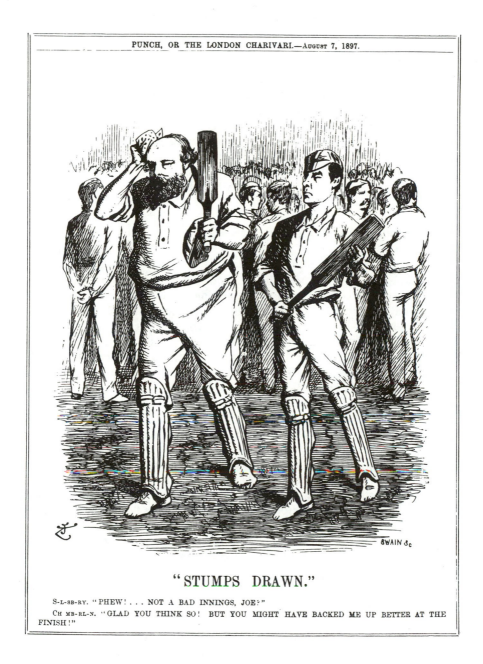

"STUMPS DRAWN."

S-l-sb-ry. "PHEW! . . . NOT A BAD INNINGS, JOE?"

Ch mb-rl-n. "GLAD YOU THINK SO! BUT YOU MIGHT HAVE BACKED ME UP BETTER AT THE FINISH!"

Fig 5.3 Joseph Chamberlain with the 3rd Marquess of Salisbury – Prime Minister 1885–6, 1886–92 and 1895–1902. [*Punch* : 1897; 7 August: 55].

has done recently, that there is no provision in the course of medical instruction at Haslar given to medical officers on joining the navy for teaching tropical diseases. On behalf of the Council of this Association, which numbers over 17,000 medical practitioners, I desire to call your attention to this defect, and to ask you if you desire further information on the subject, to be so good as to receive a deputation which shall be as representative as possible of those interested in and acquainted with the medical practice in the navy and the tropics.

I am, Sir, your most obedient servant.
ROBERT SAUNDBY, MD, LLD, FRCP,
President of the Council

The following reply has been received:

Admiralty,
16 July 1898

SIR, – Mr Goschen desires me to acknowledge the receipt of your letter of the 11th instant with regard to the question of providing special instruction in the treatment of tropical diseases to medical officers on joining the Royal Navy. In reply, I have to inform you that this subject is receiving the very careful consideration of the Board of Admiralty, who are quite alive to the importance of giving surgeons of the navy every facility for acquiring, as far as possible, the latest knowledge obtainable on the nature of the diseases in question, and the progress of scientific inquiry into the methods of of treatment.

As the Board are in agreement with the views of the Council of the British Medical Association in the matter, it appears to Mr. Goschen to be unnecessary to put the Council to the trouble of sending a deputation to represent the importance of the case to the Admiralty.

The difficulties which may have to be dealt with are mainly of an administrative character, such as to what extent, and at what periods, officers can be spared from their duties afloat for the purpose of going through special courses of instruction on shore, and in order to examine in what way the object desired can best be obtained it is the intention of the Admiralty to appoint a small departmental committee of inquiry.

I remain, yours faithfully,
W. GRAHAM GREENE

Robert Saundby, Esq., M.D.

The position at this time, regarding the almost total neglect of tropical medicine teaching in the London Medical Schools, was summarized some years later by Manson in his inaugural address when first President of the Society of Tropical Medicine & Hygiene in 1907 (chapter 8):

I once more came to London on furlough in the year 1882–3 to . . . learn the latest in medicine and surgery, especially in their application to tropical medicine. I heard plenty about the tubercle bacillus [discovered by Robert

Koch in Berlin] but, although I visited the Societies and became acquainted with many medical men of standing, I did not once hear of Laveran's important discovery of the malaria parasite. Indeed, it was not until I returned to China that I heard about it at all. I read Laveran's first book with great interest, and, as I had abundant material at my command, I set to work to find the organism he described. . . . Had there been a Society [of Tropical Medicine] in 1883, doubtless Laveran's discovery would have been a prominent subject for discussion, the technique for its demonstration would have been familiar to the Fellows, and I should have gone back to China in a satisfactory position to pursue its study under favourable conditions. I lost ten years by this.

In July 1897, Manson was appointed Medical Adviser to the Colonial Office; this was confirmed by Chamberlain on 14 July. The appointment resulted it seems from a personal intervention on the part of Chamberlain, for the application list had already been closed when Manson first became aware that the post had become vacant following the resignation of Sir Charles Gage-Brown[1,2]. Lord Lister (1827–1912), the President of the Royal Society, an admirer of Manson's theory on malaria[2], had also it seems interceded with Chamberlain on his behalf. The close association which developed between the two men was to become extremely fruitful. Successful British colonisation was recognised as only being possible if the *health* of the officials and agents of commerce was given a high priority. Chamberlain saw that efficient administration, agricultural productivity, and regular trade were being seriously impaired by 'tropical diseases'; this in turn affected his designs for 'constructive imperialism'.

Major causes of death were: malaria, blackwater fever, yellow fever, sleeping sickness, dysentery and plague[1]. Manson-Bahr[1] recalled two contemporary stories (probably anecdotal) in the context of medicine at the Colonial Office: (i) a Governor of the Gold Coast (now Ghana) asked, before sailing to take up his appointment, for a return ticket; this apparently caused a great deal of consternation because such a contingency had never before arisen (the prevalence of disease being so great in the 'white man's grave' that *return* had not previously occurred), and (ii) when applicants for certain 'far flung posts' requested further information, Colonies such as the Gilbert and Ellis Islands (now the Republic of Kiribati) could not even be found on the map! However a true narrative runs as follows: an important dispatch was sent from the Gold Coast to the Colonial Office; before it reached Whitehall, however, the secretary who drafted it, the clerk who copied it, and the Governor who signed it were all dead. The same author also quotes a popular jingle of the time:

Beware and betide of the Bight of Benin.
For few come out, though many go in.

Manson's first objective (which was wholeheartedly endorsed by Chamberlain) was to increase greatly the detailed medical information received from the Colonies; comprehensive reporting would, it was considered, produce a sound data-base, and an annual publication would be circulated in the Government service, presented to the more important libraries, and also placed on sale; appendices would consist of papers from Colonial medical officers on those diseases prevalent in their particular area(s); members of the Colonial Medical Office could thus be brought into correspondence with one another, and valuable information could be widely disseminated. Another major objective was to improve health conditions particularly in West Africa; a properly constituted West African Medical Service was therefore set up, and specially trained medical officers recruited at a higher rate of pay and emoluments. The practical results of the reorganisation would not however become evident for several years. In this project, H J (later Sir Herbert) Read (1863–1949), Chamberlain's private secretary (who later became Governor of Mauritius) took a leading role[2]. Read also played a major part in the foundation of the discipline of *tropical medicine*; his contribution has almost certainly been underestimated in the past.

Manson's changed life-style

In this new appointment Manson had to devote more time to administration than he had done since his days in Hong Kong. In 1897, he bought a cottage at Chalfont St Giles, Buckinghamshire; at this 'country retreat' he set about gardening and carpentry. In addition to his major appointments, he was in 1898 made a lecturer in Tropical Diseases to the London School of Medicine for Women – Royal Free Hospital – (this he retained until his retirement in 1912). As well as fulfilling his official duties at the Colonial Office, he was able to continue some clinical work; his very keen interest in Ross's work in India persisted. A Section of Tropical Medicine was organised for the first time at the 1898 Annual Meeting of the British Medical Association at Edinburgh; this was largely accomplished by Manson and it was here that he demonstrated some of Ross's work (on behalf of Ross) on the life-cycle of *Plasmodium* sp.

Manson made a number of powerful public addresses at this time (many focused on the need for a Tropical Medicine school in London), and in this he was backed whole-heartedly by Chamberlain. In May 1897 he had a chance meeting with P J (later Sir James) Michelli (1853–1935), Secretary of the SHS, in the residents' room at the Albert Dock Hospital; he presented him with a scheme (laid out on half a sheet of notepaper) for the setting up of a centre of instruction, in London, for the diagnosis, treatment, and prevention of tropical diseases[1]. [A more advanced version of the plan was summarized in Manson's important address at St George's Hospital in 1897 (chapter 4).] These views were also reinforced in an address delivered to the new Section of Tropical Diseases at the Annual Meeting of the British Medical Association at Edinburgh. Manson maintained that by effectively educating the Colonial Medical Officers, numerous lives of white residents in the Colonies and Protectorates would (or could) be saved; furthermore, he felt that the 'natives' also would benefit if those who ran the local hospitals and dispensaries were adequately trained in the relevant local diseases spectrum. [Over 20% of the total of British medical graduates were at that time practising in warm climates, and therefore required special instruction in the proposed discipline[1,2]]. Manson was confident that provided he could enlist the help of the SHS he could rely on Chamberlain's support[1]. A memorandum dated 2 December 1897, written by H J Read referred to a decision taken by Manson's predecessor (Sir Charles Gage-Brown) that selected junior medical officers should either attend a course of Manson's lectures at St George's Hospital, be sent to Netley (see below) for a course of instruction, or join the headquarters of the hospital of the particular colony to which they were posted to receive a 6-week course of instruction from the Principal Medical Officer. Tropical Medicine training received at Netley, and also Haslar, was in fact inadequate (especially for officers of the Indian Medical Service who required special training in parasitology[1]), and the medical officers who set off for the Colonies usually knew little of these diseases and had to gain experience 'at a terrible cost'[2].

The Royal Victoria Hospital at Netley (on Southampton Water) – staffed by RAMC officers – (Plates 29a & b) had been completed in 1863 (by special order of Queen Victoria and the Prince Consort), and was opened for soldiers invalided from the Crimea and the Colonial Empire[1]. The Army Medical School under Surgeon-General W C Maclean was also sited at Netley, and co-operation between the Army and the Indian Medical Service lasted there until 1902. The Netley Medical School was ultimately closed on 31 May 1905. The RAMC College was opened at Millbank, London in 1907 (Plate 30).

Manson considered Netley an unsuitable site for the training of Colonial Office Officials (see below); the Dreadnought Hospital, Greenwich, was more appropriate for the training of the 74 permanent medical officers in the eight British possessions in the continent of Africa[2]. It was his view that 'the atmosphere, as well as the remote situation of Netley were incompatible with the teaching of tropical medicine'[1]. As a consequence, the Colonial Office addressed a letter (2 February 1898) to the SHS suggesting that it would be a more suitable body to undertake this venture, and that training could be carried out at an enlarged Albert Dock (branch) Hospital (chapter 6). Chamberlain furthermore wrote to the General Medical Council (11 March 1898) suggesting the desirability of extending teaching in tropical medicine; as a result a memorandum was circulated to all medical teaching institutions. On 16 April 1898, a reply was received from Sir Henry Burdett, Vice-President of the SHS (who later made the facts public[4]) in which he agreed in principal with the suggestion, and included an estimate of expenses[1]:

Cost of a new wing to the Albert Dock Hospital, and school building	£13,000
Annual expenditure	£ 3047
A sum equivalent to interest at 3% per annum on a capital sum not exceeding £100 000	
Maintenance of 6 students for 10 months annually at 4 guineas weekly: Annual cost approx	£ 1000
[Proposed fees for a course of not less than 4 weeks:	
Residents per week	£ 4- 4-0
Non-residents per week	£ 2-12-6]

The *British Medical Journal* for 16 July 1898[4] summarized events so far, these being 'laid before the public' by Sir Henry Burdett, KCB, Vice-President of the SHS (chapter 6):

... Some time ago the attention of the Secretary of State for the Colonies was called to the great need of a better system of instruction for medical officers appointed to the Colonial Service in the diseases peculiar to the regions in which their sphere of work will lie. Mr. Chamberlain thereupon addressed a letter to the Committee of the Seamen's Hospital, in the course of which he stated that:

He felt confident that a marked advance would be made if some scheme could be devised by which all the newly-appointed medical officers would receive a sound and systematic training in this country before taking up their duties in West Africa. He was advised that the experience and training to be obtained by the Seamen's Hospital would be the most suitable in the present instance, and he accordingly asked for the assistance of the managing committee in the matter, by considering whether it might not be possible to so enlarge the branch hospital at the Albert Docks as to provide the necessary accommodation for the establishment of a school of tropical diseases for the benefit of the medical officers in question.

He added that The Secretary of State for Foreign Affairs was being asked whether he wished that the Protectorates in the East and West Africa under the administration of the Foreign Office should be included in the proposed scheme.

In due course the Seamen's Hospital Committee submitted to the Colonial Office a scheme for the establishment of a school for the study of tropical diseases. This has now been approved, and will shortly be an established fact . . .

The school will be open to other students than those members of the medical profession who may be sent by Government Departments, or who may wish to equip themselves for service abroad. It appears from the report of the special committee which investigated the question that 78 per cent. of the cases of tropical diseases treated by the Seamen's Hospital Society had been admitted to the branch hospital, which will now contain 45 beds. Provision will be made for from 20 to 25 students, with sleeping accommodation for about 10. There will be a fully-equipped laboratory, pathological room, museum, and every other necessary calculated to make the school efficient. The teaching staff will consist of the senior medical staff of the Dreadnought Hospital at Greenwich, as well as of the branch hospital, together with a number of teachers specially selected and attached to the new school. The school will be under the immediate supervision and direction of a medical tutor, who will attend for six hours daily. Instruction will be given to students on four days in the week for four hours each day by one or more members of the teaching staff.

The scheme appears to be well devised, and we wish it all success. Much, however, will depend on the way in which it is carried out, and particularly on the selection of the men most competent to teach what is known and to enlarge the boundaries of our knowledge. The matter, as we have already said, is one of national importance, and it would be a disaster and a disgrace if petty personal jealousies were allowed to wreck the scheme.

Chamberlain now set about getting the 'message' across to the public – who apparently did not recognise either the magnitude of the teaching problem, or the great loss of life which resulted from a failure to investigate tropical diseases scientifically. The tropics – especially West Africa – had not been designated the 'white man's grave' for nothing! The mortality during the British military occupation of the Gold Coast could probably not be equalled anywhere in the annals of British Colonial History[1]. Chamberlain wrote (14 June 1898) that for some time he 'had noted with concern the high death rate amongst Europeans in the British West African Dependencies'. In 1895 [for example] the number of European officials in the Gold Coast was 175; of these 17 died and 24 were invalided! This figure apparently did not take into account the non-official white population – amongst whom the mortality was at least as high, and who were almost entirely dependent upon the Colonial Surgeons for skilled medical advice. [In Lagos, Nigeria, available figures suggested that 46 out of 140 resident Europeans had died over a period of 15 months, and that during another period of 6 months, 72 out of a white population of 200 had perished[2].]

Encouraging results from the collaboration

Funding for the proposed school was sought, and the Royal Society made an initial grant of £300 (15 July 1898). The Government grant was to be in the region of £3500 annually, plus a further £1000 for the training of Government Medical Officers. This left the sum of £10,000 (a formidable amount) to be raised by the public together with a net income of £2000 per annum[4]. The SHS requested that a representative of the Colonial Office be on the Society Board of Management; H J Read was appointed. In order to proceed with the new school as soon as possible the SHS instructed their architect to proceed with the foundations immediately (8 July 1898). The outline plan of the proposed London School of Tropical Medicine (LSTM) had been placed before the Committee of the Board of Management of the SHS on 11 February 1898. The minutes of the Committee of Management of the SHS for 14 October 1898[5] read:

> That a sub-committee was appointed, 'consisting of Mr H J Read [of the Colonial Office and others] ... to formulate a scheme for the organisation and management of the new School of Tropical Medicine, with powers to invite the co-operation of Members of the Medical profession interested in tropical disease and bacteriology ...'

Amongst subsequent members of this committee were – Mr Perceval A Nairne (Chairman), Surg-Col O Baker, Sir Chas. Gage Brown, Thos. Lauder Brunton FRS, Dr Patrick Manson CMG, LLD, and Mr William Turner MS, FRCS. With Chamberlain's permission the committee met at the Colonial Office (and occasionally at Dr Stephen Mackenzie's residence in Cavendish Square); its work was soon completed, and its report submitted on 18 May 1899. On 10 March 1899[6], the sub-committee had made (amongst others) the following recommendations:

> (i) That the name of the School be 'The London School of Tropical Medicine' *in connection with the Seamen's Hospital Society* [my italics],
> (ii) That the first Teachers in the School and the additional Members of the Honorary Medical Staff be appointed by the Committee of Management of the Seamen's Hospital Society in consultation with the Advisory Committee,
> (iii) That an advertisement be inserted in *The Times* and Medical papers inviting applications for appointments on the Teaching Staff and the Honorary Medical Staff of the Hospital,
> (x) That there be three Sessions yearly of three months each, viz: from 1st October to 31st December, from 15th January to 14th April and from

1st May to 31st July inclusive. In addition to the practice of the Hospital, Students will be required to attend a systematic course of instruction by the Medical Superintendent during two months in each Session, and
(xi) That Students, resident and non-resident, must be qualified Medical Practitioners, or be in the fifth year of their medical studies. The School Committee shall have power to admit other applicants under special circumstances at their discretion. Students nominated by the Colonial Office shall have the first claim to residence.

The satisfactory outcome of the negotiations to date, had been announced (from Downing Street) in the *British Medical Journal* for 19 November 1898[7] and *The Lancet* for 26 November 1898[8]:

The following circular letter, signed by the Permanent Under-Secretary of the Colonial Office, has been addressed to the medical schools:

Downing Street, November 9th 1898.
SIR,

1. In the . . . letter from this Department of the 11th of March last it was stated that Mr. Secretary Chamberlain, with a view to supplementing the instruction afforded by the medical schools, was endeavouring to make arrangements for giving to Colonial medical officers special clinical instruction in tropical medicine, such as is given at Netley and Haslar in the case of medical officers of the Army, Navy, and Indian Medical Services, and which, from lack of the necessary material, cannot invariably be given at the medical schools.

2. These arrangements have now been made. The directors of the Seamen's Hospital at the Albert Docks, which offers exceptional opportunities for studying cases of tropical disease, are providing the necessary buildings and teachers for the accommodation and instruction of the medical officers who may hereafter be selected by the Foreign Office and the Colonial Office for appointments in the tropics. A substantial contribution towards the initial cost of the buildings is being made by the Government, and it is hoped that by the 1st of October, 1899, it will be possible to receive medical officers at the hospital for purposes of instruction.

3. It is proposed that, as is at present the case, candidates for medical appointments in the British Colonial Possessions shall be fully qualified before they can be put upon the Secretary of State's list, that from this list a certain number shall be selected annually to fill the vacancies which may occur in the Colonial Medical Service, that the selected candidates shall be trained for a period of at least two months at the Seamen's Hospital, and that they shall then be sent to the Colonies or Protectorates to which they have been allotted, where, when practicable, they will be attached, in the first instance, to the headquarters hospital for the purpose of gaining additional experience. In estimating the respective merits of candidates on the Secretary of State's list, regard will be had to the fact whether or not they have already received instruction in tropical medicine.

4. Judging from the replies which have been received from the General Medical Council and the medical schools, Mr. Chamberlain believes that the above arrangements will prove acceptable.

5. Although the school at the Seamen's Hospital is designed for the training of medical officers for the Government Service, doubtless there will be many other medical men, such as the medical officers of missionary societies and trading corporations, and private practitioners who propose to settle in tropical countries, who will be glad to avail themselves of the advantages which such a school can offer.

6. The Colonies are being asked to make pecuniary contributions, to collect pathological material for use in the school, and to support the scheme in every possible way. So far, then, as this Department is concerned, no effort is being spared to make the school a success, and Mr. Chamberlain feels confident that the medical schools of this country will also do what is in their power to assist the development of an institution which is likely to be of general service, and to benefit medical science not only by giving a stimulus to the investigation of tropical disease, but also by qualifying a body of men to become investigators.

7. Mr. Chamberlain is so impressed with the importance of this subject as affecting the administration and well-being of the tropical Colonies that, in addition to this scheme for providing a thoroughly efficient Colonial Medical Staff, he wishes to encourage by every means in his power scientific inquiry into the causes of tropical diseases. Accordingly, he has already, after correspondence with the Royal Society, instituted a Commission to study the subject of tropical malaria on the following lines:

8. The Royal Society has nominated two competent observers, who have already proceeded to Italy for a short preliminary study, and will afterwards go to some place in Africa, probably, in the first instance, to Blantyre, in the British Central Africa Protectorate, where it has been ascertained that there exist good opportunities for carrying out the purpose in view.

9. In addition, the Secretary of State has nominated an experienced medical officer of the Colonial Service to aid in the investigation. This officer will, in the first place, proceed to India in order to study under Surgeon-Major Ronald Ross for about two months, so as to make himself acquainted with the result of that gentleman's researches. He will then join the other two observers in Africa, where they will together pursue their studies, which will probably occupy about two years, and report from time to time to a Committee in England, nominated jointly by the Royal Society and the Secretary of State.

10. Mr. Chamberlain has been glad to learn from the replies which have been sent to the letter referred to above that arrangements already exist, or are about to be made, for giving special instruction in tropical medicine in upwards of twelve British medical schools, and he trusts that these schools, some of which (such as that of University College, Liverpool, University

College, Bristol, and the University of Durham College of Medicine at Newcastle-on-Tyne), being situated in large seaports, possess exceptional facilities for the study of tropical disease, will keep in correspondence with the School of Tropical Medicine at the Seamen's Hospital, with a view to mutual assistance and advice.

11. In conclusion, Mr. Chamberlain desires to express his thanks to the General Medical Council and the British medical schools for the warm interest which they have taken in this matter, and for the ready and cordial support which they have afforded him. He will welcome any suggestions which may be made in furtherance of the object in view.

I am, Sir, your obedient servant,
EDWARD WINGFELD.

The satisfactory progress with respect to planning of the new school at that time, was summarized in the *British Medical Journal*[9]:

The arrangements for providing a school of tropical medicine at the branch hospital of the Seamen's Hospital Society, Victoria and Albert Dock, London, E., are, we understand, making satisfactory progress. A subcommittee, consisting of Mr. Nairne, Chairman; Sir C. Gage Brown, KCMG; Mr. Macnamara, Dr. Lauder Brunton, Dr. Stephen Mackenzie, Dr. Manson, Dr. James L. Maxwell, Mr. Johnson Smith, FRCS; Mr. William Turner, FRCS; and Mr. James Cantlie, FRCS, is now engaged in drawing up a constitution for the school, and defining the curriculum. The new buildings will, it is expected, be completed by October 1st. 1899, and it is announced that Mr. Chamberlain intends to preside at a festival dinner to be held during the coming parliamentary session. A valuable collection of paintings of skin diseases and ulcers common in British Guiana has been presented to the school by Dr. D. Palmer Ross, CMG, Surgeon-General of that Colony. The paintings were executed between the years 1837 and 1842. In many instances they are remarkably accurate. We are glad to see such prompt and practical interest in this newly-founded school, and hope that Dr. Palmer Ross's example will be followed by others who may have the opportunity to contribute to the library or museum.

This was followed by a further up-date in December 1898[10]:

We have authority from the Foreign Office to state that Lord Salisbury [the Prime-Minister (fig 5.4)]* has intimated his desire that the Protectorates

---

* Robert Arthur Talbot Gascoyne-Cecil – 3rd Marquess of Salisbury, KG, GCVO, DCL, LLD, FRS (1830–1903) was Secretary for India, and President of the Indian Council 1866–67, 1874–78, First Lord of Treasury 1886–87, Secretary of State for Foreign Affairs 1878–80, 1885–86, 1887–92, 1895–1900, and Prime Minister 1885–86, 1886–92 and 1895–1902.

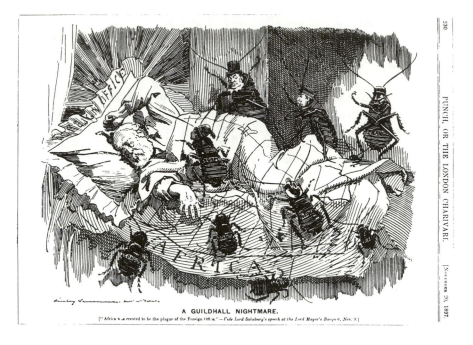

A GUILDHALL NIGHTMARE.

[" Africa was created to be the plague of the Foreign Office." — *Vide Lord Salisbury's speech at the Lord Mayor's Banquet, Nov. 9.*]

Fig 5.4 Lord Salisbury (the Prime–Minister) being tormented by the affairs of the Foreign Office, and particularly Africa [*Punch* 1897; 20 November: 230].

under the administration of the Foreign Office should participate in the benefits which will be derived from the establishment of the new School of Tropical Medicine, and that the Lords Commissioners of Her Majesty's Treasury have consented in principle to the Protectorates making the requisite contribution to the funds necessary for carrying out the scheme. We are informed that Lord Salisbury will also nominate a representative on the Board of Management of the Seamen's Hospital Society.

The enormous enthusiasm shown by Chamberlain in the foundation of the discipline – tropical medicine – is also emphasised in a later circular (28 May 1903) to the Governors of *all* the Colonies[2,11]

The great mortality amongst Europeans in such climates as those of the West African Colonies and Protectorate had not failed to attract my notice from the first as it had that of my predecessors in office, and towards the end of the year 1897, largely through the interest taken in the matter by Dr. Manson, who had succeeded Sir C. Gage-Brown as Medical Adviser to the Colonial Office, my attention was more definitely directed to the importance of scientific enquiry into the causes of malaria and of special education in tropical medicine for the Medical Officers of the Crown Colonies. In pursuance of the second of these two objects, it was clearly advisable (a) that a special training school in tropical medicine should be established, where Officers, newly appointed to the medical services of the Colonies and Protectorates, might be given systematic instruction, with special facilities for clinical study, before leaving England to take up their appointments, and where doctors already in the Service might, when on leave, have opportunities of bringing their professional knowledge up to date; (b) that all leading medical schools in the United Kingdom should be invited to give greater prominence than hitherto in their schemes of study to tropical medicine; (c) that the medical reports periodically sent from the tropical Colonies and Protectorates should be re-cast on one uniform type, designed to throw light on the diseases most prevalent in tropical countries, and to indicate the methods likely to be most successful in preventing or curing such diseases. With reference to the first of these objects, the provision of a special training school, it was considered that the Albert Dock branch of the Seamen's Hospital, which was about to be enlarged, was likely to offer the facilities required, standing as it does at the Dock gates, admitting sufferers from tropical disease direct from ships from all parts of the world, and being, moreover, within easy reach of the Colonial Office, and therefore likely to be in close touch with that Office. These considerations decided me to approach the managers of this hospital in preference to endeavouring to make whatever arrangements might be possible for obtaining the object in view, at the Royal Naval Hospital at Haslar, or the Royal Victoria Hospital for soldiers at Netley, at which latter hospital officers of the Indian Medical Service receive instruction in tropical diseases.

Such directives from Government not unexpectedly aroused the anger of the services, whose medical training took place at Netley (see above); they considered it a slight on their teaching ability (chapter 6). In response to a letter to the General Medical Council (GMC) and the leading UK Medical Schools, reiterating his views that all Medical Officers selected for appointments in the tropics should enter their careers with an adequate knowledge of the diseases which were prevalent in their particular region, replies showed that at least 12 schools were about to embark on special instruction in Tropical Medicine. The GMC adopted the following resolution:

That while the Council is not prepared to recommend that tropical medicine should be made an obligatory subject of the ordinary medical curriculum, it deems it highly desirable, in the public interest, that arrangements should be forthwith made by the Government for special instruction in tropical medicine, hygiene and climatology for duly qualified medical practitioners who are selected for the Colonial Medical Service and who otherwise propose to practise in tropical countries.[2]

Shortly after the inauguration of the first session of the School (chapter 7), Chamberlain wrote in November, 1899:

> It is clear that the work cannot stand still, and as long as those who can speak with the authority of science are confident that by human effort the rate of mortality from malaria and other tropical diseases can be greatly reduced and the strength and efficiency of Europeans resident in unhealthy climates can be sensibly increased, so long, in my opinion, ought funds to be forthcoming for carrying on what has been so well begun.[2]

Chamberlain's wholehearted support continued. He was incidentally a particularly witty and gifted speaker as the following report in which he had been replying to the toast 'The Houses of Parliament' makes clear[12]:

> It is quite true that in the House of Commons we have nowadays occasional scenes of disorder which are not very creditable to us. We have among us ill-mannered individuals who seem to be unaware of their responsibility and who try to bring contempt upon the body of which they ought to be proud. (Hear, hear.) But I am not by any means certain that that is a new state of things or that there were not in former times similar incidents and similar men. Nowadays we live in a sensational age, and, if there is anything at all out of the common, at once the evening newspapers – the *Pall Mall Gazette* or the *Star* or something or another of that kind – take possession of it, and you may be sure that it loses nothing in their hands. And so the relative importance of things is lost, and people read about 'scenes' in the House of Commons and think the whole affair is going to the dogs; and they forget that all the time, silently, slowly, surely, smoothly, and, on the whole, satisfactorily, the Government of this world-wide Empire, with its 300,000,000 of subjects of the Queen, is being carried on . . .
>
> It is a very curious thing, the types of the House of Commons are constant, although the men change. In my time I have never known the House of Commons without a funny man. (Laughter.) There is always one, and when he dies, or when he ceases to be elected, or when, for some reason or another, he retires into the background, there is another immediately to take his place. (Laughter.) . . . He is a man who has a natural taste for buffoonery, which he has cultivated with great art, who has a hatred of every Government, and of all kinds of restraint, and especially, of course, of the Government which happens to be in office. Then there is the House of Commons bore – of course, there is more than one (laughter), but there is always one *par excellence*. He is generally a man who is very clever, a man of encyclopaedic information, which he has been unable to digest himself, and which, therefore, he is always ready to impart to everybody else. Then you have the weighty man, and, gentlemen, the gravity of the weighty man of the House of Commons is a thing to which there is no parallel in the world. (Laughter.) You have the foolish man,

you have the man with one idea, you have the independent man, you have the man who is a little cracked. (Laughter.) All these men are there to-day, were there 50 years ago, will be there 50 years hence . . .

He was therefore an ideal fund-raiser, and as well as making another impressive speech presided at a Charity Dinner held at the Hotel Cecil on 10 May 1899; this raised £12,000 to meet the cost of building and equipment. *The Lancet* reported the proceedings[13]:

Between three and four hundred gentlemen attended a festival dinner of the Seamen's Hospital Society which was held in the Grand Hall of the Cecil Hotel on Wednesday evening last, May 10th.

The toasts of "The Queen", which was received with musical honours, and "The Prince and Princess of Wales and other members of the Royal Family" were proposed by the Right Hon. J. CHAMBERLAIN, M.P., the chairman.

The Marquis of Lorne proposed "The Navy, Army and Auxiliary Forces," Which was replied to by Admiral Sir Anthony H. Hoskins and the Marquess of Lansdowne.

THE SECRETARY OF STATE FOR WAR, referring to the Royal Army Medical Corps, said that the army was a small one but its liabilities were immense. The most formidable foe that the British soldier had to encounter was tropical disease. Lord Lansdowne reminded his hearers that in the Tirah campaign in round figures there were 1000 admissions to hospital from gunshot wounds and the injuries usually sustained during a campaign, while there were 11,000 admissions from fever and dysentery. Of the deaths there were 100 from wounds and injuries but nearly 600 from diseases of a tropical kind.

Mr. GARLAND SOPER, J.P., proposed "The Houses of Parliament".

Lord LOCH, in responding, asked for support for the Colonial Nursing Association.

Sir WILLIAM PRIESTLEY referred to Lord Lansdowne's interest in the Medical Department of the Army and remarked that his connexion with establishing the Royal Army Medical Corps had made him so popular with medical officers that there was a desire to have his portrait framed in every mess-room where they were assembled.

In proposing "The Establishment of the London School of Tropical Medicine and the Enlargement of the Branch Hospital of the Society in the Royal Victoria and Albert Docks," Mr. CHAMBERLAIN said that in the great work of civilisation our greatest enemy was the insidious attacks of a deadly disease which weakens where it does not kill and which shortens the lives and careers of the ablest and most energetic of those who go out to represent us in these countries. The problem before us was manifold. We had to seek out and make clear the history and origin of these diseases. We had, if possible, to find a cure for them, and with those objects we had to extend the study of these tropical diseases, and to create, it may be, a school of trained practitioners and investigators, so that in future scientific research may go hand-in-hand with practical medicine. He referred to the aid which had been given by Lord Lister and the Royal Society, to the work of Major Ross, IMS, in India and that of Dr. Patrick Manson (medical adviser to the Colonial Office) and his predecessor (Sir Charles Gage Brown), and to that of Dr. Rowell. Under the proposed scheme the accommodation at that hospital would be increased to 50 beds. When this enlargement had taken place and the necessary buildings had been erected the course of procedure would be somewhat as follows. The Colonial Office and the other offices which had dependencies in the tropics under their charge would give a preference in their selection of medical officers for those colonies and dependencies to the gentlemen who had gone through a course of special study in connexion with the subject of tropical diseases in one of the great medical institutions of the country. This course of study might extend over two or three years and be given in any of the medical institutions of the United Kingdom. After that study had been completed and the necessary certificates and degrees had been conferred it would be expected of the candidates selected that they should take advantage of schools of tropical medicine and practically learn the treatment of those diseases. Between the several institutions engaged in the same work there could be no question of jealousy and he hoped that they would always keep in close touch. After referring to the advances which science had made in the control of disease he expressed his opinion that *the man who should successfully grapple with this foe of humanity and find the cure for malaria and for the fevers desolating our colonies and dependencies in many tropical countries, and should make the tropics liveable for white men, would do more for the world, more for the British Empire, than the man who added a new province to the wide dominion of the Queen* [my italics]. All those who cooperated in securing this result, whether by their personal service or by some pecuniary sacrifice, would be entitled to share the honour and to add their names to the golden record of the benefactors of mankind.

Lord LISTER proposed, and Lord STRATHCONA and Sir P.O. FYSH responded to, the toast of "The Empire."

Sir DONALD CURRIE gave the toast of "The Health of the Chairman."

In the course of the evening subscriptions amounting to £15,800 were announced. This sum included £3500 from the Colonial Office, £2000 from the Bishop of London on behalf of the Marriott Bequest, £1000 from the India Office, £200 from the King of the Belgians, and £500 from Sir Thomas Sutherland. Lord Strathcona and Sir Donald Currie each gave £500 to endow a bed, and Sir Henry Burdett has promised to give £300 a year for three years for a travelling scholarship.

The detailed verbatim version can be found in *The Times*[14]; Chamberlain's major themes were – Heavy mortality in the tropics; investigation

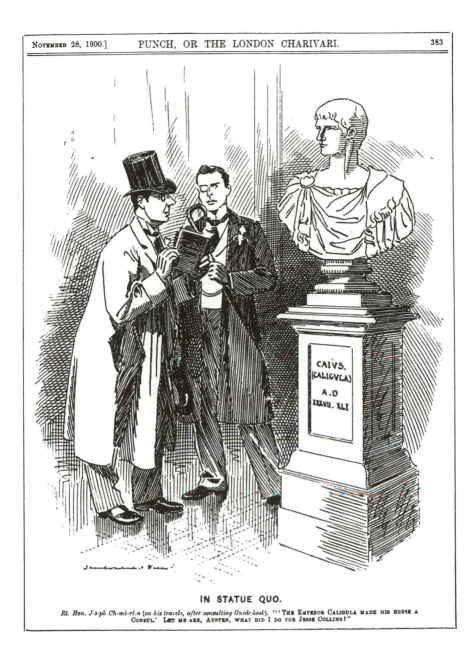

IN STATUE QUO.

Rt. Hon. J-s-ph Ch-mb-rl-n (on his travels, after consulting Guide-book). "'THE EMPEROR CALIGULA MADE HIS HORSE A CONSUL.' LET ME SEE, AUSTEN, WHAT DID I DO FOR JESSE COLLINS?"

Fig 5.5 Cartoon of Joseph Chamberlain with his son Austen [*Punch* 1900; 28 November: 383].

of tropical diseases; the selection of medical officers; and, the supply of funds. It was clear then that he equated the efforts of Manson and his collaborators with those of Cecil Rhodes (1853–1902)[15] in southern Africa, and Sir Stamford Raffles (1781–1826) in South-east Asia (Raffles had landed in Singapore on 28 January 1879 and had changed it from an 'obscure fishing village to a great seaport and modern metropolis').

There can by now be no doubt in the mind of the reader that Chamberlain (he had a reputation for great loyalty to those with whom he worked) was an extremely firm supporter of Manson, and that the entire project had become very politically motivated. If further proof is required however, the following is a reply to Manson on Chamberlain's behalf (8 December 1898) after he had already received a great deal of adverse correspondence and comment regarding his plans (chapter 6)[2]:

> Mr Chamberlain has complete confidence in your advice with regard to the School, and he does not want to be drawn into a professional dispute, which he feels sure will not interest the public. He doubts if the opposition will in any way injure the hospital, but, if you wish it, he is ready to offer to hear a small deputation to discuss the matter with you.

The colossal support which had come from Chamberlain later continued in the form of further backing from this Birmingham family of politicians. Fig 5.5 shows a cartoon of Joseph Chamberlain with his son Austen, and Plates 31a and b show plaques to commemorate the enormous support which they both rendered in the early days of the London School of Tropical Medicine. In 1914, in memory of his father, and in recognition of the work done by the school, Mr (later Sir) Austen Chamberlain* appealed for further funding, and £73,000 was received; this was divided between: the upkeep of the hospital, provision of new apparatus, and research.

---

* Sir (Joseph) Austen Chamberlain, KG, PC (1863–1937) was Member of Parliament for Birmingham West. He was the only son of Joseph Chamberlain by his first wife. He held high office in successive conservative governments, and was Secretary of State for India, Chancellor of the Exchequer, and Secretary of State for Foreign Affairs.

6

A controversial beginning for the new discipline: a major dispute within the medical establishment

Manson's personal relations with Chamberlain were always extremely cordial, but antagonism to his designs for the new school had been generated by the contemporary Medical Establishment[1]. It is therefore of interest at this point to take a look at the opposition (some of it surprisingly hostile) which Manson (always supported by Chamberlain) had to overcome in 1897–99.

The physicians at the Dreadnought Hospital, Greenwich (Plate 32) were upset by Manson's address at St George's Hospital – on 1 October 1897 (chapter 4); in it he had cast serious doubts about their ability to diagnose tropical disease(s)[1]. Following this lecture, a letter appeared in *The Lancet* during October 1897 (chapter 3) from Dr John Curnow, Senior Visiting Physician to the Dreadnought Hospital, Greenwich[2]:

To the Editors of THE LANCET.

SIRS, – In an introductory lecture at St. George's Hospital Dr. Patrick Manson gives a long list of erroneous diagnoses as transcribed verbatim from the register of the Seamen's Hospital. In the list are anasarca, rheumatism, debility, pericarditis and fits, apoplexy, locomotor ataxia, myelitis, paraplegia, tachycardia, dyspnoea, cardiac diseases, asthma and anasarca, Bright's disease, progressive muscular atrophy, and hysteria. In answer to my inquiry, Dr. Manson has informed me that they are really taken from the register of the Branch Seamen's Hospital at the Royal Albert and Victoria Docks; and he asks me, if my experience does not agree with his, that I should publish it. This branch hospital contains eighteen beds, and his vague use without qualification of the term "seamen's hospital," has led members of the profession to suppose that he is referring to this institution with its 235 beds. I can find no such errors in our register, for at the worst they are merely incomplete diagnoses, giving a prominent symptom as sufficient for admission – e.g., dropsy, oedema of legs, loss of power in legs, anaemia and oedema, &c. We have admitted eighty-seven cases in the past four years. I would add that all the medical certificates, both at the branch and at this hospital, only come from the medical officers of one of our largest shipping companies.

It is because there is such a wide discrepancy between the experience at the two hospitals that I ask you to make this correction. – I am, Sirs, yours truly,

JOHN CURNOW, MD, FRCPLond.
Seamen's Hospital Society (*Dreadnought*), Greenwich,S.E.,
Oct 27th, 1897.

Two weeks later the same journal published the following (anonymous) article[3]:

Since the delivery of Dr. Manson's address upon the necessity for improved teaching in tropical diseases sundry letters bearing on the matter have appeared in our columns and also in the lay press. The subject is no doubt of the greatest importance to a country like our own whose troops both naval and military, to say nothing of innumerable civilians, are employed all over the world, and we must allow that it would be an admirable thing if the other metropolitan hospitals and the great extra-metropolitan schools of medicine were to follow the example of St. George's Hospital and St. Mary's Hospital and institute a course of lectures upon tropical diseases. As regards the army we are not so badly off as, judging by the correspondence which has already appeared upon the matter, many people seem to think. For thirty-seven years tropical medicine has been taught at the Army Medical School, first at Chatham and afterwards at Netley, clinical material being afforded by invalided soldiers from India, China, and other tropical and sub-tropical stations in all parts of the world. All surgeons on probation from both the Army and Indian Medical Departments have to go through this course of Tropical Medicine, which lasts for four months, two or three lectures being given per week. The plasmodia of malaria are demonstrated to the surgeons, who are also taught how to search for, stain, and identify them. The amoebae of dysentery are also studied as well as the bacteriology of plague and other tropical diseases. The first professor of military medicine was Dr. Morehead, IMS and he was followed by Maclean, Boyes, Smith, Capley, and McLeod the present occupant of the chair. It is evident from this that the military and medical authorities at the War Office have not been so unmindful of their obligations with regard to this important subject as recent remarks upon the matter would suggest. With regard to the Medical Department of the Navy we see no reason why surgeons on probation from that branch of Her Majesty's forces should not be allowed, or perhaps we ought to say compelled, to attend the classes at Netley before, during, or after their time at Haslar, for although a knowledge of tropical medicine may be of slightly less importance to naval medical men than to those serving with troops on land they still see enough of the diseases in question to render instruction in them very desirable.

102

An appeal for funds by the SHS Vice-President

The controversy was seriously exacerbated by a letter from Sir Henry Burdett* which was published in *The Times* for 11 July 1898[4]:

To the editor of *The Times*

SIR, – By the unanimous request of the committee of the Dreadnought Seamen's Hospital at Greenwich I venture to ask you to kindly give publicity to the following particulars of the School for the Study of Tropical Diseases which they have organised and are about to erect and open in connexion with their branch hospital situated between the Royal Victoria and Albert Docks. As the confines of the British Empire have extended, and especially of late years owing to the development of the African continent, the Colonial Office has felt that the need for improvement in the medical service of the British colonies, especially in West Africa, called for the establishment of a school where candidates for this service can receive special training in the diagnosis, and treatment of tropical diseases before they proceed to the colonies. Heretofore an attempt has been made to give newly-appointed medical officers, whenever possible, some preliminary instruction at the headquarters hospital of the colony. Experience shows that this course cannot be followed in every case, and the arrangement has proved, on the whole, to be unsatisfactory. When these facts were brought to the notice of Mr. Chamberlain he addressed a letter to the committee of the Seamen's Hospital [chapter 5], in the course of which he stated that: – He felt confident that a marked advance would be made if some scheme could be devised by which all newly-appointed medical officers should receive a sound and sympathetic training in this country before taking up their duties in West Africa. He was advised that the experience and training to be obtained at the Seamen's Hospital would be the most suitable in the present instance, and he accordingly asked for the assistance of the managing committee in the matter, by considering whether it might not be possible to so enlarge the branch hospital at the Albert Docks so as to provide the necessary accommodation for the establishment of a school of tropical diseases for the benefit of the medical officers in question.

He went on to say: – The Secretary of State for Foreign Affairs was being asked whether he wished the protectorates in East and West Africa under the administration of the Foreign Office should be included in the proposed scheme.

Mr Chamberlain stated that the course of instruction should last for three or four months, and requested to be informed the terms and conditions on which

---

* Sir Henry Burdett KCB, KCVO (1847–1920) was an author and 'statist'. Much of his writing was about hospitals and nursing. At various stages of his career he was Superintendant of the Queen's Hospital, Birmingham, and of the Seamen's Hospital, Greenwich, and Secretary of the Share and Loan Department of the London Stock Exchange.

the committee would be prepared to make the necessary arrangements.

After careful inquiry and consideration the Seamen's Hospital Committee submitted a scheme to the Colonial Office for the establishment of a school for the study of tropical diseases, which has now been approved, and which will shortly be an established fact. The total estimated cost of the new wing, which will give the branch hospital 45 beds, in addition to the new school buildings, is about £13,000. Towards this sum the Colonial Office have agreed to contribute £3,500 on behalf of the colonies and protectorates more immediately concerned, leaving some £10,000 to be raised from the public. From carefully-prepared estimates it appears that the annual cost of maintenance, including 25 additional beds, the board of the resident students, salaries of the medical tutor and other necessary attendants, and interest on capital will be £3,000 per annum. At present the India Office has not intimated its intention of joining in the establishment of this important school of medicine for tropical diseases, but there is reason to hope that some step may be taken in this direction in the near future. Apart from any contribution form the India Office, there is therefore required a capital sum of £10,000 and a net income of £2,000 per annum, seeing that the fees to be paid by the Colonial Office for the resident and non-resident students towards the expenses of the school are estimated to produce at least £1,000 per annum. Having regarded the importance of an accurate knowledge of tropical diseases to a large number of wealthy people who, having served in the colonies are now resident in this country, or whose children are now in the colonies, and to the general sympathy which this important new departure must excite amongst all who have the welfare of the Empire at heart, it is hoped that the necessary funds will speedily be forthcoming. Contributions may be paid direct to the secretary, Mr P J Michelli, Dreadnought Seamen's Hospital, Greenwich, SE, or to the hospital account at, Messrs. Williams, Deacon, and Manchester and Salford Bank, Limited, 20 Birchin-Lane, EC.

It is important that I should state that the school will be open to other students than those members of the medical profession who may be sent by Government departments, or who may wish to equip themselves for service abroad. It appears from the report of the special committee which investigated the question that 78 percent of the cases of tropical diseases treated by the Seamen's Hospital Society had been admitted to the branch hospital which will now contain 45 beds. Provision will be made from 20 to 25 students, with sleeping accommodation for about ten. There will be a fully equipped laboratory, pathological room, museum and every other accessory calculated to make the school efficient. The teaching staff will consist of the senior medical staff of the Dreadnought Hospital at Greenwich, as well as of the branch hospital, together with a number of teachers specially selected and attached to the new school. The school will be under the immediate supervision and direction of a medical tutor, who will attend for six hours daily: instruction will be given to students on four days in the week for four hours each day by one or more members of the teaching staff. It will thus be seen that care has been taken, in co-operation with the Colonial Office, to secure that nothing shall be omitted which can tend to make this new school for the study of tropical diseases of great practical utility and value.

As I am writing, may I further point out that the branch hospital serves another valuable purpose by admitting accident cases which occur with alarming frequency in the neighbouring Albert and Victoria Docks? A recent instance, the terrible explosion on the Atlantic transport liner Manitoba, on the 6th inst., will be fresh in the public mind, though it may not be so generally known that all of the men injured in that accident were at once removed to the branch hospital. I am sure that a mention of this circumstance will tend to awaken the sympathy of many charitable people who will gladly give liberally towards the £10,000 which is now required to enable this new school for tropical diseases to be erected and paid for, and to provide ten extra beds for the reception of accident cases from the docks.

I am, Sir, your obedient servant,

HENRY C BURDETT, Vice-President of the Dreadnought Seamen's Hospital Society. The Lodge, Porchester-square, W., July 9

This letter was accompanied by a leading article[5] which was strongly supportive of its content and hence of the appeal. It also stressed the importance of *bacteriology* in this new venture, citing recent work carried out by Professor Koch. In order to stress the great importance of tropical medicine, the (anonymous) author perhaps mildly, overstated his case:

Sir John Simon [chapter 1] told us, many years ago, that a time might come when the current infections of India would be current also in Europe as a result of the increased activity of mankind and of the increased rapidity of travelling . . .

A few days later however, the author of a leading article in *The Lancet* clearly had serious doubts about the creation of Manson's proposed school[6]:

The letter of Sir Henry Burdett and the leading article based thereon in the *Times* of July 11th will bring to a focus the question of the formation of a school for studying and teaching tropical diseases in London. At the suggestion of Mr. Chamberlain the committee of the Seamen's Hospital has placed before him a scheme which practically amounts to an enlargement of the branch hospital at the Albert Docks . . . We see no provision in Sir Henry Burdett's letter for the payment of this staff of teachers. It can scarcely be expected that the physicians and surgeons attached to the Seamen's Hospital Society can undertake any more gratuitous work than they have at present. The Albert Docks is not a very accessible place [fig 6.1 indicates the position of the Albert Dock Hospital] and a visit there, with four hours' teaching, will make a serious

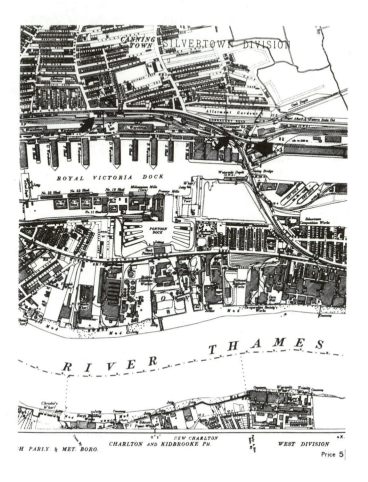

Fig 6.1 Ordnance Survey map dated 1919 (6 inches = 1 mile) showing the position of the Albert Dock Hospital (arrowed). The Royal Albert Dock is situated to the right; the two local railway stations are also indicated (smaller arrows). [reproduced by permission of the Guildhall Library, City of London].

inroad into a physician's or surgeon's daily work. The study of tropical diseases is of the utmost practical importance for colonial and military surgeons and practitioners and deserves every encouragement. Hitherto it has been best carried out at Netley and the amount of practical material in that hospital for such a study must not be ignored, although it is only at the disposal of the Indian and army medical officers. Sporadic courses of lectures in London are eminently unpractical because the students cannot watch the course and treatment of the cases illustrating the lectures. Few patients can be brought from Greenwich or the Albert Docks to a metropolitan school and few students will regularly visit either of these institutions. Sir Henry Burdett is sanguine that tropical diseases can be thoroughly studied at the docks . . . We see no statement as to the number of tropical cases which are admitted into the hospitals of the Seamen's Hospital Society. Chronic dysentery, beri-beri, and chronic malaria make up almost entirely the tropical diseases which a student may expect to see during a course of three or four months' study, and acute cases must be extremely rare, judging from the annual reports of the society. Mr. W. Johnson Smith has published the records of the cases of hepatic abscess during twenty-five years and they only amount to fifty. Bacteriological investigation in tropical diseases can be taught in the well-appointed laboratories of many of our medical schools and is a part of the Netley curriculum. Phthisis, cardiac disease, rheumatism, and renal disease figure amongst the most common cases of illness at the Seamen's as well as at other hospitals. If compulsion is exercised on applicants for Colonial medical appointments, as seems to be implied in Mr. Chamberlain's letter, of course a regular supply of students will be at once forthcoming; but if there is no compulsion we question whether many will attend at such an inaccessible situation as the Albert Docks, and we doubt whether the variety of cases is sufficient to interest and instruct them for such a long period as three or four months.

The honorary staff of the Dreadnought Hospital considered (almost certainly correctly) that they had been kept in the dark;* Burdett's letter to *The Times* had apparently appeared without their knowledge or consent[7]:

To the Editors of THE LANCET.

SIRS, – Sir H. Burdett in the *Times* of July 11th writing of a proposed school for tropical medicine, states that "the teaching staff will consist of the senior medical staff of the *Dreadnought* Hospital at Greenwich, as well as of the branch hospital, together with a number of teachers specially selected and attached to the new school." This was the first intimation of any kind that we had that such a scheme was on foot, and the statement was made without our authority or consent.

We are, Sirs, yours faithfully,
JOHN CURNOW, MD, FRCP Lond., } Visiting
JOHN ANDERSON, MD St. And., FRCP Lond., } Physicians
G.R. TURNER, FRCS Eng., Visiting Surgeon.
Dreadnought Seamen's Hospital, Greenwich, July 18th

---

* Manson's leading critics were: (i) John Curnow, MD, FRCP (1846–1902) – Physician to King's College (from 1890), Professor of Clinical Medicine, King's College (from 1896), and Dean, Medical Faculty, King's College (1883–96), (ii) John Anderson, MD, FRCP, CIE (1840–1910) – Lecturer in Diseases of Tropical Climates, St Mary's Hospital Medical School. Late, Medical Officer on the staff of the Viceroy of India, and (iii) G R (later Sir George) Turner, FRCS (1855–1941) – Surgeon to the *Dreadnought* Hospital.

These sentiments were also reflected at the quarterly Comitia of the Royal College of Physicians of London held on 27 October[8]:

> . . . The Seamen's Hospital Society [had asked] the College to nominate a representative on a committee appointed to organise a School of Tropical Medicine in connexion with their branch hospital. Dr. Curnow explained that although Dr. Anderson and himself were physicians to the Seamen's Hospital at Greenwich they had not been consulted in the matter and, having detailed some of the correspondence which had taken place between himself and the secretary of the hospital, he moved "the previous question." Dr. Anderson having made a few remarks this was carried.

The Lancet pursued its campaign, emphasising the disadvantages of the proposed site for the establishment of the new school, and questioning the amount of suitable clinical material there [9]:

> It is now generally known that at the instigation of Mr. Chamberlain it is proposed to establish an institution for the teaching of tropical medicine. A circular has been sent from the Colonial Office to the medical schools in reference to the matter, the essence of which is the following. . . . "The directors of the Seamen's Hospital at the Albert Docks, which offers exceptional opportunities for studying cases of tropical disease, are providing the necessary buildings and teachers for the accommodation and instruction of the medical officers who may hereafter be selected by the Foreign Office and the Colonial Office for appointments in the tropics. A substantial contribution towards the initial cost of the buildings is being made by the Government, and it is hoped that by Oct. 1st, 1899, it will be possible to receive medical officers at the hospital for purposes of instruction." It is proposed that, as is at present the case, candidates for medical appointments in the British colonial possessions shall be fully qualified before they can be put upon the Secretary of State's list; that from this list a certain number shall be elected annually to fill the vacancies which may occur in the colonial medical service; that the selected candidates shall be trained for a period of at least two months at the Seamen's Hospital; and that they shall then be sent to the colonies or protectorates to which they have been allotted, where, when practicable, they will be attached in the first instance to the headquarters hospital for the purpose of gaining additional experience. The circular goes on to state that although the school at the Seamen's Hospital is designed for the training of medical officers for the Government service, doubtless there will be many other medical men, such as the medical officers of missionary societies and trading corporations and private practitioners who propose to settle in tropical countries, who will be glad to avail themselves of the advantages which such a school can offer. The colonies are being asked to make pecuniary contributions, to collect pathological material for use in the school, and to support the scheme in every possible way. The Royal Society has nominated two competent observers to proceed to Italy and

then to Africa to study the subject of tropical malaria, and in addition the Secretary of State for the Colonies has nominated an experienced medical officer of the Colonial Service to aid in the investigations.

    . . . All members of the medical profession will support Mr. Chamberlain in his endeavours to increase the facilities for the teaching of that branch of medicine which is so important for the welfare of Englishmen residing in tropical countries, but we doubt whether the opinion will be so unanimous as to the suggested methods in the circular of which we have given an abstract. Our naval and army surgeons have not suffered in this respect, for the teaching at Haslar and Netley is of the very best, and at the latter place there are more cases of tropical disease than are to be found in any other hospital in Europe. At nearly all the medical schools, also, courses of lectures on tropical medicine have been delivered by medical men well qualified by experience to do so, but practical teaching, which of course is essential, has been lacking. The question therefore arises, Is the selection of the branch hospital of the Seamen's Hospital at Albert Docks a wise one? There are many objections – for instance, the size of the hospital, the difficulties of access, and the depletion of the old parent hospital at Greenwich of its most interesting material. And then arises the all important question – Are the cases of tropical diseases met with at this hospital sufficiently numerous to justify its selection as a school for the teaching and investigation of such diseases? Full details on this point would be valuable. We may refer to one disease most commonly met with in the tropics – namely, hepatic abscess. In twenty-five years at this hospital and its branch at the docks only 50 cases have been so diagnosed, and it is, of course, open to doubt how many of these were cases of ordinary subphrenic abscess [much was made of invasive hepatic amoebiasis in this controversy]. It would be profitable before any large sum of money is laid out to compare such statistics with those of other hospitals, notably those of Haslar and Netley, the London Hospital, and Guy's Hospital, in order to satisfy the minds of all as to the wisdom of selecting the branch hospital at Albert Docks for the very excellent purpose designed by Mr. Chamberlain.

    . . . If it be necessary that tropical medicine should have a school all to itself in London, why should it be placed so far away? The *Dreadnought* is much nearer and with its 235 beds is more capable of affording clinical material than is its branch with its present 18 and proposed 45 beds.

The latter theme was prominent in the following issue (26 November 1898)[10]. Lack of clinical material – not least the very low number of admissions with 'tropical liver abscess' – was again emphasised. The added criticism was that bacteriology – an important basic science in the teaching of infectious diseases – was well covered in the London teaching hospitals, and that new laboratories were unnecessary. The 'blunderbus tactics' of the SHS also came under attack:

    . . . The Branch Hospital was built as an emergency hospital and was never intended for the reception of any cases which could be allowed to cross the river. Last week we instanced the futility of such a proposal by pointing out that in 25 years only 50 cases of "tropical abscess" had been received at the hospital and on further studying the "tables of cases under treatment at the hospitals and dispensaries of the Seamen's Hospital Society in 1895 and 1896," we are at once struck with the very small number of patients suffering from "tropical diseases" who have been under treatment. Amongst the general diseases we find 73 cases of malarial fever and 2 of bubonic fever but no other recognised tropical fever. Amongst diseases of special organs or tissues there were 44 cases of beri-beri and 4 of "hepatic abscess". Where, then, are the tropical diseases? The explanation is obvious. The acute cases either die at sea before they can reach the hospital or are of an infectious nature. In the former case they will not be available for "concentration," and in the latter the port sanitary authorities would interfere to prevent such "concentration." On the other hand, the Seamen's Hospital would seem in a great measure to be an asylum for sick sailors, for there were in the period stated 221 cases of pulmonary tuberculosis, of which 73 proved fatal, and of these 1 was in the hospital over 600 days, 5 were in over 300 days, 2 over 200 days and 15 over 100 days. Whilst, therefore, fully desirous that support should be given to Mr. Chamberlain's scheme we cannot but wonder how he came to be advised to select the Branch Hospital at the Royal Albert Dock as the nucleus of the school. Further, it is intended that laboratories should be equipped at the new school for the purposes of research. But surely that is unnecessary. Laboratories already exist with every requisite appliance for such work on the Victoria Embankment, at Chelsea, and at certain metropolitan medical schools. Here qualified medical men already attend from all parts of the world, such as Uganda, West Africa, Australia, Canada &c., and diseases of tropical climates – such as malaria, leprosy, plague, cholera, Madura foot, &c. – have especially been made the subjects of original research. A knowledge of bacteriology is essential to colonial practitioners, but we doubt whether anything would be gained by the establishment of new laboratories, as is laid down in the scheme for the new school . . .

The article continued with criticism of the way in which the honorary staff of the *Dreadnought* Hospital had been treated:

. . . Sir Henry Burdett, in his letter to the *Times* of July 11th, stated that "the teaching staff will consist of the senior medical staff of the *Dreadnought* Hospital at Greenwich, as well as of the Branch Hospital, together with a number of teachers specially selected and attached to the new school."

The writer then referred to the Curnow/Anderson/Turner letter and finally, the Royal College of Physicians meeting (see above):

... a letter was read from the Seamen's Hospital Society "asking the College to nominate a representative" on a committee appointed to organise a School of Tropical Medicine in connexion with the Branch Hospital. After some remarks, however, from Dr. Curnow and Dr. Anderson, the "previous question" was carried – an act of great significance as tending to show that without further explanation the College was unwilling to be represented on the committee.

Whilst signifying its *overall* approval of Chamberlain's plan, *The Lancet*[11] continued to have serious doubts about the practicalities thereof, and became increasingly concerned at the manner in which the honorary staff of the Dreadnought had been slighted[11]:

Mr Chamberlain's scheme for the establishment of a School for Instruction in Tropical Medicine has naturally attracted a large amount of attention. ... A judicious protest against certain of these details, over most authoritative and representative signatures, has already reached Mr. Chamberlain's eye and cannot be without its influence upon a Minister so clearly desirous of doing what is right and, above all, what is best for the country. We now publish the correspondence which has taken place between the honorary medical staff of the *Dreadnought* Hospital, Sir Henry Burdett, and Mr. Michelli, the secretary to the Seamen's Hospital Society. This correspondence fully bears out our statement that the medical staff in question have received rude treatment where they might have expected particular courtesy considering the long duration – eighteen, ten, and seventeen years respectively – of their services. Dr. Curnow and Dr. John Anderson, the physicians, and Mr. G.R. Turner, the surgeon to the hospital, naturally objected to the teaching staff of the new school being formed without their previous knowledge; but, as we stated last week, the first intimation they had of what was being done was derived from a letter to the *Times*. The answer given by Mr. Michelli on behalf of the committee to a request for an explanation is simply evasive. He writes that "the statement that 'the teaching staff will consist of the senior medical staff of the *Dreadnought* Hospital at Greenwich as well as of the Branch Hospital, together with a number of teachers specially selected and attached to the new school,' was manifestly intended to convey the meaning that the members of the senior medical staff of both hospitals would have the first option of undertaking the educational work of the staff." We entirely fail to see how a positive statement can "manifestly" be taken to mean a mere proposition ...

This anonymous writer proceeded to direct the readers' attention to the following correspondence (which ran to 13 letters) which was published in the same issue[12]:

13th July, 1898

DEAR SIR HENRY BURDETT, – in your letter in the *Times* of Monday last on the subject of a proposed School for Tropical Diseases in London, you say:

"The teaching staff will consist of the senior medical staff of the *Dreadnought* Hospital at Greenwich, as well as of the Branch Hospital, together with a number of teachers specially selected and attached to the new school."

Will you be so kind as to inform me upon what authority you make this statement, in so far as it refers to the medical staff of the *Dreadnought* Hospital?

Apologising for troubling you, believe me, yours truly,

J. ANDERSON

* * *

15th July 1898.

DEAR DR. ANDERSON, – As my letter was written under instructions from the committee of the *Dreadnought* Hospital I have referred your letter of the 13th instant to them and will let you know in due course.

Believe me, yours very truly,

H. BURDETT.

* * *

The Lodge, Porchester-square, W.,
18th July 1898.

DEAR DR. ANDERSON, – With further reference to your letter of the 13th inst., I am desired to say that it is the intention of the committee of the *Dreadnought* Hospital to give the opportunity to the senior medical staff of both their hospitals to take part, if they thought well, in the work of instruction at the School for Tropical Diseases about to be established at the Branch Hospital.

Believe me, yours very truly,

HENRY C. BURDETT.

* * *

Dreadnought Seamen's Hospital,
Greenwich, S.E., 14th July 1898.

DEAR SIR, – I am directed to inform you that upon the representation of the Colonial Office, the committee of management of the Seamen's Hospital Society have resolved to establish a school for the study of tropical diseases in connexion with their Branch Hospital in the Royal Victoria and Albert Docks. This will involve the erection of school buildings and the enlargement of the hospital to 45 beds.

I have been directed to ask you to co-operate in this movement and to confer with the other members of the society's honorary medical staff, with a view to suggest to the committee of management arrangements as to the educational staff and the general system of the school. The committee will propose as far as possible to concentrate cases of tropical disease at the teaching centre.

Yours faithfully,

P. MICHELLI, Secretary.

J. Curnow Esq., MD, FRCP.

P.S. – I enclose a letter and a leader which appeared in the *Times* of July 11th in reference to the scheme.

* * *

9, Wimpole-street, Cavendish-square, W.,
16.7.98.

DEAR SIR, – I am in receipt of your letter of 14th inst., with the cuttings from the *Times* of July 11th, which I had already seen in the *Times* of that date. Would you oblige me by informing me whether Sir Henry Burdett personally, or the hospital committee, are responsible for the statement that "the teaching staff will consist of the senior medical staff of the *Dreadnought* Hospital at Greenwich," &c.? The publication of such a statement without my being asked, in a scheme of which I knew nothing before I saw it in the *Times*, seems to me most discourteous to myself and intended to convey an unwarranted impression to the public.

I also wish to know if the committee seriously propose "to concentrate cases of tropical disease" at the Branch Hospital and thus deprive the parent hospital of its one distinctive feature.

Believe me to remain, faithfully yours,

JOHN CURNOW, MD

P. Michelli, Esq., Secretary, Seamen's Hospital Society

* * *

Dreadnought Seamen's Hospital,
Greenwich, S.E., 21st July, 1893.

DEAR SIR, – In reply to your letter of 16th inst., I am directed to say that Sir Henry Burdett's letter was written upon information supplied to him by the committee of management, and the statement that "the teaching staff will consist of the senior medical staff of the *Dreadnought* Hospital at Greenwich, as well as of the Branch Hospital, together with a number of teachers specially selected and attached to the new school"; was manifestly intended to convey the meaning that the members of the senior medical staff of both hospitals would have the first option of undertaking the educational work of the school.

Yours faithfully,

P. MICHELLI, Secretary.

J. Curnow, Esq., MD, FRCP,
9 Wimpole-street, Cavendish-square, W.,

* * *

Dreadnought Seamen's Hospital,
Greenwich, July 18th.

To the Editor of The Times [1898; 20 July: 12].

PROPOSED SCHOOL FOR TROPICAL DISEASES.

SIR, – Sir H. Burdett in your issue of July 11th, writing of a proposed School for Tropical Medicine, states that "the teaching staff will consist of the senior medical staff of the *Dreadnought* Hospital at Greenwich, as well as of the Branch Hospital, together with a number of teachers specially selected and attached to the new school." This was the first intimation of any kind that we had that such a scheme was on foot, and the statement was made without our authority or consent. – Yours faithfully,

JOHN CURNOW, MD, FRCP, $\left.\right\}$ Visiting
JOHN ANDERSON, MD, FRCP, Physicians
G.R. TURNER, FRCS, Visiting Surgeon.

* * *

9 Wimpole-street, W.,
25.7.98.

DEAR SIR, – I cannot accept your letter of the 21st inst. as a satisfactory explanation of the position. Sir Henry Burdett's statement that "the teaching staff will consist of the senior medical staff of the *Dreadnought* Hospital at Greenwich, &c.," is quite positive, and is an unauthorised statement. It will not convey to the readers of the *Times*, who I may point out are asked for subscriptions in aid of the committee's scheme, that it manifestly means "that the members of the senior medical staff of both hospitals would have the first option of undertaking the educational work of the school." Such an explanation should be publicly given in the *Times* by either Sir H. Burdett, who has apparently been misinformed, or by the committee.

As you have not answered my second question I must ask it again and I will put it in the following form. Has the committee decided to concentrate as far as possible the cases of tropical disease which alone give its distinctive character to the *Dreadnought* Seamen's Hospital at Greenwich, and has this course of action been determined on without consulting either Dr. Anderson or myself?

Faithfully yours,

JOHN CURNOW, MD

P. Michelli, Esq., Secretary, Seamen's Hospital Society.

* * *

Dreadnought Seamen's Hospital,
Greenwich, S.E., 28th July, 1898.

DEAR SIR, – In reply to your letter of the 25th inst., it appears that you and your colleagues have already taken the most efficient method of undeceiving the readers of the *Times* by your letter explaining that the senior staff of the *Dreadnought* were not consulted on the question of their joining the educational staff before Sir Henry Burdett's letter was written to the *Times*, and that the statements therein were made without their authority or consent. It does not, therefore, seem that any good purpose could be served by reiterating the fact, even if the *Times* would accept a second disclaimer.

Your question with regard to the tropical cases at Greenwich is rather one for the committee than for me to answer, and I will take care that your letter is laid before the Board at their next meeting.

Yours faithfully,

P. MICHELLI, Secretary.

J. Curnow, Esq., MD, FRCP, 9, Wimpole-street, W.

* * *

Oct. 10th 1898

DEAR SIR, – Referring to the proposed School of Tropical Medicine at the Victoria and Albert Docks and Mr. Michelli's letter of July 14th, we think our letter to the *Times* of July 20th was a plain statement of facts. We see nothing to regret on our part, and if there is any meaning in plain English, Sir Henry Burdett's words can have but one interpretation, i.e., that the senior staff of the *Dreadnought* were to be on the teaching staff of the proposed school.

On July 15th he wrote Dr. Anderson that his letter to the *Times* was written under instructions from the committee of the *Dreadnought*; a committee, we would remind you, who had not had the courtesy to let us know that such a scheme was on foot, still less to ask for our co-operation until some five days after the vice-president's letter appeared in the lay press and he had been asked for explanation by Dr. Anderson.

We beg to ask the committee, as Dr. Curnow has twice already asked the secretary, whether they have decided to concentrate the cases of tropical diseases at the Branch Hospital and have done this without consulting the visiting physicians of the parent *Dreadnought* Hospital.

It is impossible for us to give any answer to a request for co-operation until we have been put in full possession of the details of the proposed school.

– Believe us, yours faithfully,

J. CURNOW
J. ANDERSON
G.R. TURNER.

The Chairman of the *Dreadnought* Hospital Committee.

* * *

Dreadnought Seamen's Hospital,
Greenwich, S.E., 17th Oct., 1898.

DEAR SIRS, – I am instructed to acknowledge the receipt of your letter of the 10th inst. which was laid before the general committee at their meeting on Friday last.

The committee regret that you still feel aggrieved by Sir Henry Burdett's letter which was published in the *Times* of July 11th.

They also much regret that you do not feel able to signify your wish to co-operate with them in carrying out the scheme of H.M. Secretary of State for the Colonies for the establishment in connexion with the society's Branch Hospital of a school for the study of tropical diseases.

The details of the scheme must necessarily remain open for consideration by the committee which will be appointed to manage the school.

I am, dear Sirs, yours faithfully,

P. MICHELLI, Secretary.

115

John Curnow, Esq., MD, &c.
John Anderson, Esq., MD, &c.
G. Robertson Turner, Esq., FRCS, &c.

* * *

9, Wimpole-street, Cavendish-square, W.,
29th Oct., 1898.

DEAR SIR, – We beg to acknowledge the receipt of your letter of the 17th inst.

It is true we are aggrieved by the entirely unauthorised statement contained in Sir Henry Burdett's letter published in the *Times* of July 11th last; but we are still more so by the committee's want of courtesy in not asking the opinion of the senior medical staff of the *Dreadnought* Hospital at any time during the inception of their scheme before the letter was written, and for which lack of courtesy no apology has been offered or regret expressed.

The question as to the concentration of tropical cases at the Branch Hospital and consequent starvation of the parent hospital at Greenwich in its one distinctive feature has not yet been answered, although three times asked, and we press your committee for a definite reply upon this point, after the receipt of which we will not trouble them with further correspondence.

We are, dear sir, yours faithfully,

JOHN CURNOW.
J. ANDERSON.
G.R. TURNER.

The Secretary, *Dreadnought* Seamen's Hospital, Greenwich.

* * *

Dreadnought Seamen's Hospital,
Nov. 28th, 1898.

SIRS, – Not having received any reply to the question we pressed upon you in our letter of Oct. 29th last we are sending the correspondence that has taken place between us to the press for publication. In doing so we wish to remind you that we have performed the medical and surgical work of the *Dreadnought* Hospital for eighteen, ten, and seventeen years respectively.

We are, Sirs, yours faithfully,

JOHN CURNOW.
J. ANDERSON.
G.R. TURNER.

The Secretary, *Dreadnought* Seamen's Hospital, Greenwich.

The following week, *The Lancet* published a further leading article in which the correspondent (who seems to have been a Royal College of Physicians man!) considered that Netley (chapter 5), and neither the *Dreadnought* nor the Albert Dock Hospital was the correct venue for the proposed school[13]:

> ... One of the main objects of the new school is to afford opportunities for candidates for colonial appointments to study tropical diseases and we believe that Netley, with its staff of teachers who have practical experience of tropical diseases and its admirably equipped bacteriological laboratory, together with the number of patients recently returned from tropical countries, would afford every facility for the purpose. Building, equipping, and maintaining at an enormous cost a new school at the Royal Albert Dock would simply be to duplicate what already exists and if the public were duly informed of these circumstances we very much doubt if the necessary funds would be forthcoming. The [Seamen's Hospital Society] memorandum goes on to say, "There is no reason to suppose that the War Office would allow medical men of every class [i.e., civilians, medical missionaries, &c.,] to study at Netley." We may reply that "civilians, medical missionaries, &c.," can, if they so desire, obtain ample instruction at the various medical schools and laboratories already in existence, whilst we believe that an arrangement might well be made between the Colonial Office and the War Office whereby the colonial medical officers might undergo a course of instruction at Netley.

The policy of the committee of the London School of Tropical Medicine is certainly curious, for in reply to the objection "that the concentration of tropical cases at the Branch Hospital will operate to the detriment of the parent hospital – the *Dreadnought*," they simply remark, "Concentration of cases of tropical disease at the Branch Hospital is certainly desirable, but patients suffering from tropical diseases and applying for admission to the *Dreadnought* Hospital would still be admitted and treated there." This practically admits the intention to deplete the *Dreadnought* Hospital of cases of tropical disease. The third objection selected for answer is the all-important one – namely, "that the clinical material offered at the Branch Hospital is insufficient and that the hospital is difficult of access." We have already given statistics, derived from the printed report of the Seamen's Hospital Society, which conclusively prove that the material of both the parent and the branch hospitals is not sufficient to justify the proposal to expend large sums on new buildings for the purpose of establishing a school. The total number of beds is to be only 45, whilst at Netley there are 1000. The memorandum states that the number of cases of tropical diseases under treatment at the Branch Hospital during the year ended Nov. 30th last was 81 (our figures were taken from the report 1895–96), and that of this total 31 were suffering from malaria; and then come the words, "These cases alone are sufficient to justify the establishment of a school there." Are they? All connected with general hospitals know that numerous cases of malaria, amply sufficient for instruction and investigation, are treated every year in the wards of such hospitals without the incurring of any special public expenditure.

The fourth objection attacked by the memorandum is "that it is unnecessary to build laboratories as it is proposed, seeing that at

many places in London there are now fully-equipped establishments."
The only answer offered is, "Every teacher of clinical medicine must
be fully aware that to separate the laboratory from the ward is highly
prejudicial to successful work." We very much doubt whether "every
teacher of clinical medicine" would agree with this. A microscope with
a few simple reagents might be kept in a room near the ward, but the
laboratory, every clinical teacher would think, is better some distance
away.' . . . 'Professor Crookshank's communication [see below] strongly
supports our view that new bacteriological laboratories are unnecessary.
Finally in the memorandum the personal element is introduced. For this
portion of the controversy there can be no doubt that the committee of the
Seamen's Hospital Society is to blame. The letters published last week as
well as those in our present issue show that an apology from the committee
to the honorary staff of the *Dreadnought* Hospital is the least amend which
can be made.

It is much to be regretted that the Royal College of Physicians of London
was not approached in the first instance and asked to advise as to the
foundation of the school. Looking to the manner in which the scheme has
been introduced we cannot but feel that if every portion of it is managed in
the same way as the attempted formation of the teaching staff has been, the
Managing Committee will at once lose the confidence of both the medical
profession and the public.

The main thrust of Crookshank's letter[14] was that adequate *bacteriological*
facilities were already in operation at King's College Hospital and the
Institute of Preventive Medicine; it would be a serious mistake therefore,
to duplicate these laboratories at the Albert Dock Hospital:

To the Editors of THE LANCET.

SIRS, – In referring to the subject of a proposed School of Tropical
Medicine in your issue of Nov. 26th you remark that laboratories already
exist on the Victoria Embankment at Chelsea and at certain metropolitan
schools. A "Colonial Physician," writing in the *Daily Chronicle* (Nov.
29th), supports the suggestion of a new laboratory by stating that the
existing institutions exist for "a variety of quite different uses." . . . As
regards the laboratories at King's College let me say most emphatically
that they differ very materially from those attached to some of our metropolitan medical schools. Twelve years ago these laboratories were founded
and equipped for *teaching and research*. They were opened to all comers
and special facilities were granted to colonial and foreign practitioners both
for obtaining instruction and for carrying on original research. More than
1000 qualified medical practitioners, many of them holding high positions
in the colonial, naval, Indian, and army medical services, have entered for
instruction in the laboratory. The list of registered names includes those
of practitioners and medical officers from Egypt, West Coast of Africa,
Uganda, the Cape, British Guiana, Jamaica, Trinidad, Straits Settlements,

India, Ceylon, China, Japan, Queensland, New South Wales, Canada, New York State, Michigan, Ohio, Missouri, Indiana, California, Florida, Chili, and Buenos Ayres. Several workers in the laboratory have been specially trained with a view to combating plague, cholera, yellow fever, madura disease, actinomycosis, cattle plague, pleuro-pneumonia, and other diseases prevalent in our colonies and in foreign countries. The Colonial and War Offices have recognised the laboratories by granting leave of absence in order that their officers might be trained in King's College.

The course of instruction consists of (1) lectures and practical instruction in all that relates to the knowledge which we at present possess of the causation and prevention of diseases of man and animals attributed to bacteria and other micro-parasites; (2) Advanced technical instruction in the methods of original research, thereby encouraging further researches in the colonies by competent observers. A thorough knowledge of these diseases cannot be imparted in a small clinical laboratory attached for convenience to the wards of a hospital. In the first place, there would be no opportunity for learning anything about the epidemic diseases of animals. It will at once be admitted that the services of colonial health officers and colonial practitioners would be of increased value if they were qualified (especially in the absence of any veterinary surgeon, or by co-operation with them) to advise upon the best means of stamping out tuberculosis, actinomycosis, cattle plague, pleuro-pneumonia, surra, Loodiana disease, &c., and also if they were competent to undertake original researches in connexion with diseases of animals, especially those communicable to man. In the second place, I would point out that cases of leprosy, yellow fever, cholera, plague, madura disease, and many other tropical diseases are very rarely imported to England, and therefore instruction at the bedside, supplemented by examination in a clinical laboratory would be very irregular and inadequate. For training students in these diseases reliance must be mainly placed upon the pathological and bacteriological investigation of morbid specimens and materials supplied from the colonies and the study of cultivations. To collect such material requires time, and to constantly carry on cultivations necessitates a large, well-equipped laboratory and a well-trained staff. The teachers should be ready at all times to give instruction and, indeed, willing to practically devote the whole of their time to teaching and research. Such a laboratory can only be provided and maintained at very great cost, and the establishment of a new laboratory on this scale would only provide for work for which provision has already been made at King's College and the Institute of Preventive Medicine. It would not supply any want, but it would enter into competition more especially with the teaching at King's College and thus undermine the work which has been carried on for twelve years. The effects of this would be severely felt. . . .

All candidates for colonial medical appointments should be required to attend and be "signed up" for the following:

1. A special course of clinical instruction in tropical medicine. This

course might be given at the Seamen's Hospital and in co-operation with the metropolitan hospitals. An arrangement might be made with the metropolitan hospitals by which candidates for the colonial service were granted a circular ticket giving them the privilege of being shown in the wards any cases of interests to colonial practitioners.

2. A course of lectures on tropical medicine and hygiene, delivered at the proposed School of Tropical Medicine and the Seamen's Hospital or any other medical school recognised by the Colonial Office as providing adequate training in this subject.

3. Lectures and practical instruction for not less than six weeks in a bacteriological laboratory or institute which is recognised by the Colonial Office as fully equipped with the materials and teaching staff necessary for giving the instruction required.

. . . Those already holding appointments in the colonial service and those engaged in private practice in the colonies would derive very great benefit if they were to take advantage of these lectures and practical studies and thus keep themselves in touch with the most recent views and with current research. Encouragement might be given to those on leave from the colonies by the creation of colonial scholarships or studentships entitling the holders to free attendance on the same course of instruction demanded from candidates for the colonial service.

I am, Sirs, yours faithfully,

EDGAR M. CROOKSHANK, MB Lond.
King's College, London, Dec. 5th, 1898.

Further lengthy correspondence (5 letters) was also published in this issue of *The Lancet*, and the controversy showed no sign of abating[15]:

We have not thought it necessary to print at length a memorandum which has been issued by the Seamen's Hospital Society with the idea of answering certain objections which exist to the projected School of Tropical Medicine, because the memorandum was not sent to us – for reasons best known to the committee of the society. . . . We publish below a letter which has been addressed to Mr. Michelli, the secretary of the Seamen's Hospital Society, by Sir William Broadbent* in acknowledgement of the receipt of the memorandum:

84 Brook-street, Grosvenor-square, W.,
Dec. 7th, 1898.
DEAR MR. MICHELLI, – You have done me the honour to send me

---

* Sir William Henry Broadbent, Bt, KCVO, MD, LLD, DSc, FRS (1835–1907) was consulting physician to St Mary's Hospital and Physician Extraordinary to Queen Victoria. He was later Physician in Ordinary to King Edward VII and King George V.

a copy of the memorandum issued or to be issued by the committee of the Seamen's Hospital and I feel bound to make one or two observations upon it.

It is implied that because the first four of the contentions have been carefully considered by the Secretary of State for the Colonies they may be regarded as *choses jugées*. But the Secretary of State would be guided by the information laid before him, and if this information was imperfect or one-sided his approval was obtained under false pretences.

The personal matter of the injustice and discourtesy to the medical staff of the *Dreadnought* is said . . . to have nothing whatever to do with the merits or demerits of the scheme. But this discourtesy entirely prevented certain aspects of the question from being brought to the notice of the Secretary of State and made the data on which he based his judgement imperfect and one-sided.

How little any conclusion formed by the committee is entitled to respect is made clear by the memorandum itself. "It may be mentioned," it says, "that the visiting staff of the *Dreadnought* have been invited to co-operate," leaving it to be understood that this invitation was part of the original scheme, whereas it was not sent till it had become an insult.

This *suggestio falsi* is aggravated by the circulation with the memorandum of a copy of Sir H. Burdett's letter from which the passage in which he states that the senior medical staff of the *Dreadnought* would form part of the teaching staff of the school is omitted. A committee capable of such a suppression of truth material to the issue and of such a suggestion of what is calculated to mislead is, in my opinion, totally unworthy of confidence.

Yours faithfully,
W.H. BROADBENT.

* * *

We have received from Mr. G.R. Turner, the surgeon to the *Dreadnought* Hospital, the following letters for publication. They complete the story told by the letters published last week and confirm our opinion that the honorary medical staff of the *Dreadnought* Hospital have been treated with marked discourtesy by the committee.

49 Green-street, Park-lane, W.,
July 19th, 1898.

DEAR SIR, – I have conferred with Drs. Curnow and Anderson on the subjects mentioned in Sir H Burdett's letter to the *Times* which by your direction was sent to me. I was astounded to hear from them that this letter was the first notice they had of the project for a school for tropical medicine in which their services and possibly mine were to be used as members of the teaching staff. Had I, a surgeon, been the only one of the visiting staff kept in ignorance of the matter I should not have supposed that any intentional discourtesy was meant, nor can I think even now that it has been more than a blunder on the part of the Managing Committee to direct the publication of their intentions in the *Times* newspaper before conference of any kind with those so closely interested as the honorary visiting staff of the *Dreadnought* Seamen's Hospital. As a member of that senior staff mentioned by Sir H Burdett I should like much to know the constitution of the sub-committee which reported that 78 per cent. of the cases of tropical disease go to the Branch Hospital; by whom was it decided what cases were tropical and what not; and whether this report may be inspected and shown to be accurate and true (a very necessary proceeding before asking the public to subscribe to the erection of buildings and the attempted formation of a school in a very out-of-the-way and inaccessible situation); by whom were the already elaborate plans for this proposed school drawn up; and did their author or authors know that the visiting staff of the *Dreadnought* Hospital were in absolute ignorance that such a scheme was on foot?

I have written thus freely because as a surgeon these matters do not nearly concern me, and I cannot help feeling that my medical colleagues have been treated with a marked lack of the ordinary consideration to which all of us honorary officers are entitled, and I trust that the Managing Committee will able to give us some explanation.

Believe me, yours faithfully,

(Signed) G.R. TURNER.

To the Chairman of the Committee,
Seamen's Hospital, Greenwich.

* * *

3, Crosby-square, Bishopsgate, E.C.,
July 20th 1898.

SEAMEN'S HOSPITAL.

DEAR SIR, – I write a line to acknowledge the receipt of your letter of July 19th, 1898.

I am sorry to learn that the senior medical staff of the *Dreadnought* Hospital take exception to portions of Sir Henry Burdett's letter relating to the proposed establishment at the Branch Hospital of a school for the study of tropical diseases which was published in the *Times* of July 11th.

The questions asked by your letter are rather for the Committee of Management than for me personally as chairman to reply to. I will take care that your letter is brought before the committee at their next meeting.

I am, dear Sirs, yours faithfully,

(Signed) PERCEVAL A. NAIRNE.

G.R. Turner, Esq., FRCS, 49 Green-street,
Park-lane, W.

* * *

49 Green-street, Park-lane, W.,
July 21st, 1898.

DEAR SIR, – Thank you for your letter of July 20th. The senior medical staff of the *Dreadnought* Hospital – I believe I may speak for us all – take exception to the elaboration and publication of a scheme for a school in which it is stated they will teach before any of them had heard a word on the matter. It is not, I think you will agree with me, customary or considerate to make statements about the co-operation of honorary officers in work the existence of which they know nothing about. This Sir H. Burdett has done by the direction of the Managing Committee and it is against this that I most vigorously protest. It is not, I will only say, usual for managing committees to ignore the honorary staff as we have been ignored. It looks, although I can hardly believe it, that we have been purposely kept in the dark. – Believe me,

yours faithfully,

(Signed) G.R. TURNER.

Percival A. Nairne, Esq.

* * *

Dreadnought Seamen's Hospital, Greenwich, S.E.,
Sept. 15th, 1898.

DEAR SIR, – Your letters to the chairman of July 19th and 21st have been laid before my Board.

The committee feel that their relations with the medical staff in the past are a sufficient answer to the suggestion that any discourtesy or want of consideration towards them in connexion with the society's reply to the Secretary of State's proposal for the establishment by the society of a school for the study of tropical diseases was intended.

The committee regret that any expression in Sir Henry Burdett's letter published in the *Times* of July 11th should appear to you and to some of your colleagues to have represented that you and they had engaged to take part in the educational work of the school. Sir Henry Burdett (with the committee) probably felt no doubt that the educational work would in the main be taken charge of by the medical staff of the society's hospitals, but the committee do not read his letter as a pledge that each member of the staff would join in the educational work.

The committee have read with much regret the joint letter of Dr. Curnow, Dr. Anderson and yourself, published in the *Times* of July 20th, and in some of the medical papers a few days later, which they feel must tend to injure the success of the project into which the committee have entered at the invitation of the Secretary of State. They will be glad to know whether they are to infer from it that the writers have renounced all connexion with the proposed school and upon this point they ask for a definite reply at an early date.

Yours faithfully,

P. MICHELLI, Secretary.

G. Robertson Turner Esq., FRCS,
49 Green-street, Park-lane, W.

No less than 15 distinguished physicians (including the doyen of the IMS Sir John Fayrer (chapter 2)), – 3 of them Fellows of the Royal Society and 11 Fellows of the Royal College of Physicians – then joined the correspondence in *The Times* and *The Lancet*. They reiterated much of the criticism which had already been aired, and felt strongly that the

Dreadnought Hospital's staff had been abysmally treated[16]:

To the Editor of the TIMES [1898; 15 December: 7].

SIR, – The proposed scheme for affording additional instruction in tropical medicine has attracted attention to a subject with which the medical profession entirely sympathise. That physicians and surgeons who propose to practise in hot climates should have an opportunity afforded them for the special study of tropical diseases is no doubt most desirable not only on the ground of humanity, but also as a duty to British subjects resident in the tropics. Having regard, however, to the scheme as detailed in the Colonial Office circular, dated the 9th ult., there are several points bearing on its practicability and prospect of success which require careful consideration before it is finally adopted.

The scheme is very costly . . . Fees from students would partly defray the yearly expenditure, but it is doubtful whether such sums can be procured from either or both sources.

A memorandum and circular are now being circulated by the Seamen's Hospital Society which state that the school is intended for medical graduates only. Of these candidates for the Colonial Medical Service will form a part and it is anticipated that missionary societies, trading corporations, and private practitioners connected with the tropics will avail themselves of the opportunities offered by the proposed school. The number of students expected to be forthcoming is not stated, and it is well to consider whether additional facilities to those already existing are required before incurring the contemplated heavy expenditure.

The candidates for the Colonial Medical Service could be instructed at Netley where the Royal Victoria Hospital affords more material for clinical instruction than can be obtained anywhere else and has a staff of teachers practically acquainted with tropical diseases as well as an excellent bacteriological laboratory. There seems to be no reason why these candidates should not go through a four months' residential course at Netley and obtain the advantages which its hospital and school now afford to candidates for the Army and Indian Medical Services. It appears to us that candidates for the Colonial Medical Service might fairly be required to pass through this course as a qualification for appointment.

Medical men connected with missionary societies and trading corporations, along with those who in a private capacity propose to practice in the tropics, have open to them for the special study of these diseases the London and provincial schools of medicine where the subject is already taught. Many of these are provided with bacteriological laboratories and all that is required for academic teaching. For clinical work the material afforded by the *Dreadnought* and its Branch (the former is much more accessible) is available for those residing in London, while those resident in the provinces have valuable opportunities in this respect at such ports as Liverpool, Newcastle, Bristol, and other places. It must not be overlooked that the diseases of hot climates are included in the lectures on the practice of medicine given at every medical college and school in the kingdom.

It appears therefore that sufficient means of instruction already exist and the large initial outlay and costly maintenance of the proposed school and hospital are consequently uncalled for.

In the published correspondence between the honorary medical staff and the committee of management of the *Dreadnought* Hospital it is stated in Mr. Michelli's letter, dated July 14th, that "the committee will propose, as far as possible to concentrate cases of tropical disease at the teaching centre." We are informed that this has been already done to some extent, for the Albert Docks branch has detained patients who were originally intended to be passed on to Greenwich and the parent institution has therefore been depleted in order to feed its branch. This seems to be very undesirable in the case of the *Dreadnought* with its past traditions, and the more so because the cases of tropical disease in that hospital have been used already for teaching purposes in connexion with one of the London schools.

It is, we think, unfortunate that the Secretary of State for the Colonies did not consult such an authority as the Royal College of Physicians as to the best method of giving effect to the scheme before it was made public, and it is much to be regretted that the Committee of Management of the Seamen's Hospital Society neglected to consult their senior visiting medical staff on a matter so seriously affecting themselves and the usefulness of the hospital at Greenwich.

We are, Sir, your obedient servants,
Wm. ROBERTS, MD, FRS
DYCE DUCKWORTH, MD, LLD,
Physician and Lecturer on Medicine, St. Bartholomew's Hospital.
J. FAYRER, MD, FRS,
Consulting Physician, Charing-cross Hospital.
WILLIAM M. ORD, MD Lond, FRCP,
Consulting Physician to St. Thomas's Hospital.
W.S. CHURCH, MD, FRCP,
Senior Physician, St. Bartholomew's Hospital.
W.R. GOWERS, MD, FRS,
Consulting Physician, University College Hospital.
I. BURNEY YEO, MD, FRCP,
Senior Physician to King's College Hospital and Professor of Medicine
in King's College.
FREDK. T. ROBERTS, MD, FRCP,
Professor of Medicine at University College;
Physician to University Hospital.
ERNEST SANSOM, MD, FRCP,
Physician to the London Hospital and Lecturer on Clinical Medicine to
the London Hospital.
THOMAS BUZZARD, MD, FRCP,
Physician to the National Hospital for the Paralysed and Epileptic.
W.B. CHEADLE, MD, FRCP,

Senior Physician to St. Mary's Hospital and Lecturer on Clinical
Medicine.
THOS. WHIPHAM, MD, FRCP,
Physician to St. George's Hospital.
W. CAYLEY, MD, FRCP,
Physician to the Middlesex Hospital.
G. FIELD BLANDFORD, MD, FRCP,
Lecturer on Psychological Medicine, St. George's Hospital.
F. De HAVILLAND HALL, MD, FRCP,
Physician to the Westminster Hospital.
Dec. 14th.

In December, *The Times* carried a leading article[17] which was clearly
precipitated by the letter from Roberts *et al*. It pointed to the 'unexpected
amount of opposition [to the Chamberlain-Manson plans] amongst the
medical profession'. It continued 'it is impossible not to inquire why
two great schools of medicine – that of Guy's Hospital, and that of the
Royal Free Hospital, which is limited to female students, and which finds
its most important work in educating lady doctors for India – should be
unrepresented.' A further point was that 'of the ten hospitals no less
than four are represented by their 'consulting' physicians'. Nor, with
one exception was there anyone who has 'of late years contributed in
any remarkable degree to that increased knowledge of the causation of
tropical disease.' 'As for Mr Hutchinson's 'Polyclinic' (see below) . . . it
may, we think be dismissed from serious consideration in regard to this
particular matter.' The leader writer considered that 'The result has been
a correspondence not without animus on either side, and certainly marked,
on the side of the officials of the *Dreadnought* Hospital, by an unfortunate
tardiness in admitting that they had been entirely in the wrong.'

The issue of *The Lancet* which also carried the letter by Roberts, *et al*
contained yet more correspondence (led by Curnow) on the pros and cons
of the project and the unsuitability of the Albert Dock Hospital[18]:

To the Editors of THE LANCET.

SIRS, – In your issue of last week you referred to the memorandum
issued by the Seamen's Hospital Society in support of the scheme proposed
for the New School of Tropical Medicine as a question of general policy.
I wish to examine it from another standpoint. I would incidentally remark
that the memorandum and the appeal for subscriptions have not been sent
to either Dr. Anderson, Mr. G.R. Turner or myself.

I am writing as the senior visiting physician of the *Dreadnought* Seamen's Hospital, whose experience of its medical work goes back more than
twenty years, to the time when Sir Henry Burdett was the secretary, and
is probably more complete than that of anyone living except Mr. Johnson
Smith, the principal medical officer. I have continued my associations with

the hospital for this long period partly from a desire to see tropical cases, partly from the old traditions of the *Dreadnought*, and partly from the opportunities it afforded me to show students and medical men specimens of tropical disease. The scheme of the committee of management of the Seamen's Hospital Society will, if carried out, effectually destroy all these.

I think that the scheme promulgated by the Committee of Management is unnecessary, most unwise, and extravagant. £13,000 in July has expanded into £16,000 in December. I shall also show that the arguments urged in its support are misleading. The scheme in the appeal of the society merely mentions a bacteriological laboratory, pathological laboratory, lectures, &c.; but the details are clearly stated in Sir Henry Burdett's letter to the *Times* of July 11th.

. . . Before the bacteriology of tropical medicine can be studied a general knowledge of bacteriological methods and of ordinary bacteriological diseases must first be learnt, and this can easily be obtained in the many bacteriological laboratories which now exist in London and elsewhere. . . . [This] laboratory is obviously unnecessary, and the sum for furniture, fittings, &c., for a new school of from 20 to 25 students – viz., £400 – if this is to include a bacteriological laboratory and its equipments, is almost too ridiculously inadequate to be referred to.

I have carefully looked over the list of the names of the gentlemen forming the Advisory Committee, and I can only find two (excluding the chairman and deputy chairman) who can be in the slightest degree conversant with the medical work of the *Dreadnought* Seamen's Hospital. Dr. Robert Barnes was its physician in its best old days and Mr. Johnston Smith is the principal medical officer (resident). It will be news to all the others that there exists at present in the Seamen's Hospital an excellent little museum, rich in pathological material, started in the days of Busk and George Budd, and which only needs a curator for its further development. I may venture to say that with the exceptions above named no one on that Advisory Committee has ever crossed the threshold of that museum.

For the teaching of tropical medicine in London the essentials which are needed are a working laboratory for the examination of blood, sputa, excreta, &c., and an electrical room such as are in existence at every properly equipped general hospital and such as are evidently contemplated at Liverpool. These should be established at both the parent hospital and the Branch Hospital and would probably come much nearer to the modest expenditure (£350) annually required at Liverpool [chapter 7] than to that asked for in the proposed scheme. The calculation that £1,000 will be contributed annually in fees by students sent by Government is too absurd for serious attention unless the boarding and lodging of the ten students are included. But that these rooms will be constantly filled seems doubtful if the new school is so easy of access as is urged by the committee.

From these remarks on the general scheme I now pass on to a consideration of the reasons put forward in the memorandum sent out by the Seamen's Hospital Society.

1. The small number and but little variety of the cases of tropical disease treated in the society's hospitals have been clearly pointed out. We are told that the "building called the 'Dreadnought' at Greenwich which formerly was the infirmary of Greenwich Hospital is not the property of the Seamen's Hospital Society but is held by them from the Lords Commissioners of the Admiralty subject to six months' notice." This of course would obviously be a fatal objection to such a scheme as that indicated in Sir H. Burdett's letter, but considering that the society has been in possession for twenty-eight years the establishment and proper fitting up of a working laboratory and electrical room would not seriously embarrass the society's architect. Indeed, I find [in] its latest report, published only this year, that since the society has occupied the premises it has much improved the building at Greenwich, a chapel has been added, and the entire drainage of the hospital has been renewed. The building of the chapel necessitated a very extensive alteration of the Somerset ward of the hospital. I think, therefore, that even on the insecure tenure put forward by the committee the necessary alterations for its proper conduct as a hospital might be carried out without incurring the displeasure of the Lords Commissioners of the Admiralty. I venture, however, to ask, Is the whole truth disclosed in the statement that it is held from the Lords Commissioners of the Admiralty at six months' notice? for I find the following statement in "An Account of the Origin and Progress of the Seamen's Hospital Society," published . . . in the same report: "After four years' endeavours on the part of the committee to effect so desirable an object the Lords Commissioners of the Admiralty in the year 1870, under the powers afforded them by the 'Greenwich Hospital Act' of the previous session, granted the society a lease for 99 years of the infirmary (and adjoining Somerset ward) at Greenwich Hospital at a nominal rental in view of the loan of the ship, with the attendant expense of the external repairs, fittings, and ship's stores." I leave it to the Committee of Management to reconcile the two statements.

2 and 3. These can be taken together. The relations of the Branch Hospital to the parent institution at Greenwich are sufficiently clear from a paragraph in . . . the committee's report for the year 1889.

It is intended that the branch shall be in telephonic communication with the hospital at Greenwich and that the beds shall be used for the retention of urgent or special cases, all others being transferred by ambulance to Greenwich.

There is a special ambulance and a room for it at the Branch Hospital which was opened in 1890.

The manner in which this intention has been carried out since the present honorary physician was appointed in 1892 is clearly shown by the following figures. In 1892 the number of cases of malaria and dysentery – typical tropical diseases – treated at the Greenwich Hospital were respectively 65 and 36. In the past year, 1897, they have fallen to 32 and 25. If this is not a depletion and starving of the parent institution I should like to know what is. It is, moreover, admitted in the memorandum that 31 cases of malaria were treated at the Branch Hospital during the year ending Nov. 30th last. Does anyone conversant with malaria believe that the bulk of these cases could not have been taken safely and without harm across the river to the parent institution in accordance with the expressed intention of the founders who publicly appealed for subscriptions on the lines quoted above? If this policy had been honestly adhered to by the visiting physician and the present Committee of Management no such enlargement of the hospital as is now proposed would have been necessary. The ambulance does not now carry across any tropical cases except it be someone who is expected to undergo a protracted convalescence. This starving of the parent hospital of tropical diseases is rapidly bearing fruit on its medical side, for this is being more and more turned into an asylum or infirmary for chronically-diseased and incurable sailors. A census of my wards at the end of last month showed that in my 33 beds there were patients who had been there for 671, 444, 408, 266, 212, 193, 163, and 139 days, and for whom no benefit can be expected.

I would submit that it is very unfortunate that Mr. Chamberlain's most excellent wishes should not have been placed before a representative body like the Royal College of Physicians of London who would probably have nominated a committee to report on the subject. Such a committee would have carefully considered the question in its whole bearing and a comprehensive scheme would have been laid before the Right Honourable the Secretary of State for the Colonies. It must necessarily have included the work of the existing bacteriological laboratories, of the parent hospital at Greenwich as well as of its branch, and of any other medical institutions with sufficient tropical cases of disease, such as Liverpool, Leith, &c., to afford facilities for such clinical teaching. All tropical cases do not come into the Albert Docks, and other institutions should be recognised partially or entirely as teaching centres for colonial surgeons as well as the proposed new school. It would seem that Mr. Chamberlain has only had the opportunity during the inception of the scheme of obtaining the somewhat one-sided views of the medical adviser to the Colonial Office and of the Committee of Management of the Seamen's Hospital Society. The result is that he is recommended to enlarge and extend the work of the Branch Hospital, to which the colonial medical adviser is the sole physician, to build a new school there, and to make a two months' course at that school compulsory on every aspirant to the Colonial Medical Service. The injurious effects of the carrying out of the scheme on the parent hospital and other institutions have apparently but little troubled its framers.

I presume that my remembrances of these past years and my knowledge of these unpalatable facts were considered sufficient reasons why I and my colleagues were deliberately excluded from the conferences of the committee.

Another instance of disingenuousness is shown in the appeal for funds and should be mentioned. In the face of our published correspondence they actually circulate this paragraph:—

The educational body of the school will include not only members of the staff of the Seamen's Hospital Society, on which are to be found men who have themselves practised in the tropics, but . . .

Two members only of the medical staff – Dr. Manson and Dr. John Anderson – have practised in the tropics. Dr. Manson may be the educational staff. I have yet to learn that Dr. Anderson has signified his willingness to join. Can any statement be more misleading? Apologising for the length of this letter which, I hope, clearly explains the situation,

– I am, Sirs,
yours faithfully,
JOHN CURNOW, MD, FRCP Lond.,
Senior Visiting Physician to the Seamen's *Dreadnought*
Hospital, Wimpole-street, W., Dec. 12th, 1898.

And this was followed by a letter from the Secretary of the SHS to Sir William Broadbent[19]:

Dreadnought Seamen's Hospital, Greenwich, S.E.,
Dec. 14th, 1898.

DEAR SIR WILLIAM BROADBENT, – I have to acknowledge the receipt of your letter of Dec. 7th. I understood it to have been written as an official communication and therefore brought it before the Committee of the Seamen's Hospital Society at their meeting on Dec. 9th.

You state that the action of the Committee "prevented certain aspects of the question from being brought to the notice of the Secretary of State and made the data on which he based his judgment imperfect and one-sided" and that thus "his approval was obtained under false pretences." This statement the Committee maintain has no foundation. There has certainly been no false pretence and the use of such a term is indefensible. The Committee believe that all aspects of the question have been put before the Secretary of State and fully considered by him. If in your view this is not so the Committee cannot doubt that Mr. Chamberlain is still open to consider the matter from any fresh aspect in which it can be put before him. You further state broadly that the Committee have made a suggestion falsely in saying that the visiting staff have been invited to co-operate. The Committee much regret that you should have permitted yourself to make such a statement and they protest not only against the language but against so strained an interpretation of the memorandum. The correspondence which the *Dreadnought* visiting staff have published shows clearly at what stage they were asked to co-operate and nothing has been written in the memorandum to lead to the conclusion that they were invited to co-operate at an earlier date than is disclosed by the correspondence. Whether the invitation when sent was an insult or not is a question on which the public will form their own opinion. It was not so intended by the Committee and they do not gather that the visiting staff have so viewed it.

The Committee observe that you object to the omission from Sir Henry Burdett's letter, as issued with the memorandum, of the passage against which the *Dreadnought* visiting staff so strenuously protested. The letter was reprinted in such a form as to show that a passage had been omitted. The Committee recognised that after the protest of the visiting staff the paragraph objected to must not be republished, but they saw no occasion to abstain from publishing the rest of the letter. We can hardly suppose that the visiting staff will join in your protest against the omission of the paragraph in question.

The Committee cannot but feel astonishment at a charge of such dishonourable acts as "suppression of truth material to the issue and suggestion of what is calculated to mislead" being made against them by a leading physician. Such charges as these are most regrettable and unfounded and, the Committee fear, will not tend to the amicable adjustment of the difficulty which has arisen and which the Committee greatly regret and are anxious to do everything in their power to remove.

Believe me to be, yours faithfully,

P. MICHELLI, Secretary.

Sir Wm. Broadbent, Bart. MD, FRCP, FRS, &c.,
84 Brook-street, Grosvenor-square, W.

Mr Jonathan Hutchinson* now joined the debate in a letter to *The Times* (15 December 1898)[20]. He pointed out that the tropical school was being founded at the same time as a 'Polyclinic' at Gower Street [in which he had a personal interest]; both institutions, he continued, were being funded by wealthy benefactors – many of whom would be the same individuals. He strongly favoured a proposal that: 'Seamen . . . do not suffer solely nor chiefly from tropical disease, nor are 'tropical diseases' the whole of what the British colonial surgeon needs to be familiar with'. He considered the Albert Dock extensions expensive, and there was the problem of inaccessibility from Harley Street. Overall, he felt that the two schools would 'rival in their work'; although the Seamen's Hospital could be developed, he felt that the teaching should be carried out at the 'Polyclinic'.

The controversy regarding the proposed Albert Dock Hospital project continued to the end of 1898 (and beyond). *The Lancet*'s correspondent again extolled the virtues of Netley[21]:

. . . The Royal Victoria Hospital is a large military hospital to which sick and wounded soldiers are relegated from all parts of the world wherever

---

* Mr (later Sir) Jonathan Hutchinson, FRCS, MD, LLD, FRS (1828–1913) had been Professor of Surgery at The London Hospital College, and President of the Royal College of Surgeons 1889–1890.

soldiers are stationed and numerous cases of malarial disease in all its forms and dysentery are nearly always forthcoming, together with diseases of the liver including abscess of that organ. An excellent bacteriological laboratory, microscopes, and all appliances for the scientific investigation of disease are available, together with a pathological museum. Practical instruction is systematically given in the microscopical examination of the various fluids and tissues of the body, including of course the examination of the blood for the detection of the plasmodium malariae. The instruction is afforded by men practically acquainted with tropical disease and there are always present and doing duty in the hospital wards medical officers who have had foreign service and experience in various parts of the world. Of course the distance of Netley from London would be prohibitory to its being used by residents in London, but why should not candidates for the Colonial Medical Service be required to go through a course of instruction in tropical medicine and remain at Netley whilst doing so? There is no reason, moreover, why such candidates should not confine themselves to this work without entering upon that connected with the more purely military course, unless they desired to do so in the direction of practical hygiene which would be very much to their advantage. If Netley Hospital does not offer all the varieties of tropical disease that could be desired it nevertheless affords a larger amount of tropical disease and more facilities for studying that subject than could probably be obtained elsewhere. For all those who were not seeking to enter the Colonial Medical Service but were desirous of practising in the colonies there would still remain open to them for clinical study the Seamen's Hospital at Greenwich and its Branch, as well as the metropolitan hospitals and such bacteriological laboratories as that at King's College. It is, we think, to be regretted that, instead of having years ago selected Netley as the site for our largest military hospital with its Army Medical School, London was not chosen for the purpose. The school might then have formed a teaching institution for a united medical service and for all medical officers in the employment of the State. The hospital and its attached school would then have been more largely available for all concerned and the hospital might have been fully utilised as such all the year round which is not, we believe, the case with the Royal Victoria Hospital at Netley. It is obviously too late, however to think of this now; but that is no reason why its sphere of usefulness should not be enlarged and developed in the public interest and in that of the Government.

This leader might well have been precipitated by Sir William Broadbent who apparently wrote personally to Chamberlain in December 1898 favouring Netley and not the Albert Dock Hospital (see below).

Not content with the coverage of these viewpoints in *The Times* and *The Lancet*, the controversy also raged in the *British Medical Journal*[22]:

SIR, – Professor Crookshank's letter [see above] on the proposed school of tropical medicine amounts, when analysed, to a vigorous opposition to any consolidated "one-roof" scheme, and he definitely proposes that the intending student should have to chase his subject about London, much as he does at present, if he does it at all. If Professor Crookshank were commissioned to start a brand-new King's College medical school, which type would he choose? I think I could make a correct guess.

. . . He begins by a description of the completeness and excellent quality of the instruction supplied in his own bacteriological laboratories at King's College in reference to many parasitic diseases, and especially those found in the various Colonies. Let it be so, and what then? Professor Crookshank immediately goes on to remark that "a thorough knowledge of these diseases cannot be imparted in a small clinical laboratory attached for convenience to the wards of a hospital." Of course not. But he cannot seriously mean us to draw an inference that a "thorough knowledge" of these diseases can be imparted in a large laboratory such as that he describes at King's College, or in any other. Let him ponder over what a "thorough knowledge" of a disease means.

Professor Crookshank next states it as his opinion that "the services of colonial health officers and colonial practitioners would be of increased value if they were qualified . . . to advise upon the best means of stamping out tuberculosis," etc., "and also if they were competent to undertake original researches in connection with diseases of animals, and especially those communicable to man." Certainly. But allow me, as a colonial practitioner from one of the colonies enumerated in Professor Crookshank's long list, to offer as additional opinion that the services of *English* health officers and practitioners would probably be of "increased value" if they also were all similarly competent. It would indicate a very creditable standard of knowledge.

Next, Professor Crookshank points out that some diseases are very rarely imported into England, and says that therefore instruction at the bedside supplemented by examination in a clinical laboratory would be very irregular and inadequate, and that for such diseases study in a large and well-equipped laboratory is to be mainly relied on. Sir, a man *must* have a good laboratory training to have a decent understanding of microbial diseases, and the necessity is not confined to those of the tropics. What about diphtheria, typhoid, tuberculosis, and pyogenic infection? Every modern practitioner, whether for the tropics or not, ought to have at least the six weeks' course of bacteriology which Professor Crookshank advises.

But what sort of laboratory instruction will such a place as King's College afford on malaria, filariasis, dysentery, distomiasis, and ankylostomiasis? The idea of properly demonstrating the phases of a malarial organism, or the peculiarities of a filaria, in a non-clinical laboratory must show itself as absurd to such a man as Professor Crookshank. And yet he decries the clinical laboratory, or seems to. I am certain that he is under a misapprehension if he thinks the existence of a good clinical laboratory a menace to the prosperity of the general laboratory of the university type. In my opinion, exactly the reverse is the case. If a man has not already learnt how necessary is a course of systematic general bacteriology he will not see much of a clinical laboratory without having it impressed on him. The laboratory of the university type and the clinical laboratory are complementary, not competitive, and each has its own place in the teaching function. Because, in a clinical laboratory chemical examinations of urine are carried out, do we hear the Professor of Chemistry complain? Does the Professor of Pathology cry out because morbid tissues are examined, or necropsies performed? How many Professors of Bacteriology grow pale because Widal tests are made, or throat swabbings cultivated there? – I am, etc.,

C.E. CORLETTE, MD
Selwood Place, S.W., Dec.13th.

* * *

This was followed by another lengthy letter from Dr Curnow!:

SIR, – In your issue of December 3rd you were good enough to express the hope that a frank apology should be given by the Committee of Management of the Seamen's Hospital Society, and frankly accepted by the staff. That apology has not been made, but last week an appeal for subscriptions and a memorandum (published in your columns) were widely circulated among the profession, but they were not sent to either Dr. Anderson, Mr. J.R. Turner, or myself, the senior visiting staff of the /Dreadnought Hospital. I am compelled to make some remarks on this memorandum and the appeal, as an explanation of my action towards the proposed scheme. . . .

This letter from Dr Curnow then proceeded with a duplicate version of the text of his letter to *The Lancet* of the same date (see above)[18].

Before 1898 came to an end, *The Times* published four more contributions on this matter in its correspondence columns. Surgeon Lt-Col Baker IMS (retd)[23] supported the Albert Dock project. He considered 'It is very doubtful if the Government would throw the school at Netley open to all comers . . . Moreover, the patients at Netley consist entirely of Europeans suffering from disease in its more chronic forms; whereas at the Seamen's Branch Hospital natives of tropical countries, as well as Europeans coming from all parts of the world, are received with diseases in their more acute stages.'

A further letter from Curnow, Anderson and Turner[24] considered that 'One serious effect [that the Branch Hospital] is likely to have is that of diverting money from longer established hospitals, which are mainly supported by voluntary contributions and are in sore need of all the support they can get.' Dr R Howard[25] had recently studied malaria at the

Royal Albert Dock Hospital prior to leaving for Central Africa as medical officer of the Universities' Mission on Lake Nyasa; he supported the work of the hospital – especially the examination of malaria films. And finally, Dr C E Corlette[26] (see above) strongly supported the Branch Hospital project, and in so doing summarized the various objections outlined in the letter from Roberts et al[16].

Involvement of Manson in the correspondence

The vitriolic correspondence in The Lancet became even more heated (and personalised) and the Medical Advisor to the Colonial Office now became the centre of a personal attack by Curnow and his colleagues[27]:

> To the Editors of THE LANCET.
>
> SIRS, – The "honourable apology" of the committee of the Seamen's Hospital Society is obviously insufficient and is followed by a confused attempt at explanation and extenuation which makes it practically no apology at all. Such as it is it has not reached the visiting staff in any shape or form except as a publication in the British Medical Journal, and it has been published in that paper only.
>
> The committee state in the British Medical Journal that they do not contemplate the transfer of all tropical cases to the Branch Hospital. At least four times previously they have refused this information to the visiting staff of the Dreadnought. There are other matters at issue between the committee and us than the premature publication of Sir Henry Burdett's letter and the unauthorised statements contained therein. As some of the visiting staff of the Dreadnought were intended to be teachers in the proposed school it was obviously improper and open to misconstruction for the committee to be in consultation with the physician of the Branch Hospital without the knowledge of his assumed future fellow medical teachers of the Dreadnought, both of them much senior to him in the service of the society. Even the statement of the committee that they have been in full and constant consultation with the visiting staff of the Branch Hospital cannot be allowed to pass.
>
> The ophthalmic surgeon, who probably would have told us of what was going on, was like ourselves excluded from all information. His name was lately published in the list of the advisory committee without his consent, and it has now by his request been removed from it.
>
> The committee quote an extract from Mr. Chamberlain's correspondence with them. It would be more satisfactory to have it in extenso. Are we to understand that the offer of public money came from the Colonial Office solely to increase the accommodation of the hospital to which the medical adviser to the Colonial Office is attached, that the committee deliberately kept their visiting officers of the Dreadnought in ignorance of their scheme until it had been decided to accept this offer, and to become responsible for the expenditure of this public money? If so, was this done with only one

possible teacher of tropical medicine then at their disposal – the medical adviser to the Colonial Office himself?

The committee in their memorandum have referred to the assumption by this gentleman of the title of physician to the Seamen's Hospital, Greenwich (235 beds), when he was physician to the Branch Seamen's Hospital, Victoria and Albert Docks (18 beds), and say that we objected to his being so described. Dr. Manson really so described himself in Kelly's "London Medical Directory," 1895, Churchill's "Medical Directory," 1896, in the list of contributors to Davidson's "Hygiene and Diseases of Warm Climates," and in the *British Medical Journal*.

There is abundant evidence in the minute-book of the Seamen's Hospital Society and elsewhere to show that he was elected a physician to the Branch Seamen's Hospital at the Victoria and Albert Docks on the same day that Mr. Gunn was elected ophthalmic surgeon to the Seamen's Hospital Society. To this mistaken action of Dr. Manson's we took exception and for it he apologised. The matter has not hitherto in this controversy been publicly mentioned by us, although it might have ultimately become necessary, as we understand that this was the reason the committee deliberately refused to let us know of the proposed school.

Because the physician to the Branch Seamen's Hospital, Victoria and Albert Docks, was asked in 1896 why he described himself as physician to the Seamen's Hospital, Greenwich, the visiting staff of the latter are to have no voice in matters closely concerning them in 1898. Such has been the judgment of a committee that Sir William Broadbent has written "is unworthy of confidence." Resenting this criticism, they say they do not gather that the visiting staff have viewed their invitation as an insult or would join in Sir William Broadbent's protest. The visiting staff most cordially join in this protest against the treatment they have received and against the omission of parts of Sir Henry Burdett's letter. They regard the latter proceeding as unfair and misleading.

As the explanatory memoranda of the committee were not sent to any except a carefully selected *clientèle* from which we were excluded, it more than ever behoved the committee to omit nothing in the letter bearing on the present attitude of the visiting staff of the *Dreadnought*.

We are, Sirs, yours faithfully,
JOHN CURNOW, MD, FRCP
JOHN ANDERSON, MD, FRCP
G.R. TURNER, FRCS
Dec. 20th, 1898.

A reply from Manson was published the following week[28]:

To the Editors of THE LANCET.

SIRS – The letter in your issue of last week . . . might lead readers to infer that in various publications I had deliberately assumed a title to which I had no claim, that knowing that this description was untrue I had designated myself "Physician to the Seamen's Hospital, Greenwich." In self-defence I am constrained to ask you to allow me space to make the following statement.

In 1892 I was appointed a physician to the Seamen's Hospital Society. My duties, I was informed, were sole charge of the medical cases in the society's Branch Hospital, Albert Docks; to visit convalescents at the Dreadnought Hospital, Greenwich, when transferred there from the Branch Hospital; to take part in the meetings of the society's honorary visiting staff. In discharge of these duties I visited the Seamen's Hospital, Albert Docks, twice a week, and the Seamen's Hospital, Greenwich (*Dreadnought*), once a week, and attended most, if not all, of the meetings of the medical staff to which I was summoned. At the time of my election I was not informed that my office carried with it any particular title; but as I performed all the duties of a hospital physician at both of the Seamen's Hospitals I naturally inferred that I was a physician to both of these hospitals and that I had a perfect right to designate myself as such. Accordingly, and in conformity with medical custom, I called myself, or was called in various publications, sometimes, "Physician to the Seamen's Hospital, Greenwich", sometimes "Physician to the Seamen's Hospital, Greenwich, and Seamen's Hospital, Albert Docks."

Some three years ago I was pained and surprised to be informed by the secretary of the Seamen's Hospital Society that my colleagues (as I regarded them) at the *Dreadnought* (Seamen's Hospital, Greenwich) had collectively and officially represented to him that I had assumed a title to which I had no right and that he had been asked officially to request that I should discontinue the practice. If I am not mistaken (unfortunately I have destroyed the correspondence) I was requested to write to the medical press and publicly intimate that I was not a physician to the Seamen's Hospital, Greenwich, and that I had no right so to describe myself. I protested. After some correspondence, in the course of which I intimated that I considered that my colleagues might have spoken to me privately if they thought I was in error or considered themselves aggrieved, I expressed regret if I had unwittingly arrogated to myself a title to which I had no claim. In consequence of the want of consideration shown me by my colleagues at the *Dreadnought* I have ceased to visit there, feeling that my seniors did not care to be associated with me, and myself not caring to be associated with those who, I considered, had treated me with scant courtesy, not to say fairness or friendliness.

At the time of the correspondence referred to I did consider, as I still consider, that I had a perfect right – in fact as much right as either Dr. Curnow or Dr. Anderson had – to designate myself "Physician to the Seamen's Hospital, Greenwich." I regret now that, shrinking from a petty squabble and for the sake of peace, I gave way on what at the time seemed to me a most trivial matter.

I am, Sirs, yours faithfully,

PATRICK MANSON.

Queen Anne-street, Cavendish-square, Dec.28th 1898.

Following this, the seemingly petty correspondence drifted on and *The Lancet* published further letters in its first issue for 1899[29]:

To the Editors of THE LANCET

SIRS, – Dr. Manson's impressions as to his position on the staff of the Seamen's Hospital Society as set forth in his letter in THE LANCET of Dec. 31st are so mistaken that we are again obliged to draw his attention to the written records on the subject.

On April 9th, 16th, and 23rd, 1892, advertisements appeared in the medical press (THE LANCET and *British Medical Journal*) for a visiting physician to the Seamen's Hospital Society's Branch Hospital, Victoria and Albert Docks. Dr. Manson was a candidate for this post. He was selected on May 4th by a sub-committee of which we were members and duly elected on May 13th to the appointment he sought. Reference to the minute-book to which we referred him clearly shows this. It was some considerable time after Dr. Manson was appointed to the Branch Hospital that the physicians of the *Dreadnought* as an act of courtesy to him allowed him the use of 6 beds in their wards for cases which had been under his care at the Branch. They both lent him 3 beds, little supposing that this concession would lead him to assume the title of "Physician to the Seamen's Hospital, Greenwich."

The annexed letter from us to Dr. Manson (Jan. 21st, 1896) clearly put before him his real position, yet after his apology (copy of which is enclosed) he now writes: "At the time of the correspondence referred to I did consider, as I still consider, that I had a perfect right – in fact, as much right as either Dr. Curnow or Dr. Anderson had – to designate myself 'Physician to the Seamen's Hospital, Greenwich.'" The profession must judge whether it is "in conformity with medical custom" for a physician elected to one hospital to describe himself as physician to another and whether the officers of the latter have not cause for remonstrance if such is repeatedly done.

We are, Sirs, your obedient servants,

JOHN CURNOW.
JOHN ANDERSON.
G.R. TURNER.
Jan. 3rd, 1899.

* * *

[Copy of Letter from the Staff of the Seamen's Hospital to Dr. Manson.]
Dreadnought Seamen's Hospital, Greenwich,
21st January, 1896.

DEAR DR. MANSON, – With reference to your letter to Mr. Michelli of the 18th Dec. last, a copy of which has been sent to one of us and which we should have replied to sooner but for the Christmas holidays, we wish to draw your attention to the terms of your appointment as shown in the minute-book of the Seamen's Hospital Society.

On May 4th 1892, a sub-committee met to recommend a physician to the Branch Seamen's Hospital at the Royal Victoria and Albert Docks and an ophthalmic surgeon to the Seamen's Hospital Society. In the same minute-book (May 13th, 1892, . . .) it is noted that you were elected to the office of physician to the said branch hospital and Mr. Gunn ophthalmic surgeon to the Seamen's Hospital Society. We also wish to call your attention to the 74th official report of the Seamen's Hospital Society (copy enclosed) in which you are styled Physician to the Royal Victoria and Albert Docks' Hospital and to the official note-paper in which a distinction is clearly drawn between the *Dreadnought* Seamen's Hospital, Greenwich (235 beds), and the Branch Seamen's Hospital, Royal Victoria and Albert Docks (18 beds).

It appears clear to us from the foregoing that you should not allow yourself to be described as "Physician to the Seamen's Hospital, Greenwich," as has lately been done in the list of contributors to Davidson's "Hygiene and Diseases of Warm Climates," the *British Medical Journal*, Kelly's London Medical Directory, 1895, and Churchill's Medical Directory, 1896. If there is still any misunderstanding we shall be happy to meet you and discuss the matter. We are forwarding a copy of this letter to Mr. Michelli.

We remain, yours faithfully,

(Signed)   JOHN CURNOW,   } Visiting Physicians.
JOHN ANDERSON,

G.R. TURNER,   Visiting Surgeon.

* * *

[Copy of Letter from Dr. Manson to Mr. W. Johnson Smith.]

21, Queen Anne-street, Cavendish-square,
4th Feb., 1896.

DEAR MR. JOHNSON SMITH, – Many thanks for your very courteous letter.

Your interpretation of mine to Mr. Michelli is correct. Therein I explained how I came to call and allow myself to be called "Physician to the Seamen's Hospital, Greenwich," a mistake I shall be careful to avoid in future. Please accept and convey my apologies to the medical staff. Yours very truly,

(Signed)   PATRICK MANSON.

On 6 January 1899, a letter from Dr John Anderson[30] was published in *The Times*; he published actual figures for admissions of 'tropical cases' to Netley. *The Lancet* commented as follows[31]:

. . . Full statistics were furnished enumerating the number of patients suffering from tropical disease who were admitted during the years from 1892 to 1898 (to Nov. 30th) inclusive. The figures show that whilst the clinical material for teaching beri-beri is clearly insufficient (this being naturally due to the fact that Europeans rarely suffer from this disease), the advantages offered in other forms of tropical disease are much greater than in any other hospital in Europe. The number of cases of ague and remittent fever in 1897 were 176 and 25 respectively, and in 1898 were 402 and 83. The advocates of the establishment of the proposed school for tropical medicine at the Branch of the Seamen's Hospital at the Albert Docks have made a *point d'appui* of the fact that during the year ending Nov. 30th last 31 cases of malaria were admitted into that hospital. This number should be compared with those quoted above. Again, in *The Lancet* of Nov. 19th last we mentioned that in twenty-five years only 50 cases of hepatic abscess had been treated at the Seamen's Hospital, whilst at Netley in 1897 there were 33 instances of this disease, and in 1898 (to Nov. 30th) there were 86 cases of "inflammation of the liver" and 20 of "other hepatic diseases." We may also draw attention to the number of cases of "simple continued fever" and of "Mediterranean fever" [brucellosis] which were under treatment. The figures quoted by Dr. Anderson add strong support to our contention that although every assistance should be given by the profession to Mr. Chamberlain's scheme, yet the size of the hospital at the Albert Docks (and we are not forgetting the proposed extension) and the number of tropical cases admitted do not justify the proposed large expenditure. We do not deny that it affords a most valuable additional place of study for medical men preparing to reside abroad, but we do protest against the laying out of large sums of money when there already exists such a well-equipped and in every way suitable establishment as Netley.

Chamberlain's decision

A letter which, in effect, clinched the issue was written on behalf of Chamberlain himself and published in *The Lancet* in January (1899)[32]:

WE have been requested by the Secretary of King's College to publish the following letter from the Secretary of State for the Colonies to the Principal of King's College:–

Downing-street, Jan.7th, 1899.
SIR, – I am directed by Mr. Secretary Chamberlain to inform you, with reference to the letter from this office of Dec. 23rd last, that he has carefully considered your letters of Nov. 22nd and Dec. 5th and their enclosures and that he has come to the conclusion that in selecting candidates for the Colonial Medical Service preference should be given (other things being equal) to those doctors who have received such bacteriological or similar special training as King's College provides, but that when candidates have been definitely selected they should be required to attend at the School of Tropical Medicine which is being established at the Albert Docks Branch of the Seamen's Hospital (fig 6.2) and to go through the complete course of instruction which is now being settled by a special committee of experts appointed for the purpose.
2. Mr. Chamberlain considers this arrangement to be the one best suited to the requirements of the Colonial Medical Service, and he trusts that the

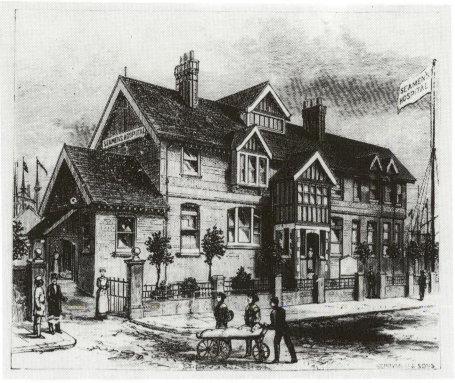

Fig 6.2 The Albert Dock ('Branch') Hospital during the 1890s [reproduced by permission of 'The Wellcome Institute Library, London'].

medical authorities at King's College will co-operate as far as possible in giving effect to it.

3. Mr. Chamberlain desires me to express his thanks to you and to Professor Crookshank for the great interest which you have shown in this scheme for extending the study of tropical medicine and also for the suggestions which you have been good enough to put forward.

I am, Sir, your obedient servant,

(Signed) H. BERTRAM COX.

The Principal, King's College.

In the same issue, *The Lancet* devoted yet another leading article to the subject and outlined Chamberlain's proposed scheme for Schools of Tropical Medicine in general[33]. The leader writer applauded Chamberlain's decision not to go ahead with a fully equipped general *bacteriological* laboratory at the Albert Dock Hospital; it also outlined the merits of the proposals for the Liverpool school (chapter 7):

. . . This is noticeable as the first public departure of the Secretary of State for the Colonies from the elaborate and expensive scheme put forth by

141

Sir Henry Burdett in his letter to the *Times* of July 11th, for obviously now no fully equipped general bacteriological laboratory will be needed but merely one for the purposes of clinical investigation and research in tropical diseases. A large waste of public money will thus be avoided. The necessary requirements for such a school have been clearly laid down by Principal Glazebrook and Mr. Adamson, President of the Southern Hospital, Liverpool. . . . We would again point out that the diseases treated at the Albert Docks Hospital are all brought from India, China, and other Eastern countries, and with the exception of beri-beri (which is almost exclusively brought into England by the native sailors and firemen employed by the Peninsular and Oriental and the British India Steamship Companies) their number and variety are in no way to be compared with those which are treated at Netley. Mr. Chamberlain's colonial surgeons must therefore be trained at a disadvantage with the officers of the Indian and Army Medical Services. If the committee of management of the Seamen's Hospital Society had arranged for the reception of tropical cases at the *Dreadnought* Hospital on the lines adopted by the Liverpool Southern Hospital it would have been quite unnecessary to issue such an appeal to the subscribing public as they have issued. The ambitious scheme which is shown in their proposed enlargement of the Branch Hospital as an adjunct to a lavishly planned school of tropical medicine might have given place to one of modest dimensions and equal utility.

Despite what was in fact a *fait accompli*, correspondence continued, albeit at a slacker pace; much of it was supportive of the Albert Dock scheme, but some opposition continued to be aired[34-36]. The issue had thus stirred up unprecedented controversy and even anger, both in the medical and national press. The final say came not surprisingly, from Chamberlain himself in a parliamentary statement[37]:

. . . It was well known [Mr Chamberlain said], that all the colonies, and especially the West African colonies, were subject to peculiar diseases of a most distressing and very often of a fatal character. . . .

. . . One cause [of this high morbidity and mortality] was the insufficient and improper nursing, and the remedy, he was most happy to say, was now being undertaken by a private association called the Colonial Nursing Association, which was sending out to all these colonies trained European nurses to deal with the sick patients who required their attention. A second difficulty had been that of finding medical practitioners who were acquainted beforehand with these peculiar diseases; the diseases themselves were very peculiar and it was almost impossible to give clinical instruction to medical practitioners who were going out to the coast in these particular diseases. It was suggested to him by the very able and well-known medical gentleman who was the Colonial Office adviser in all these cases, Dr. Manson, that they might establish a graduates' class, and that just in the same way as they had a school of musketry at

Hythe to which military men were always sent for a month or a couple of months' training before they went to their foreign appointments, so they might have a school of tropical medicine somewhere in the country to which all the medical men sent to these countries should go for two months before leaving, and in which they might have clinical and practical instruction in the cure of these particular diseases. Dr. Manson considered that the *Dreadnought* Hospital offered the best opportunity for dealing with these matters, as it so happened that many sailors went there who came home from the colonies suffering from these diseases, and there was more opportunity for efficient study provided there than at any other hospital. They had considered very carefully the alternative advantages of Netley and Haslar, but they came to the conclusion that it would be very much better to take advantage of the *Dreadnought* Hospital. Accordingly, arrangements had been made for erecting the necessary buildings for the accommodation of the medical men who would go through this probationary course and they hoped also in a short time to have accommodation there for nurses who equally required a similar training. That would cost a considerable sum annually and a considerable sum for first expenditure. That sum would be provided partly by private subscriptions in this country, partly by contributions from the colonies, and partly by this small grant – for it was really a small grant – which the Chancellor of the Exchequer had been good enough to give him for the purpose. He should say that up to the time when they made this proposal he did not think it had been made by anybody else, but the moment it was made there was some disturbance in the minds of the medical officers of different institutions, who all thought their institutions ought to have been or might have been selected instead of the one actually selected. He believed, though he could not speak confidently, that they had satisfied these gentlemen, so far, at all events, as they had seen their complaints, by assuring them that to such cases as King's College Hospital, for instance, or the Liverpool School, or other cases in which special training in tropical diseases was given, they would give a preference in the selection of officers for these colonies. But they did not intend to give up the further security that after these gentlemen had been selected they should undergo this probationary course of two months at the *Dreadnought* Hospital before they finally left.

– Dr FARQUHARSON, after expressing approval of the arrangement, asked whether the vote would be an annual one. – Mr CHAMBERLAIN explained that the present vote was for the cost of the buildings. He had been in communication with the Royal Society and the Royal Society had made a grant which the Government proposed to supplement. A Commission had been appointed by the Royal Society to inquire into the cause and cure of malaria. That Commission would visit Egypt to study the experiments which had been made there and would then go on to India. They would afterwards probably go to Nyassaland [now Malawi], where there was a permanent station, to make examinations on the spot, and would wind up in West Africa. – General RUSSELL said he had suffered

143

greatly from West African fever and he had found that there was scarcely a medical man in London who knew anything about it. – Mr LAWRENCE, one of the representatives of Liverpool, said he was sorry to find that that city was not to benefit by this grant and suggested that having regard to the trade with West Africa carried on in Liverpool there should be a hospital established there for the study of tropical diseases. – The vote was shortly afterwards passed by the Committee.

Resignation of Drs Curnow and Anderson, and Mr Turner

In March 1899 *The Lancet* carried, perhaps by now not surprisingly, the following notice[38]:

> We are informed that Dr. Curnow, Dr. John Anderson, CIE, and Mr. G.R. Turner, have signed a joint letter resigning their posts as physicians and surgeon, respectively, to the Seamen's Hospital Society, but offering to continue the performance of their duties until their successors are appointed. Mr. Donald Gunn, the ophthalmic surgeon, has also resigned his post.
> . . . [This has] thus left the *Dreadnought* Seamen's Hospital, Greenwich, without any honorary medical staff.

In June 1899 the names of their successors were announced[39]:

> SIX of the appointments advertised as vacant on the staff of the Seamen's Hospital Society have been filled up as follows:– Physicians: Dr. R. Tanner Hewlett and Dr. Guthrie Rankin. Surgeons: Mr. James Cantlie and Mr. J. Brian Christopherson. Ophthalmic surgeon: Mr. L. Vernon Cargill. Superintendent and medical tutor of the London School of Tropical Medicine: Mr. David Charles Rees.

The whole sad saga leading to the resignations of the three devoted members of the *Dreadnought* staff was summarized by *The Lancet* in April 1899[40]:

> THE resignation of the honorary medical and surgical staff of the *Dreadnought* Seamen's Hospital at Greenwich affords a remarkable illustration of the results of the mismanagement of the affairs of a hospital which must occur sooner or later when it is solely under the control of a lay committee and when there are no members of the medical or surgical staff (consulting or visiting) on the committee. The visiting staff which does the work of the hospital and supervises the well-being of the patients is kept in ignorance of important matters of policy and even of points of detail with regard to which it is of the utmost value to the proper administration of the hospital that it should be at once informed and should be able to express its opinion. With a medical staff represented on a committee it would be

impossible for that committee to initiate and carry out such a discourteous line of conduct as that which the present committee of management of the *Dreadnought* Seamen's Hospital has thought fit to adopt towards its visiting staff.

. . . although the physician to the Branch Hospital (who is also the medical advisor to the Colonial Office but a junior in standing) was consulted, the members of the senior visiting staff of the *Dreadnought* were never, individually or collectively, asked for their opinion. The committee do not see that there is any "want of courtesy" in this procedure. We think that the medical profession will hold a very different opinion from that entertained by the committee. On July 11th of last year Sir HENRY BURDETT published a letter in the *Times* giving the details of a fully-matured scheme for the new school and the extension of the Branch Hospital, and appealing for public support; his letter contained the statement that "the teaching staff will consist of the senior medical staff of the *Dreadnought* Hospital at Greenwich," &c., whereas that staff did not know that any such scheme was even being contemplated. Sir H. BURDETT subsequently said that his letter was written under instructions from the committee of the *Dreadnought* Hospital, so that he repudiates any personal responsibility for the statement. The visiting staff wrote to the *Times* to point out that this statement was made without their authority or consent. A long and somewhat bitter correspondence then ensued, inasmuch as no apology or expression of regret was forthcoming from the committee for its lack of courtesy in not consulting the visiting staff. We understand that no apology has even yet been offered to the staff. A memorandum full of controversial and incomplete statements, which was published in a contemporary in December last and which should evidently have been sent to the visiting staff, merely intensifies the lack of courtesy. The staff therefore could do nothing but resign, as it was impossible for them any longer to carry on the work of the hospital under such circumstances. Moreover, the value of the appointment has been seriously diminished. Cases from the Victoria and Albert Docks are to be concentrated at the Branch Hospital and not to be conveyed across the river as in the days when the Branch Hospital was founded, and so the parent hospital is to be largely deprived of its historic cases and turned into a sailor's infirmary or asylum.

The judgement of the heads of the profession on the conduct of the committee of management is on record. Sir WILLIAM BROADBENT, in a letter published in the *Times* of Dec. 7th[41], sums up his objections to a memorandum and appeal for public monetary support, which were sent to him by the committee of management, in the following forcible paragraph: "A committee capable of such a suppression of truth material to the issue and of such a suggestion of what is calculated to mislead is, in my opinion, totally unworthy of confidence." The Royal College of Physicians of London has twice refused to take part in the carrying out of the scheme notwithstanding the appeals of the committee of management who plaintively plead, when they give no answer to the questions asked by the visiting staff, that they object to being so catechised. The Royal College of Surgeons of England has withdrawn its representative. A school of tropical medicine, or even more than one, will be of great advantage to Englishmen who intend to practise abroad, but it is much to be regretted that this one is started on a narrow and personal basis instead of being founded on lines approved by the official bodies representing the profession and thus securing their hearty co-operation and support. Moreover, we are sorry to see that the students of the Liverpool School of Tropical Diseases will have to attend a two months' compulsory course at the London School of Tropical Medicine seeing that the former institution has facilities for affording instruction in West African diseases and that cases of these diseases very rarely reach London.

7

Foundation of the London School of Tropical Medicine (LSTM), and a'rival' institution at Liverpool

Despite the 'trials and tribulations' outlined in chapter 6, the Manson-Chamberlain project rapidly blossomed. The SHS administration certainly lost no time in implementing the new scheme; enlargement of the Albert Dock Hospital proceeded apace.

The following two notices appeared in *The Lancet* for 2 September 1899[1]:

THE LONDON SCHOOL OF TROPICAL MEDICINE, ALBERT DOCK.

This school, which is in connexion with the hospitals of the Seamen's Hospital Society, has been founded under the auspices of the Colonial Office and is intended to supply colonial medical officers with the advantages that are enjoyed by the workers at Netley and Haslar. The scientific side of the work will, we are sure, be thoroughly well done, but there is some doubt as to the amount of clinical material that will be available.

The winter session will commence on Monday, Oct. 2nd, when the new school will be formally open for students. A travelling Scholarship of £300 will be offered to students of the school. Lectures on Tropical Medicine, Tropical Hygiene, and Surgery in the Tropics will be delivered during the winter, summer, and autumn sessions, and the laboratory, museum, and library will be open daily.

Clinical instruction will be given daily in the wards of the hospital and special arrangements are to be made for the accommodation of those who may desire to reside on the premises. For prospectus, syllabus, and other particulars apply to the secretary, Mr. P. Michelli, Seamen's Hospital, Greenwich, S.E.

INSTRUCTION IN TROPICAL MEDICINE AT KING'S COLLEGE, LONDON.

It was at first believed, when the Colonial Office were publicly associated with the School of Tropical Medicine to be established at Albert Dock, that the officers selected for the Colonial Medical Service would have to receive their instruction solely at the Albert Dock Branch of the Seamen's Hospital, but early this year a letter from Mr. Chamberlain to the Principal of King's College, London, which we published in THE LANCET, showed this to be a wrong inference. The Colonial Office state that in selecting candidates for the Colonial Medical Service preference will be given to those medical men who have received such bacteriological or similar special training as King's College provides, but that when candidates have been definitely selected they will be required to attend at the School of Tropical Medicine which is being established at the Albert Dock Branch of the Seamen's Hospital. This is a considerable departure from the position first put before the public, as now no fully equipped general bacteriological laboratory will be needed at Albert Dock but merely one for the purposes of clinical investigation and research in tropical diseases. A large waste of public money will thus be avoided, while it is open for any medical school, metropolitan or provincial, to offer to intending colonial practitioners instruction that will count later in their chances of selection for an appointment. Information with regard to the bacteriological courses at King's College, London, under the supervision of Professor Crookshank, can be obtained on application at the College.

According to plan, the school was opened to students on 2 October 1899 – a day short of Manson's 55th birthday![2] At that time, the new wing of the Albert Dock Hospital was also approaching completion. Plate 33 shows the London School of Tropical Medicine (LSTM) in 1899. Expenditure on the school and hospital had amounted to £5758 and £5947 respectively; a good public response to the various appeals had been forthcoming, and subscriptions had been received from as far afield as Russia, Finland, the Netherlands, Norway, Sweden, Denmark, Spain, Austria, Hungary, Germany, Italy, Portugal, China and India[2].

Structurally, the school and hospital (Plate 34) were separated by about 50 yards and were connected by a covered corridor. Plate 35 shows the interior of the main ward – in which Manson's clinical teaching took place; above the beds some of the endowment plaques can be seen – Plate 36a–d show details of four of these. The laboratory (Plate 37) and class-rooms were close to the wards[2]. A library was provided. The students lived on the premises; there were 12 bed-sitting rooms on the third floor of the school, together with dining and smoking rooms. Although open primarily to medical graduates, there were also some veterinarians.

The full course lasted three months; three took place each year. At the end of each course there was an examination and a certificate was issued to those who passed with ≥ 60%. The first Medical Superintendent acted as tutor; there were two demonstrators who were former members of the class – they were on duty during laboratory demonstrations and classes – who assisted students with their microscopic work. The Medical Tutor was Dr D C Rees – who had started on the preparation of specimens for teaching purposes in June 1899[2,3]; he was responsible for drawing up the syllabus and for organising the courses of lectures. The teachers at the school (they had been appointed in May 1899) were: Dr Patrick Manson, Prof R Tanner Hewlett, Dr Andrew Duncan, Col Oswald Baker, Prof W J Simpson, Dr L W Sambon, Mr James Cantlie, Dr Malcolm Morris (a dermatologist) and Mr E Treacher Collins (an ophthalmologist)[2].

At the opening of the school (there was no formal ceremony), Mr (later Sir) Perceval Nairne (1841–1921), Chairman of the SHS presided. Professors Alphonse Laveran, William Osler, and Guido Baccelli had all declined invitations to give an inaugural address[4]; it seems likely (although not well documented) that this was a result of the widely publicised controversies surrounding the venture. 'Only the Members of the Committee of Management, the Members of the Honorary Medical Staff and the members of the Advisory Committee were invited'[7]. The first formal address was in fact given by Sir William MacGregor on 3 October 1900[5] (chapter 8). A formal opening was postponed therefore until the hospital buildings had been completed; the gathering which assembled was however 'large and influential'[6]. Manson's address emphasised the need for such a school and dealt with the various criticisms which had been raised (see below). This address (2 October 1899) was apparently read on Manson's behalf by Mr (later Sir) James Cantlie (Plate 38)[7] – the reason(s) for his absence is not clearly stated in the minute book. A brief account of the opening of the LSTM has survived[6]; the anonymous writer was clearly impressed with the overall standard of the new facilities; he continued:

> . . . With the advantages to be derived from a thorough acquaintance of both the theoretical and scientific aspects of tropical medicine, let us hope that [the future medical practitioner in the tropics] will not only make a good practitioner in his tropical home, but also that he will endeavour to advance scientific medicine by seriously attacking some of the many problems that are awaiting solution in those regions, and which it is impossible for others less instructed to attempt. The lament of most who have hitherto practised in the tropics has been the impossibility of carrying on observations on subjects of the highest importance because of the defects in their early training. There has been no lack of material ready for investigation, but the knowledge of methods has been wanting, and theories have had to take the place of facts. Exceptions only prove the rule. The work of Manson and others has been carried on under peculiar difficulties, and the results form but a microscopic portion of that immense mass of scientific truths which has been and is still waiting to be revealed.

The impetus of research, strong in general medicine, has happily been extended to tropical medicine by the efforts of these pioneers. The result is even visible to-day. Theories are beginning no longer to pass counter for facts, and the impulse is to examine even the most cherished doctrines in the light of observation and experiment. This impulse, however, is impotent without proper direction, and is but likely to lead further astray. For illustration we have only to compare the observations and experiments of Ross on the blood and its relations to malaria before he was trained in modern methods, with those of a later date. In the former case they were misleading, while in the latter they are invaluable and pregnant with the most far-reaching results. No better example could be given of the necessity and of the advantage of a practical training in the subjects which will be dealt with in the Tropical School. In the tropics, as elsewhere, the most approved and best methods have to be employed if the best results are to be obtained. These are to be learnt at the school . . .

And the writer concluded with these glowing comments:

. . . Opened under favourable auspices, everything connected with the school bids fair for its future success. . . . All concerned in the movement have good reason to be congratulated. The Seamen's Society is especially to be congratulated on its efforts being crowned with success. A special meed of praise is due to Mr Michelli, the secretary, whose indefatigable labours have in no small measure contributed to the success of a scheme which was promoted in the Colonial Office and had as its support the powerful influence of Mr. Chamberlain. We trust that in time the School will develop, as it should, into an imperial centre of scientific learning in tropical medicine worthy of the empire.

A later SHS minute states: 'since the opening of the School 73 students had entered their names upon the books, including 21 this session . . . 7 were from the Colonial Service, 1 in the Service of the Foreign Office, 1 in the Japanese Navy, 1 in the Chinese Customs, and 11 private students, 3 of the latter being women graduates'[8]; Manson's introductory address to them contained the following comments[9]:

I have been deputed by my colleagues to welcome you to the London School of Tropical Medicine. It is hardly necessary for me to say that we are glad to see you. You are welcome for many reasons, but more especially because you are the first instalment of what we hope will grow in the course of years into a numerous and important band, a band that shall not only leave its mark in the history of tropical medicine, but shall exercise an influence for good in the development of the empire. You are welcome, also, because your presence here is substantial evidence that an idea, long cherished by some of us, has taken firm root in the country, and has at last grown into a vigorous plant, which, we trust, will become by-and-by not only vigorous but also fruitful . . .

In outlining some of the problems he had encountered, he continued:

> There are, or there were, some who, while fully recognising the necessity
> for a school of tropical medicine, have cavilled at the selection of this
> particular place as its site. Some have said that the Albert Docks Hospital,
> twenty to twenty-five minutes from Fenchurch Street Station, is too far
> from the centre of London; others that the clinical material likely to
> available is inadequate; others that there are better places elsewhere;
> others that tropical medicine is already efficiently taught at the military
> school at Netley, and that therefore a second school is unnecessary. One
> and all of these objections have already been fully and satisfactorily met. I
> have no intention of reopening the subject. Suffice it that the school at the
> Albert Docks is to-day an accomplished fact; that the student who finds
> the distance from London too great a tax on his time can be lodged within
> the walls of the school – a privilege which I am pleased to see has been
> fully availed of; that the hospital, which, ere another session is over, will be
> much enlarged, affords a good and sufficient supply of tropical cases, quite
> enough for much useful practical work; that Netley has not been opened
> to the public, and were it opened, in consequence of the remoteness from
> the metropolis it certainly could not and would not be used by many who
> could and will come to a school in or near London. The objections I have
> mentioned were carefully considered at the time of the inception of this
> scheme, and the distinct verdict of those who had worked longest and
> hardest to carry the scheme into effect was that, *all things considered*,
> although it may not be in every respect an ideal spot, the Seamen's
> Hospital at the Albert Docks is by far the most suitable place in the
> United Kingdom for a school of tropical medicine. However this may be,
> and whatever may be said or thought about the site, about the curriculum,
> or about the clinical material, we – that is my colleagues and myself –
> have determined to make the best of the opportunities provided for us
> by the Colonial Office, the Seamen's Hospital Society and the public, in
> the conviction that if we work hard and earnestly, and pull together, this
> school will sooner or later prove a great boon to many, and, we believe,
> play no unimportant part in advancing tropical medicine, and in helping
> our countrymen to carry out some of the duties imposed by circumstances
> on our race; that is to say, that it will attain the object for which it was
> established.

In stressing the importance of a special training for the practice of
medicine in the tropics Manson used the following simile:

> . . . A scientific Aberdeenshire agriculturist may be a successful grower
> of turnips in Aberdeenshire; but without special training and experience
> I suspect, notwithstanding all his science, he would be a failure as a
> coffee-planter in Ceylon. Just so with medicine . . .

151

He referred also to the influence of environment and climate on the aetiology of disease:

> It is well to remember that pathology is, in the main, but the study of a certain fauna and flora – a fauna and flora that inhabit the human body – and the study of the reaction of the human body in the presence of these organisms. In the main, the etiology of disease is but a branch of natural history. Climate, that is, temperature, influences pathology mainly, if not only, inasmuch and so far as it influences the distribution of the pathogenic flora and fauna which, just as in the case of the ordinary fauna and flora, are markedly regulated by atmospheric conditions. . . . The geographical limitations of the animal parasitic diseases are undoubtedly, in many instances, determined by atmospheric temperature. But although high temperature may be an indispensable and ultimate determining factor in their distribution, temperature does not usually operate directly on the causal germ; its operation is usually an indirect one, acting probably through many channels . . .

Manson also dwelt on the topical theme (always very close to his heart) that intermediate hosts were essential for the life-cycle of many human parasites:

> Most entozoa require at least two hosts, a definitive and an intermediary; without both the germ would die out. Thus in malaria we know, thanks to the recent revolutionising discoveries in which Ross played so brilliant a part, that a particular genus of mosquito is the necessary definitive host, whilst man, and possibly other mammals, fill the less dignified rôle of intermediary. Recent investigation would suggest the conclusion that without insect definitive and mammalian intermediary there would be no malaria. Consequently, wherever one or the other is absent there is no malaria. Wherever there are no mosquitos of the appropriate kind there the disease cannot be acquired. One indispensable biological condition for the mosquito in question is a high atmospheric temperature. This is a principal reason why malaria is a disease more especially of the tropics, but also of the warm season in higher latitudes.
>
> The same or similar explanations hold good for the geographical distribution of those great groups of tropical diseases included under the terms filariasis, dracontiasis, endemic haematuria, endemic haemoptysis, and a crowd of others already known, and probably also of many as yet unrecognised, or, if recognised, etiologically imperfectly understood diseases.
>
> The peculiar distribution, therefore, of a large class of tropical diseases depends, in the first place, on the fact that they are entozoal diseases; in the second place, that the entozoa concerned require intermediary or definitive

hosts; and, in the third, that one or other of these hosts requires a high atmospheric temperature – in other words, are natives of warm climates only . . .

The importance of zoonotic disease (to this day inadequately appreciated and under recognised) was also addressed:

> . . . that the lower animals, especially, I would add, those that are intimately associated with man, play an important part in the transmission of human disease, is only now becoming properly appreciated. In this matter I would point out that, for once in a way, science is vastly in advance of practice. Our sanitarians and the public do not fully recognise all that the community of interest, as regards disease germs, of man and beast means in the spread of disease. At all events if they do understand it they certainly do not act as if they appreciated it.

Emphasising the dominance of parasitology in the forthcoming course, he told his students:

> . . . In this school, although the bacterium will not be neglected, necessarily a large share of your time will be occupied with animal parasites, a subject which I fear has not been sufficiently studied hitherto in our medical schools. One of our principal objects will be to make you thoroughly familiar with all the tropical disease germs so far as they are known – bacterial, protozoal, and helminthic; to teach you how to demonstrate these germs, how to grow them, and how to kill them; in other words, how to study them scientifically and practically, that is, from the standpoint of natural history and of practice. We feel assured that this is the only way to arrive at sound methods for the prevention and treatment of the diseases these germs give rise to, as well as for fostering and securing the further advance of tropical medicine.

Manson (Plate 39) continued by thanking those who had contributed to the establishment of the new school:

> . . . To the Secretary of State for the Colonies (Mr. Chamberlain) we are under very great obligations. Without his initiative, and without his sympathy and active support, the hopes of some of us would not have been so speedily and so effectively realised. Apart from philanthropic and scientific considerations, as a piece of practical statesmanship, I confidently predict that the future will prove that of the many public measures Mr. Chamberlain has instituted and advocated this school is by no means the least important or the least promising.

He concluded this introductory talk by reminding his audience that funding would remain a major issue in the future:

> . . . The present generation of teachers may be willing to work for nothing; we have no right to assume from this that our successors will be content to work on the same terms. The school requires an endowment. We look to that good fairy the public, which has already been so generous, and for whose generosity we are so deeply grateful, to provide this . . .

Manson's words seem convincing enough. However there were, from the outset, difficulties in giving a precise identity to the newly established discipline – 'clinical tropical medicine'. Was it a new (separate and distinct) medical specialty, or essentially a scientific pursuit (based on recent developments in human parasitology) with a clinical 'spin-off'? The truth of the matter was that it was an essential component in the development of British economic and social imperialism – it was in fact one of the essential 'colonial sciences'. This was underlined in a paper read by Manson to the Royal Colonial Institute in April 1900 [*J R Col Inst* 1900; 31: 307–337]: *This school strikes, and strikes effectively at the root of the principle difficulty of most of these colonies – disease. It will cheapen government and make it more efficient. It will encourage and cheapen commercial enterprise. It will conciliate and foster the native* [my italics].

After a mere nine months the new school buildings had already proved too small[10], and within eighteen months the SHS committee noted that although £20,000 had been spent on the LSTM, the buildings and facilities were already inadequate for the numbers wishing to take the course(s). A resolution was passed that the Colonies should again be canvassed for financial support[11].

The 'rival' school at Liverpool

The Liverpool school had in fact opened about 6 months before that in London[12]. Despite the fact that the idea of a Liverpool School of Tropical Medicine was conceived later, the plan of action developed more rapidly and the building was opened to students on 21 April 1899[2]. The initial momentum originated in Chamberlain's circular to the GMC and the leading British Medical Schools (11 March 1898) and his letter to the Governors of the Colonies (14 June 1898)(see also chapter 5). The time-scale of the first appointments was impressive by any standard[12,13]: 20 January 1899 – Dean appointed; 7 February – Demonstrator in tropical pathology (Dr H E Annett); 10 April – Lecturer in tropical medicine (Major Ronald Ross, IMS); 22 April – school officially opened by Lord Lister; May 1899 – teaching started. Unlike the LSTM it was not Chamberlain's 'brainchild' and it did not receive Government support – a source of some irritation (and perhaps even anger) at the time. It owed its inception to the initiative of Mr (later Sir) Alfred Jones KCMG (1845–1909). Alfred Jones had been born at Carmarthen on 24 February 1845. He was a prominent local figure in Liverpool (an important seaport) and he was an energetic leader in the development of Liverpool's overseas trade with the West African Colonies; he was in control of the Elder Dempster shipping line – which traded with the Canary Islands and West Africa where he had a thriving business in bananas, groundnuts and oil nuts[2]. Together with several Liverpool merchants – who were at that time extremely wealthy (and generous) he provided both the initiative and finance for the foundation of the Liverpool School. The other major figure to be involved was Dr (later Sir) Rubert Boyce, FRS. In December 1898 *The Lancet* reported[14]:

> Mr. Chamberlain's scheme for the teaching of tropical diseases to colonial surgeons, wherever the school may be located, has already borne practical fruit. Mr. Alfred Jones of Liverpool has offered £350 annually to establish and maintain a laboratory in Liverpool for the study of tropical diseases and the scheme will be carried out by a joint committee of the Royal Southern Hospital and of University College. A laboratory for immediate investigation will be built opposite the hospital, whilst prolonged research will be carried on in the pathological laboratory of University College, under the direction of Professor Boyce. A large number of cases from the West Coast of Africa are taken into the wards of the Royal Southern Hospital, as Liverpool, being the centre of the African trade, is in constant communication with West Africa. We again have to congratulate Liverpool on the munificence of her citizens and would direct the attention of medical men about to practice in any capacity on the West Coast of Africa to the opportunity that is being afforded them for obtaining invaluable information.

In support of the project, the Principal of University College, Liverpool, had received the following letter from Dr. (later Sir) Michael Foster (1836–1907), Secretary of the Royal Society[12]:

The Royal Society,
Burlington House,
London, W.
18th November, 1898.

My Dear Glazebrook,

I think the idea of starting something at Liverpool about Tropical Diseases in connection with the College, most admirable. The opportunities of studying Tropical Diseases are greater at Liverpool than anywhere else in England, excepting perhaps London.

You have to arrange:

1. For teaching.
2. For Investigation.

No. 2 wants, I think, more support than No. 1.

If you have a ward, say at the Southern Hospital, one of the physicians might take charge of it, and give lectures, clinical at the Hospital, and general say at the College – I suppose you might give him a title.

For investigation you do not, I think, need a separate Laboratory at College, but a small Clinical Laboratory at the Hospital itself. At this Clinical Laboratory ordinary observations would be made; any prolonged research would be carried on at the Pathological Laboratory of the College, there is room enough there.

The next point, I am in doubt about. I am inclined to think that the Pathology of Tropical Diseases should belong to the *Professor of Pathology*, who should, by virtue of this have some connection with the Tropical Diseases Ward in the Hospital, have access to the cases, &c. But he would need an assistant Pathologist, specially told off to take care of the Pathology of Tropical Diseases, a young man, qualified, *not* a student, say at a salary of £250 or so. He, under the Professor, should have command of the Clinical Laboratory, and free access to cases; whether he should give Lectures or Demonstrations only might be arranged between him and the Professor.

This system of a Pathologist working with the Physician or Surgeon in Clinical charge of the sick is being very largely worked with great success in America, and this Tropical Disease seems to offer an opportunity for it.

I have talked with Lord Lister, and he generally approves of what I have proposed, at least, thinks it most desirable that the Hospital and College should lay hold of Tropical Diseases.

I myself feel very strongly that it is an opportunity of *study* of these diseases.

When the experts on Malaria sent out to Africa get to work on the West Coast, as they will in time do, it will be a great advantage to have an Institution for Tropical Diseases already in work at Liverpool. The experts abroad can work with the men at home.

Ever yours truly,
M. FOSTER.

A meeting was convened at the offices of Messrs. Elder, Dempster & Co., by Mr. Jones on 23 November 1898[12]. The following were present:

Alfred L. Jones; William Adamson, President of the Royal Southern Hospital; RT Glazebrook, FRS, Principal of University College, Liverpool; William Alexander, MD, FRCS, Senior Surgeon of the Royal Southern Hospital; William Carter, MD (Lond.), FRCP (Lond.), Physician to the Royal Southern Hospital, Professor of Therapeutics, University College, Liverpool; Rubert Boyce, Holt Professor of Pathology, University College, Pathologist Royal Infirmary, Bacteriologist to the Liverpool Corporation, and Consulting Pathologist Royal Southern

Hospital.

Mr. Jones was appointed Chairman, and Mr. Adamson, Vice-Chairman. The following Resolutions were unanimously passed:

1. That the gentlemen present form themselves into a Committee, with the approval of their various boards, for promoting the study of Tropical Diseases and to consider the best means of carrying out Mr. Alfred L Jones' intentions in the munificent offer he has made to further the above object.'

2. 'That Mr. Charles W. Jones (of Messrs. Lamport and Holt) be asked to serve on this Committee.'

It was decided that the above resolutions should be printed, and that Mr. Jones would hand a copy to the Rt. Hon. Joseph Chamberlain, Secretary of State for the Colonies. The Committee recommended that before the next meeting, the Professional Members should meet together to consider and suggest the best means for carrying out these objects.

A second meeting of the Committee was held on 12 December 1898. A letter (1 December 1898) from Lord Ampthill (of the Colonial Office) to the Chairman was read[12]:

Dear Mr. Jones,

I have shown your letter of the 28th ult. with regard to the School of Tropical Medicine, which you have started in Liverpool, to Mr. Chamberlain. He was much interested and very glad to hear of the important work you have thus commenced.

You are no doubt aware of what Mr. Chamberlain has been doing himself with regard to the establishment of a School of Tropical Medicine at the Seamen's Hospital, and he considers it a great advantage that Liverpool should be co-operating on similar lines.

If it would interest you, I should be very glad to send you particulars of the Colonial Office scheme and information as to what has been done already, but I dare say that you have learnt all that is essential from the newspapers.

Yours very faithfully,
AMPTHILL.

A letter (1 February 1899) from the Colonial Office was read to a subsequent Committee meeting in which it was stated that Chamberlain was very glad to learn that it had been decided to establish this School, but regretting that the Government could not grant any financial aid; however, in the selection of candidates for medical appointments in the Colonies, preference would be given to those who had received instruction in tropical medicine, such as that provided by the Liverpool School. However, a further letter from Chamberlain (23 February) stated that at present all doctors appointed to the Colonial Service must be attached to the Albert Docks' Hospital for at least two months. The Committee resolved to: (1) write to the Colonial Office and express regret that Mr. Chamberlain did not see his way to dispense with the latter condition in the case of students from the Liverpool School; and (2) approach the Colonial Office on the subject later.

On 20 March 1899, Professor Boyce announced that Lord Lister had written stating that he intended to approach Mr. Chamberlain on behalf of the School, and it was therefore resolved to postpone further action in the matter pending receipt of information concerning the result of Lister's initiative[12].

However, Government funding was not forthcoming (Chamberlain's reasons were doubtless complex) and there can be no doubt that this led to a significant souring of relationships (some of this rivalry still exists) toward Manson and the London School of Tropical Medicine. *The Lancet* summarized the inauguration of the Liverpool School[15]:

This school was inaugurated under fortunate auspices on April 22nd of this year by Lord Lister. 'At the annual dinner of the Royal Southern Hospital on Nov. 12th, 1898, Mr. Alfred L. Jones, a prominent Liverpool citizen and West Africa merchant, made an offer of £350 a year to start a school in Liverpool for the study of tropical diseases. The offer was made in the presence of Professor Rubert Boyce of University College, Liverpool, and Dr. William Alexander of the Royal Southern Hospital'. Mr. William Adamson, 'the president of the Royal Southern Hospital, accepted the generous offer on condition that University College, Liverpool, and the Royal Southern Hospital should be united in the undertaking. This condition was cordially acquiesced in by Professor Glazebrook', at that time the principal of the College. 'The great interest subsequently taken in the project by Mr. Alfred L. Jones, aided by the indomitable energy of Professor Boyce, resulted in subscriptions and donations coming in from all quarters towards the expenses of the proposed school. To those two gentlemen, warmly supported by the committee and medical staff of the Royal Southern Hospital, is due the establishment of the Liverpool School of Tropical Diseases. The management of the school is in the hands of a strong committee, of which Mr. Alfred L. Jones is the chairman and Mr. William Adamson . . . the vice-chairman. The committee also consists of duly appointed representatives of University College, Liverpool, the Royal Southern Hospital, the Liverpool Chamber of Commerce, the Steamship Owners' Association, and the Ship-owners' Association. A sum of over £1700 has already been promised, partly in annual subscriptions and partly in donations, in support of the school', but more pecuniary support is urgently needed if the practical work already begun is to be maintained at its excellent level. 'A large floor in the Royal Southern Hospital has been set apart for tropical cases. This floor includes a cheerful ward containing 12 beds, now fully occupied, also an extensive laboratory for the examination of blood, urine, faeces, &c., and furnished with the apparatus applicable to modern research'. Professor Boyce superintends 'the pathological department of the school, with Dr. Annett as pathological demonstrator. The committee have been fortunate in securing the services of Major Ronald Ross, IMS, as special lecturer on tropical diseases. ... The number of malarial cases treated in Liverpool in 1898 amounted to 294. In the previous year ... there were 242 cases of malaria, 14 of beri-beri, 30 of dysentery, and 39 of tropical anaemia. With the means of instruction in the varied forms of tropical diseases thus afforded there will be no need for Liverpool students to proceed to London to obtain that which is ready to hand at their own doors'. The authorities of the Liverpool School of Tropical Medicine have lost no time in getting to real work.

Very shortly after its inauguration (in April 1899), the Liverpool School set up a series of 'expeditions'; the first embarked for Sierra Leone in July 1899 and 11 more had been carried out by the end of 1903. Worboys in reviewing them retrospectively considered that these crusades were basically 'entrepreneurial activities', each being financed by subscription, whilst the School promoted itself as a consultancy[16]. The School survived therefore by subscription, and there was no year-to-year stability.

In June 1899, Ross gave his inaugural lecture; in this he committed himself to the *practical* application of his malaria researches; he envisaged extirpation of the mosquito as the solution to the malaria problem. Ross had thus embarked on the 'sanitation' (or hygiene) tack which was to dominate much of the work of the Liverpool School for the forthcoming century.

Foundation of the Schools in London and Liverpool

Ross' account some years later (in 1914) of the origin of the discipline – tropical medicine – and of the foundation of the two schools of tropical medicine differs in various details from most contemporary accounts.[17]:

... The history of its origin [tropical medicine] has not always been correctly given. The movement really commenced with the work of the old parasitologists rather than with that of the bacteriologists, and from the first was divided into two classes – first, the identification of pathogenic organisms; and, secondly, the determination of their life-history. To the first class belong the discoveries of many animal parasites, especially certain filariae, trypanosomes, spirochaetes, the malaria parasites, the leishmania, and many allied parasites of animals. But while these distinguished discoveries were of great importance in zoology and medicine, they did not directly help the sanitarian until the life-histories were worked out. This branch of the subject really commences with the discovery of *metaxeny*, or change of host, especially by Küchenmeister in 1851–53. A little later Leuckart extended the general law to intermediary hosts among the Arthropods, and Fedschenko, following his instructions, determined the life-history of *Filaria medinensis*, or the guinea-worm, in *Cyclops* (published in 1869). This work was followed by a succession of discoveries which extended the same law to many parasites, namely, the development of *Filaria bancrofti* in mosquitos by Manson (1877); the discovery of the *Piroplasma* of cattle by Smith and Kilborne, and of its carriage by ticks (1889); the similar discovery of Bruce regarding the tsetse fly disease of cattle (1894); my solution of the malaria problem (1891–99); the determination of the carriage of yellow fever by *Stegomyia* (1900); the carriage of plague by rat fleas and of relapsing fevers by ticks, and similar discoveries regarding many diseases of animals. These advances have evidently opened an entirely new chapter in the sanitation of tropical countries, inasmuch as they showed us how the most important diseases of such countries may be reduced.

I think it was especially the work of Bruce and of myself which led in 1899 to the foundation of the two schools of tropical medicine in Liverpool and London [my italics]. Mr. Chamberlain then issued a circular suggesting that this study might be taken up at the principal British ports. It is important to note that in other countries the whole of the movement would have been paid for by Government, as, for example, was the case in regard to the Tropical School of Hamburg; but Mr. Chamberlain's scheme suggested that the English schools should be paid for chiefly from private contributions. The Liverpool School was started in accordance with this idea, chiefly by the late Sir Rubert Boyce, the late Sir Alfred Jones, and the African merchants of Liverpool; and the London School had a similar origin under the influence of Manson and Mr. Chamberlain himself.

I was appointed the chief lecturer of the Liverpool School at its commencement in 1899. It was evident that we had a great campaign before us; and my first effort was to organize an expedition to Freetown, Sierra Leone, for the purpose of attempting to apply my researches on malaria to the actual prevention of the disease by the method of mosquito reduction, which I had already carefully considered in India . . .

Another part of the work done was to found permanent centres for teaching the new discoveries, which, of course, meant the endowment or payment of teachers, the provision of buildings, the collection of museums, the publication of special journals, and the maintenance of experts to advise on Government committees. With regard to the teaching of students, it was always apparent that in Liverpool we could never hope for as many students as our friendly rival, the London School, could obtain, and therefore we made expeditions and research our principal line of effort. Nevertheless, Liverpool laid down funds for a permanent institution on the lines indicated above and this with much less support from Governments than the London School has received . . .

Ross then proceeded to focus on the work of the Liverpool School which from the early days was clearly far more 'sanitation-oriented' than the essentially clinically based one in London:

> Summed up, the work of the school has been of great imperial significance. At the time we started, our administrators in the tropics were certainly not keen either upon sanitation or upon medical science. Doctors were generally called "pills," were supposed to know all about the cure of disease by intuition, and were allowed little or no power, even in connexion with sanitation. Frankly, from my experiences of tropical sanitation since 1881, this was in a shockingly bad state. Scarcely any intelligent attempt was made to deal with the great problems regarding the housing of the poor, conservancy, drainage, and water supply. Tropical towns were chiefly collections of slums with an enormous death-rate. Little or no investigation was being done except by a few individuals (at their own expense). When we ventured to express an opinion on sanitary matters we were told to mind our own business, and the same spirit has not entirely died out even yet. But the principal power for good of a school such as ours, practically independent of Government, and consisting of a non-official medical staff, has lain in its capacity for boldly drawing attention to these defects. We have not hesitated to speak out on these matters, and the experience given to us by our expeditions has fully justified us in doing so . . .

But a particular concern remained, and this was funding. In the case of Liverpool, Ross concluded, by again emphasising the lack of financial support which the School had received from Government ('the revenues from the Colonies and the British Exchequer'):

> . . . Numbers of the lecturers and other officials receive nothing or next to nothing, and the payment of the junior posts no longer tempts the best men. And this is for a movement which has probably done, and will do, more for our Empire and the tropics than the work of any number of our highly paid and pensioned "proconsuls" put together! But then we are only "pills"! . . .

From the outset, therefore, the staff of the Liverpool School seem to have taken exception to Manson's dominance over the tropical scene, together with the fact that the LSTM was supported by Government and the Royal Society, and therefore obtained more research grants. Although founded later it became the undisputed centre of British 'tropical medicine'. Such sentiments were expressed by Lt Col (later Sir) David Bruce (1855–1931), who had carried out pioneering work on brucellosis in Malta and had been involved in the investigations on African trypanosomiasis[16]. Another critic who took a similar line was Professor G H F Nuttall of Cambridge. According to Worboys[16], the Liverpool School was from the outset moving in a direction opposite to that of its London counterpart; it also 'became more and more independent, and soon had little connection with the Liverpool medical community.'

8

The Albert Dock years: 1899 – 1920

The day of small nations has long passed away. The day of Empires
has come.

Joseph Chamberlain (1904)

Although there were practical disadvantages of considerable magnitude –
the distance of the School and Hospital from central London produced
enormous inconveniences – the early years of the *clinical* tropical medicine centre, with the British Empire at its zenith, were undoubtedly its
most successful ones. Although at the 'hub of road, rail and sea traffic'[1];
the hospital was sited 9 miles from the centre – in a most unattractive
part of London. The rail journey from Fenchurch Street to Connaught
Road station took 30 minutes, but this service was infrequent and the
alternative station – Custom House – (which took somewhat longer and
which remains in use today) meant a lengthy walk to or from the LSTM.
As Manson-Bahr has pointed out[1], there were no local attractions; 'only
one hostelry was available in the neighbourhood, and to most students
the 'Connaught Arms' offered no rosy charms'; students who came
to the school had to lead a 'monastic existence', and work! It was
also apparently impossible to see a show in London and return the
same night.

During the first year, 120 students (9 of them women) passed through
the school[2]; table 8.1 gives the annual attendance figures for 1899 to 1911,
and table 8.2 shows the provenance of the students from 1899 to 1905.
Amongst the tropical diseases seen during the first 15 months were: 55
cases of acute malaria, 4 chronic malaria, 29 beri-beri, 7 guinea-worm,
and 4 plague. Table 8.3 gives the diagnoses of the 'tropical' cases seen at
the LSTM up to 1903. Plate 40 shows the admission books of the Albert
Dock Hospital in the early twentieth century. After 4 years of existence,
the school was recognised as a 'unit' within the University of London[1].
In 1912, the much needed extension to the LSTM was completed and was
opened by King George V (1865–1936) thanks to yet another appeal for
funds (see below); Plate 41 shows the extension soon after completion.

The school was to attract a succession of eminent speakers to give

Table 8.1 – Attendance figures at the
London School of Tropical Medicine: 1899–1911

Numbers of Students attending each Course since the Foundation.

YEAR	1ST SESSION Jan.– April	2ND SESSION May–July	3RD SESSION Oct.– Dec.	TOTAL FOR YEAR
1899	–	–	27	27
1900	24	27	23	74
1901	19	28	28	75
1902	27	31	33	91
1903	26	31	31	88
1904	37	41	37	115
1905	28	24	42	94
1906	21	32	42	95
1907	24	37	29	90
1908	30	37	45	112
1909	34	52	59	145
1910	40	53	44	137
1911	37	58	64	159
	347	451	504	1302
			Grand Total	1302

Table 8.2 – Provenance of students attending courses at LSTM
between its inauguration and 1905[1]

Colonial office	220
Foreign office	18
IMS	22
Other government departments	32
Army	5
Navy	12
Missionary Societies	63
Private students	192
Total	564

Table 8.3 – Diagnoses of 'tropical cases'
admitted to the Albert Dock Hospital between 1899 and 1903[1]

Acute malaria	128
Chronic malaria	22
Blackwater fever	6
Sleeping sickness	1
Filariasis	8
Guinea worm infection	17
Bilharziasis	11
Dysentery	101
Liver abscess	16
Hepatitis	10
Plague	4
Sprue	6
Leprosy	6
Beri–beri	76

the major lectures. Sir William MacGregor (chapter 2), one of the most distinguished of Colonial administrators, gave an address – 'On some problems of tropical medicine' – on 3 October 1900[3]:

... If this branch of medicine is neglected, then the sufferer from the tropics will be a certain loser, but not always the only one. At the present moment, however, many of us are very specially interested in this school in relation to the medical services of our more unhealthy tropical colonies. It is probably the case that not a few of those who have so far passed through this institution were already familiar with many tropical diseases, knew them by experience, and understood how to treat them. To students of that category the clinical studies of these maladies here is not nearly so important as is the training to be had to fit them to investigate tropical diseases on the spot, on the most advanced systems known to medical science and with a full knowledge of what has already been done in these matters in this country and elsewhere. Any average medical officer who has sufficient training in making investigations of this kind will soon master the practical details of all tropical diseases in his district, provided that he is given time, the necessary instruments, and proper accommodation. The best and most proper place for making such researches is undoubtedly the tropics themselves. It must be patent to every person who thinks at all on the subject that the training of medical officers to carry out investigations of this kind is of the utmost importance to each colony, to the empire, and to humanity at large. We all know, or ought to know, what has been done in this field by such men as my late highly esteemed friend Dr. Bancroft of Brisbane; by the distinguished Dr. Patrick Manson, the inspiring genius of this school; by the father of Strachan's disease, the present chief medical officer of Lagos; and by many others who have practised medicine in the tropics. These men had no specialised opportunities given them; they had not the advantage of any systematic training such as is offered now at this school. We are therefore justified in expecting a great deal from the younger men who now come forward here to learn at once the most suitable and the most advanced methods of conducting original investigations in the great and rich tropical field . . .

But I can tell you that this training and preparation will not yield all that we are justified in expecting from it without the cooperation of the Secretary of State for the Colonies and of colonial administrators. The trained medical officer must have time and opportunity granted to him. That the Colonial Secretary will in every possible way encourage and suitably recognise the researches of medical officers may safely be taken as granted. It is, however, at times a very difficult matter for an administrator so to arrange service affairs as to be able to grant to medical officers the time so necessary to carry on scientific investigations of this kind without their being submitted to grave or destructive interruptions. Colonial administrators and others in high authority have not always in the past lent to the head of the medical department the support required by him. They have not always given to their chief medical officer the confidence that Alexander the Great extended to his. . .

MacGregor's address which marked the first anniversary of the School's existence, proceeded to give an overview on the contemporary state of knowledge regarding most major tropical diseases affecting residents of a tropical country; also, his vast experience of administration in many of these countries (chapter 2) came to the fore.

The opening address a year later was given by Lord Brassey; fund-raising (see below) was again high on the list of priorities[4]:

. . . Experience had shown that the demand for instruction in tropical medicine was much greater than had been originally anticipated. During the last session it had been found necessary to refuse several students, and some four or five had been compelled to postpone their attendance until the next session. To carry on the work efficiently further funds were required to enlarge the school and to place it in a sound financial basis. The importance of the health of Europeans in the tropics could not be over-estimated, especially to a country like ours that depended for colonial prosperity upon the efficiency of our fellow-countrymen in tropical countries. A healthy community gave continuity of administration to the Government, diminished sick leave through improved conditions of health, and conduced enormously to efficiency of administration. In commercial operations it was all important that those who conducted them should not be too often away on account of sickness. Sir Francis Lovell was about to proceed to the tropics on behalf of the Seamen's Hospital Society to make known the advantages of the London School of Tropical

Medicine, and to endeavour to raise funds on its behalf. The school needed a sum of £100,000, but large as that sum was it was yet a small one for the great British Empire with so great a stake in the tropics.

[Following this address] Dr. PATRICK MANSON said the object of the school was to educate medical men who proposed to practise in the tropics. Another function was to attempt to advance the science of medicine in regard to tropical diseases. Mainly through the assistance of Mr. Chamberlain and of the managers of the Dreadnought Hospital the initial financial difficulties and professional opposition had been overcome. The number of students was so numerous that they could not admit them because the accommodation was too scanty. A growing institution should not be choked by a superfluity of work thrown upon it. There was a danger that students coming to them and finding no room might go elsewhere or give up the idea of special education in tropical diseases. The students were no callow youths – they were men of experience, many of them with grey hairs. The space at their disposal did not suffice to accommodate the students. They wanted enlarged laboratories, a lecture-room, a museum, and a library. . .

Manson's talk was followed by one given by the Dean:

Sir FRANCIS LOVELL, CMG (1844–1916), late Surgeon-General of Trinidad, said that he had undertaken an expedition to the tropics on behalf of the Seamen's Hospital Society in order to provide funds to enable that society to put the London School of Tropical Medicine in a more satisfactory financial position. It was absolutely necessary that funds should be forthcoming, and it was felt by the Seamen's Hospital Society that an appeal should be made to those resident abroad. He had offered to the society to go abroad to induce the English residents in the East and in other tropical parts to contribute towards the objects which the school had in view. It had been decided that he was to go to India, to Ceylon, to the Straits Settlements, to China, to Japan, to New Zealand, and to Australia. He would return home probably by way of the United States and Canada. His intention was to raise funds to enable the society to put the London School of Tropical Medicine on such a footing as would make it worthy of its name as a teaching body in the great city of London.

Manson gave a further up-date on the state of the School in December 1903[5]:

. . . Sir Patrick Manson said that since the school opened on Oct. 3rd [sic], 1899, over three hundred students had passed through its portals. During the first two years (six sessions) they had had 149 students; during the last two years (six sessions) they had had 178 students. In the earlier days of the school's existence many of the students came for one or two months only. Now a large proportion of the students remained during the full course of three months. When they left the majority of the students had a genuine practical grasp of their subject. They had seen and most of them had applied for themselves the most recent methods of diagnosis, and as far as teaching and opportunity could insure they were qualified for medical work in the tropics – qualified both to practise their profession and to advance the science of tropical medicine. Where two or three men took a languid interest in tropical disease some five or six years ago, a whole army of eager investigators had arisen, mainly composed of men educated or inspired by the London and Liverpool schools of tropical medicine. This multiplication of investigators had already borne remarkable fruit. Without alluding to what had been done in Liverpool he could point out not a few notable triumphs by men from the London school, although the school had been in existence for only just over four years. . . .

In referring to beri-beri Sir Patrick Manson said they did not despair of getting light on this disease. Dr. C.W. Daniels [Plate 42], their late superintendent, had been placed in charge of the research laboratory at Kuala Lumpur, and in the Federated Malay States beri-beri was rampant. Perhaps no country in the world, he thought, was so likely to benefit by recent advances in tropical medicine as the British colonies and protectorates in the Malay Peninsula, for beri-beri was a terrible drag on the mining and agricultural industries there. . . .

After paying an eloquent tribute to the energy and unselfishness displayed by Sir Francis Lovell in his work for the school, Sir Patrick Manson concluded by an appeal for public support. At the present time, he said, the school had certain schemes of investigation before it for some of which they wanted money, for others men and money. They wished to furnish their museum and library on a scale adequate to the needs of the school. In short, they wanted £100,000, or as much of that sum as they could get. Any one of the discoveries which he had mentioned, said Sir Patrick Manson, was worth the sum he had named ten times over, apart from the education which the school had supplied to its students. They had given the public a great deal more than they had ever received, or would ever be likely to receive, and therefore they had no hesitation in asking for something more on account. The teachers were strictly honorary, their pay was so small that the laboratory microscopes were sometimes required to see it. They had the approval of those best qualified to judge of the work the school had undertaken – viz., the medical profession, whose hearty practical sympathy was peculiarly gratifying to them. Finally, Sir Patrick Manson said that 'he who gives to the London School of Tropical Medicine lends to humanity.'

On the motion of Sir WILLIAM S. CHURCH, seconded by Sir F. YOUNG, a vote of thanks was heartily passed to Sir Patrick Manson for his address.

In September 1905 *The Lancet*[6] again stressed the growing importance of a knowledge of tropical medicine, but not only for those doctors working in tropical countries; medical graduates taking appointments on board ships were equally relevant, and the steamshipping companies should insist, it was claimed, that their medical officers were familiar with the 'ordinary problems of tropical disease.' The importance of research was also stressed:

A feature of recent research in the investigation of tropical diseases is the necessity for the aid of the botanist, the zoologist, the bacteriologist, and the parasitologist in arriving at a real knowledge of the many serious endemic and epidemic ailments which beset the dwellers in warm countries, be they Europeans or natives. So many diseases have been proved of late years to be carried by certain insects that for their complete elucidation an exact knowledge of many apparently insignificant animals, their habits, their anatomy and geographical distribution, is an absolute necessity. Details of the fauna and flora of the area in which a disease flourishes have become essential to the conscientious investigator, and the study of these in their bearing on disease is imperative now that we have decided not to treat tropical diseases in the empirical fashion handed down to us in so many directions. Hitherto much biology has possessed little more than an academic interest for students of medicine, and the tendency has been to disassociate biology from the instruction provided at our medical schools. The effect, however, of the methods of investigation followed during the past few years has been to bring the subjects of botany and zoology to the forefront and the medical investigator finds that the immediate help of biological experts is required at every step. The Schools of Tropical Medicine at London and Liverpool have each instituted lectureships on parasitology, and the London School has in addition created a lectureship for the subject of helminthology alone. For students whose bent is towards biology there has hitherto been little to encourage them in the particular branch of study they found most congenial, for beyond a few chairs in our universities, mostly very poorly endowed, there have been few appointments open to them. All this will be changed, is indeed already being changed, and the biologist apparently will be as requisite a coadjutor in the field of scientific investigation of disease as the chemist and bacteriologist. The commercial value of biology has been recognised, and we are glad to know that the lectureships in parasitology and helminthology, to which we have alluded, have been endowed. The endowments are not large, but such as they are they form tangible proof of the direction of public opinion. These facts should encourage men with tastes for what is known as "pure science" in contradistinction to practical medicine to qualify in medicine, for without a full course of medical instruction their value as investigators of disease from the biological standpoint is seriously hampered. There can be little doubt that in every large medical school at no distant date, a lectureship in parasitology will be instituted, so that there will be a demand for men specially qualified in this branch of study for some time to come . . .

The writer then referred to the lectureships in tropical medicine which had by then been instituted in most British universities and medical schools:

> . . .but the subject is not compulsory and as a rule [the student] finds that he has quite enough to do to attend those classes which bear directly upon the subject in which he is likely to be examined. Tropical medicine is therefore a post-graduate study and in all probability will remain so for a long time to come. Medical men entering the navy and army will find that excellent courses of instruction are given at Haslar and the Staff College in London, and those who resolve to enter the Colonial service, or who intend engaging in private practice in warm climates, are provided with well-equipped laboratories and a staff of teachers at London and Liverpool. Diplomas in tropical medicine are obtainable at the Universities of Cambridge and Liverpool. At Cambridge the authorities accept certificates of instruction from any recognised school of tropical medicine, but at Liverpool only the pupils of the University are allowed to take the diploma. At the London School of Tropical Medicine and at several universities certificates of having passed an examination in tropical medicine are obtainable.
>
> At the University of London the subject of regulations for the degree of MD in tropical medicine is being considered. Candidates must have taken the MB, BS degrees of the University and must produce proof of having attended for not less than one academical year at a school of tropical medicine satisfactory to the University, or of having been engaged for two years in hospital, official, or private practice in tropical or sub-tropical regions. The examination at the University is to consist of one paper in Medicine; one paper in Tropical Medicine (including general and operative treatment); one paper in the Pathology of Tropical Disease and in Tropical Hygiene; an essay on one of two subjects in Tropical Medicine (including pathology and hygiene); a clinical examination; and a laboratory examination . . .

In October 1905, *The Lancet*[7] devoted a leading article to an assessment of the LSTM, and tropical medicine in general in the light of the opening address for that session which had been given by Dr G H F Nuttall, FRS (1862–1937) (lecturer in bacteriology and preventive medicine at Cambridge)[8]:

> The committee of the London School of Tropical Medicine [opened] the nineteenth session with an introductory lecture followed by a dinner of past and present students in imitation of many of the older medical colleges. The committee did wisely in securing as lecturer Dr. G.H. Nuttall, who is one of the examiners for the Cambridge diploma in tropical medicine and hygiene, which he and others recently persuaded the Senate of the Univer-

sity to establish. Instead of referring, as his hearers perhaps expected, to his own researches in protozoology, he preferred ... to point out some of the obvious needs of the Tropical School. In mentioning the peremptory need of further research work he reminded his audience that science workers are little valued financially in this country and teachers are constantly distressed by finding that students, gifted with scientific training and special powers of research, have unwillingly to drift away to the practice of medicine in order to gain a living wage. The lecturer's early training in America and Germany caused him not unnaturally to compare scientific work in those more fortunate countries with the difficulties put in the way of research workers here. In the United States it seems hardly necessary for scientific institutions to be State-aided because in all the big cities there are millionaires able and willing to endow schools, colleges, and research laboratories. All German universities and many towns in Germany are provided by the State with institutes of hygiene, while the salaries of teachers are provided for by special grants. Even the poorer Italian universities are equipped with institutes of hygiene for scientific research and teaching purposes. We must allow that the hygiene laboratories of Edinburgh and Manchester in this country compare favourably with some of their foreign rivals but it is sad to be reminded that neither at Oxford nor at Cambridge is there as yet any adequate provision for research work or experimental work in preventive medicine. All help in this country must come from the general public, who have not yet learned that money given to scientific workers sometimes proves a valuable commercial investment. Benevolent people give money to hospitals during their lifetime and by legacies, but little is done for the endowment of teaching chairs and, as we have often pointed out, most teachers of science in this country receive miserably inadequate salaries. If it were not for this Great Britain and her colonies would be able to employ our own countrymen instead of having to borrow scientific men from abroad. The knowledge of tropical disease is growing every year and the students are becoming in consequence more and more weighed down by the amount which they have to learn during a course which only lasts three months, and the time must shortly come when those responsible for the teaching of tropical diseases will have to consider whether the session should be prolonged. *But all this costs money and the Imperial Government, though appreciative of the value of work in preventive medicine, is not yet moved to subsidise it. . .*

An extremely comprehensive survey of parasitology was given by Manson in a Huxley lecture at Charing Cross Hospital in October 1908[9]. In an address entitled 'The Nation and the Tropics' delivered in October 1909 at the LSTM, Professor William Osler, FRS (1849–1919), Regius Professor of Medicine at Oxford – gave a remarkable overview of medicine in relation to tropical exposure[10]:

... The tropical world has been appropriated, and this country has a burden of tropical population six times greater than the other three [colonising countries] combined. A few comparatively small districts remain either independent, or as yet unexplored, as Abyssinia and parts of Polynesia . . .

It is no light burden for the white man to administer this vast trust. It is, indeed, a heavy task, but the responsibility of Empire has been the making of the race. In dealing with subject nations there are only two problems of the first rank – order and health. The first of these may be said to be a speciality of the Anglo-Saxon. Scarlet sins may be laid at his door – there are many pages in the story of his world-exodus which we would fain blot out; too often he has gone forth in the spirit of the Old Testament crying "The sword of the Lord and Gideon." But heap in one pan of the balance all the grievous tragedies of America and of Australasia, the wholesale destruction of native races, all the bloodshed of India, and the calamities of South Africa, and in the other pan put just the one little word "order," which has everywhere followed the flag, and it alone makes the other kick the beam. Everywhere this has been the special and most successful feature of British rule. We are entering upon a phase in which the natural results of this stable government upon the subject races are shown. Just as at home the fate of the rich is indissolubly bound up with that of the poor, so in the dependencies the fate of the strong and the weak cannot be dissevered; and whether he will bear or whether he will forbear, the brother's keeper doctrine of the strong, helpful brother must be preached to the white man. The responsibility is upon the nation to maintain certain standards which our civilisation recognises as indispensable on the supposition that our Western ideas are right; but we have to meet the fact that the ways of the natives are not our ways, nor their thoughts our thoughts; and yet we place them in such a position that sooner or later they become joint heritors with us of certain civil and social traditions and aspirations. It is in India and the Philippines that the political problem looms large, but no matter how large or how formidable it must not be allowed to interfere with the great primary function of the Anglo-Saxon as a policeman. There may be a doubt as to the grafting of our manners, and still greater doubt as to the possibility of inculcating our morals; a doubt also as to the wisdom of trying everywhere to force upon them our religion; but you will, I think, agree that the second great function of the nation is to give to the inhabitants of the dependencies, Europeans or natives, good health – a freedom from plague, pestilence, and famine. And this brings me to the main subject of my address, the control of the tropics by sanitation.

After a masterly historical review on progress in the field of communicable disease in Britain during the nineteenth century, and in the understanding of tropical infections in the previous 25 years, Osler continued:

I have indicated briefly to you the pressing necessity to take up the heavy burden of securing health in the tropics. To make our knowledge effective, to make it as effective as Dr. Gorgas has done at the Isthmus of Panama, as Ross has done at Ismailia, is the problem which to-day confronts us. Enough has already been accomplished to indicate a successful plan of campaign. Two things are necessary. First, organised centres from which the work may proceed; a model of this sort is the "Sleeping Sickness" Bureau under the auspices of the Royal Society. The work which it has done and which is under progress shows the value of central organisation. Similar central bodies have already dealt with plague and malaria, but these organisations should be placed on a permanent basis and unified in some way under a central Tropical Institute, the different departments of which would be in touch with its workers all over the world. . . .

Is it likely that the white man can ever thrive in the tropics except as a sort of exotic, as he is at present in the West and East Indies? As the nations of the north and south increase and multiply, doubling every century, will he find an outlet by settlement in the tropics, or will he simply use them as Rome did Egypt, as a granary? It cannot be said that so far the European has been a success as a settler in the tropics, since no white colony has ever prospered below 30 degrees of northern latitude, but has he ever had a chance? In contact with brown and black races, which have become inured to heat, tolerant of parasites, and more or less immune to the worst of the tropical diseases, he has so far never had an opportunity to show of what he might be capable when placed in really sanitary surroundings. The 8000 whites now at the Isthmus work eight hours a day in the burning sun, and they with their wives and children thrive and enjoy a health quite as good as dwellers in any town in the United States. Heretofore man has never met nature on equal terms; now science has taught him how to be master, but the knowledge is so new and so recently made effective that we have not the data from which to make a clear judgment. How far the introduction of tropical diseases has accounted for the decadence of Greece has been discussed by W.H.S. Jones and Ronald Ross, who seem to have made out a good case, but given a white race living in the tropics for two generations, and free from malaria and parasitic anaemia, would it show the hardy vigour at present the characteristic of the Anglo-Saxon? Time alone will tell. Personally I doubt it. Man is a lazy animal, and the best thing that ever happened in his history was when Adam's wife ate the apple and they both were turned out of a tropical Eden to earn their bread by the sweat of their brows. As Sir Charles Dilke has remarked, the banana is the curse of the tropics, and when have ever "the blossom-fed Lotophagi" done anything for the race? The most successful attempt has been in the English West Indies, but commercial conditions have been adverse, and to-day the negro may be said to possess the islands where the white man lives it is true, but hardly thrives . . .

Other notable Introductory Addresses over these years were given by[1]: Sir Charles Bruce (1904), Col Kenneth Macleod (1906), and Sir Lauder Brunton (1907).

A growing emphasis on hygiene

It is now clear, I think, that although the importance of clinical medicine and the basic sciences (parasitology and bacteriology) were considered essential to the training of a doctor working in a tropical country, sanitation was coming increasingly to the fore. Preventive medicine had after all been an extremely important theme in the reduction of disease prevalence in nineteenth century Britain (chapter 1). Ross and other members of the Liverpool School of Tropical Medicine had in fact taken this approach for some time; this is further borne out by the following account published in 1914[11]:

> The first of two Chadwick public lectures was delivered by Sir Ronald Ross, KCB, FRS, at the London School of Economics on Dec. 4th, Sir James Crichton-Browne (Chadwick trustee) being in the chair. The lecturer pointed out that the relations between administration and public sanitation had not been completely discussed. The older theory of government, well enunciated by David Hume, was that government had "no other object or purpose but the distribution of justice." This idea had now been abandoned in favour of the view that government should do everything possible for the prosperity of its subjects. The lecturer then traced the history of tropical sanitation. Civilisation had been excluded from large tropical areas such as tropical Africa, largely because grave tropical diseases were present which had not been investigated until recently. The causes and prevention of many of these maladies were now understood; but the question still remained whether public administration could utilise the preventive measures suggested by science. Examining the history of this question, the lecturer pointed out that in the old days medical and sanitary matters were originally in the hands of the priestly caste, many of whose religious injunctions were really of a sanitary nature. In the Middle Ages little attention was given to sanitary matters, and epidemics often provoked ridiculous attempts at prevention. The modern history of tropical sanitation began from the time when the European nations commenced colonisation. About the middle of the last century sanitation in Europe began to approach its modern growth and naturally affected tropical sanitation.

The following anonymous contribution, published in *The Lancet* for 1919, refers to a series of preventive medicine lectures – aimed at expatriates

174

living in a tropical environment[12]:

> The value of a sound knowledge of first aid in tropical medicine on the part of their representatives in Africa and other hot countries is being recognised by the heads of many business firms; as the outcome of this interest Sir James Cantlie, Principal of the College of Ambulance, has inaugurated a series of lectures on Tropical Ailments and Their Prevention. The lectures will be given by medical men who have made a special study of tropical diseases. The first lecture was delivered on March 31st by Sir James Cantlie on Personal Hygiene. On April 2nd Professor W.J.R. Simpson spoke on Tropical Sanitation. He described the climate of the belt lying between the tropics of Cancer and Capricorn; the hottest places were situated in the regions of the tropics, and the variations of climate depended on altitude as well as latitude. Houses intended for Europeans should not be built near native dwellings, because in places where mosquitoes abounded the infection of malaria and yellow fever was carried from the natives to the Europeans. The site should be dry and away from marsh land, as the latter, though appearing suitable in summer, might be inundated during the rainy season. Buildings should be erected on a slope, if possible; a two-storeyed house was more healthy than a bungalow, but either should be built on a raised platform 6 feet above the ground. If built on pillars of a lower height the smaller space below the house was apt to become a harbour for rubbish. Solid arches might be used as an alternative method of construction. In both cases the buildings should be approached by a few steps. Ceilings should be high or the house would become hot and disagreeable. Between the ceiling and the roof there should be a good air space with ventilating screens of mosquito netting to prevent the entrance of bats. Verandahs 10 or 12 feet wide should be provided in order to keep the walls cool and to allow the occupants to enjoy the cool air in the later part of the day. Sanitary offices should be constructed in towers at the back of the house. Houses could also be kept dry by surrounding them with a sloping platform with a drain close to the walls of the house or verandah. This platform should terminate in a stretch of Indian or Bramah grass, which grows very short and allows the water, which might otherwise lie in pools, to evaporate quickly. Between the grass and the drain there should be a belt of sharp gravel to prevent the approach of snakes. There should be no trees near the house, and this applied especially to banana or bamboo plants, as they held moisture and harboured the larvae of mosquitoes. Houses built round a courtyard possessed certain advantages: the rooms could be well ventilated and protection by mosquito screens was easier. The servants' quarters should be away from the house; the kitchens should be well detached and approached by a covered passage; the servants' quarters should be inspected periodically, as rubbish was likely to collect and become a breeding-place for mosquitos. Cleanliness in the kitchen should be insisted upon. In malarious districts some part of the verandah should be mosquito-proof, netting at least 20 strands to the inch being necessary, and ventilation effected by electric fans. In some cases

the whole house would have to be mosquito-proof. Milk should always be boiled as the natives made a practice of adulterating it with water which was generally contaminated. Water should be boiled and filtered, and care taken to see that the filter was acting properly; he had frequently found defective filters being relied upon. With the exception of the tank storage of rain water, no water-supply in the tropics was safe. Servants would often dip water out of the filter before it had passed through the filtering candles. Salads were dangerous on account of the possibility of their contamination by the faecal matter which was used on the fields. Fruits which grew above the ground were safe, but anything that grew close to the ground or under it should be avoided or special care taken in cooking it. The lecturer said that he always advised young men going to the tropics to take 5 gr. of quinine on arrival and, in malarious districts, to take 5 gr. immediately after the morning meal. It was his practice to have 5-gr. tablets on the breakfast table, so that they might not be forgotten. It was always necessary to sleep under a mosquito net.

Much of this advice is of course not far removed from that which is being given some 70 years later!

The Great War – 1914–1918: a major disruption

The war came as a mighty blow to the LSTM which by 1914 had been in full swing. Student numbers plummeted, but with the exception of a brief period in 1918 the courses continued; in 1916 the student total was down to 25 (the lowest on record) and in 1917 only a single doctor (from Bombay) presented himself[1]. However, much fighting took place in countries where tropical diseases abounded. Dysentery was a major problem amongst the troops in the Mediterranean, Gallipoli and the Middle-east; malaria proved to be a major menace in Salonika, Mesopotamia, Palestine and East Africa. Morbidity and mortality from tropical disease in fact outnumbered that inflicted by the enemy by 30 to 1![1]; therefore tropical experts were in great demand. Officers were trained in protozoology by Dr C M Wenyon and Dr C Dobell and thence dispatched to many 'fronts'. Many members of the staff served overseas[1]. Dr (Lt Col) R T Leiper (1881–1969) investigated schistosomiasis in Egypt. Dr A Balfour (who was to become the first Director of the London School of Hygiene and Tropical Medicine) undertook malaria control in Alexandria and Salonika. Wenyon, together with Balfour and Dr J C G Ledingham, toured several fronts and gave advice on tropical infections. Dr F W O'Connor joined the laboratory service in Egypt and Salonika. Dr H M Hanschell served with the Navy at Haslar and in Central Africa. Dr H B G Newham was appointed Consulting Physician to the Forces in East Africa. Colonel

176

A Alcock was briefly called up and served as a surgical specialist to the Indian Military Hospital, Woolwich. The School therefore became seriously depleted of staff.

Offers were made to the War Office to admit naval and military personnel to the Hospital, and/or to use the hostel for convalescent officers. Some felt that the School should organise itself into a unit for 'overseas service in the tropics'. Later in the war, the hospital became filled with officers and men suffering from dysentery and malaria from the Mediterranean area and Gallipoli.

On the night of 19 January 1917, a TNT explosion occurred at the nearby Brunner and Mond's works in Silvertown. This almost wrecked the hospital and school; the windows were all shattered[1]. A large number of casualties from the explosion were brought into the hospital and it became a temporary First Aid Post. [The explosion is commemorated to this day by a wall plaque recording the endowment of a Silvertown cot (Plate 43a)]. HM King George V visited the LSTM on 10 October 1917, and early in 1918 Queen Mary accompanied by the Prince of Wales and Princess Royal also paid a visit.

When the regular courses were suspended in 1917 (see above) Colonel S P James IMS (retd) organised a course of lectures for Army Medical Corps Officers. Later, the India Office used the Hospital and School as a depot for Indian Army personnel invalided from Egypt, Gallipoli, India and Mesopotamia. Dr G C Low (1872–1952) was placed in charge – with the rank of Major, IMS.

In January 1919, Sir Havelock Charles put forward a resolution that the School should move to central London (chapter 9); it was felt that as a result of the war, there would be a great increase in the number of individuals suffering from tropical diseases. The 59th session of the School commenced on 15 January 1919 with 7 students; by March conditions were laid down for admission of the School to the University of London.

Funding the LSTM; the struggle for support intensifies

Despite the Government grant (which included generous contributions from the colonies) the school remained very heavily dependant on voluntary contributions. However, in its first two years the school had a working profit of £200; students' fees formed a major source of income. The overseas visits by the Dean, Sir Francis Lovell, KCMG also helped (see above); during one of these (to India) in 1902 for example, he received donations amounting to £10,000 – Bombay having 'answered the appeal with great warmth but very little has been got from Calcutta'[13]. Chamberlain presided at a second highly successful banquet at the Hotel

Cecil; the first had been on 10 May 1899 (chapter 5), and this one which was held on 10 May 1905 raised £11,000. *The Lancet* reported in a leading article[14]:

> The banquet held on Wednesday evening with the object of relieving the London School of Tropical Medicine from a heavy burden of debt has drawn public attention, mainly through Mr. Chamberlain's forceful speech, to the affairs and performances of a most deserving scientific institution. Although it has been but a few years in existence the school has done excellent work and has established some striking facts . . .

and after a summary of some of its achievements, especially in research, continued:

> Formerly the medical officer proceeding to his work in tropical climates had first of all to learn it in those regions; now he can proceed thither having first mastered the elements of this portion of the medical art. England is the great colonising country of the world; how great, then, is the necessity for the various deadly diseases to be understood fully by those of her sons who proceed to the colonies, the home of these diseases. We cordially wish this school and its staff the fullest measure of success that will doubtless in the future accrue to their endeavours. But in order to insure this object funds are necessary and we feel sure that the British public, once it is alive to the great benefits which the school is conferring, will not be backward in supplying them. As the Duke of Marlborough has stated in a public appeal, an increasing number of our kith and kin are annually required to carry on the work in the tropics, where the white man's burden is the heaviest, and it is undoubtedly a matter of Imperial importance that a knowledge of the etiology and treatment of the diseases to be met with in the tropics should be obtained. The London School of Tropical Medicine should not be hampered in its work by the shackles of debt and we are glad to learn that since Wednesday evening its coffers have been enriched by upwards of £10,000.

Chamberlain, who had relinquished the post of Colonial Secretary in 1903 (his successor was Alfred Lyttelton) remained a very strong supporter of the school[15]:

> After the usual loyal toast, Mr. Chamberlain proposed 'The London School of Tropical Medicine' and said that when he was invited to preside at this dinner he could not resist the temptation to repeat the experience of six years ago when he presided at a similar banquet at the establishment of the London School of Tropical Medicine. Now he came back to rejoice in their past success and to inquire into their future, his interest in tropical medicine being unexhausted and unbounded. He regarded it as a privilege as well

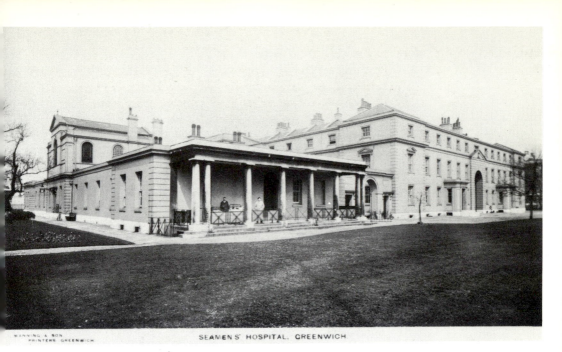

SEAMEN S' HOSPITAL, GREENWICH

32. *Dreadnought* Hospital, Greenwich - early 20th century

33. London School of Tropical Medicine - October 1899

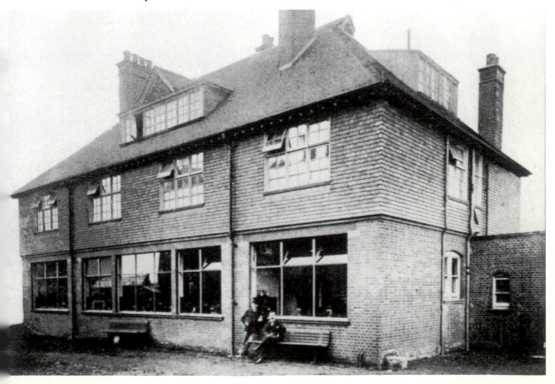

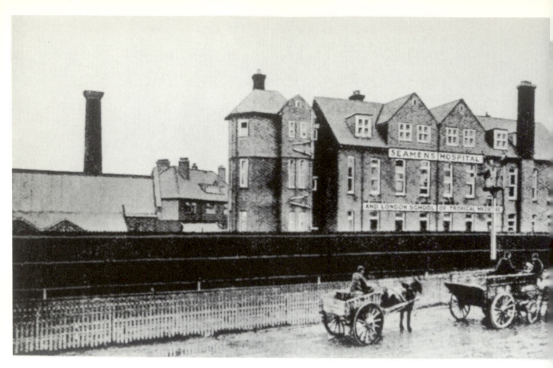

34. The London School of Tropical Medicine and Albert Dock Hospital - 1899

35. Interior of the 'Top Ward' of the Albert Dock Hospital - 1899

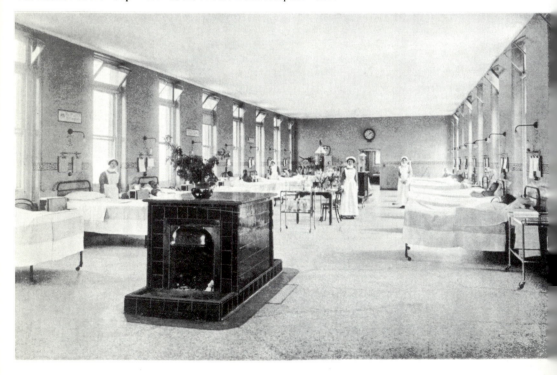

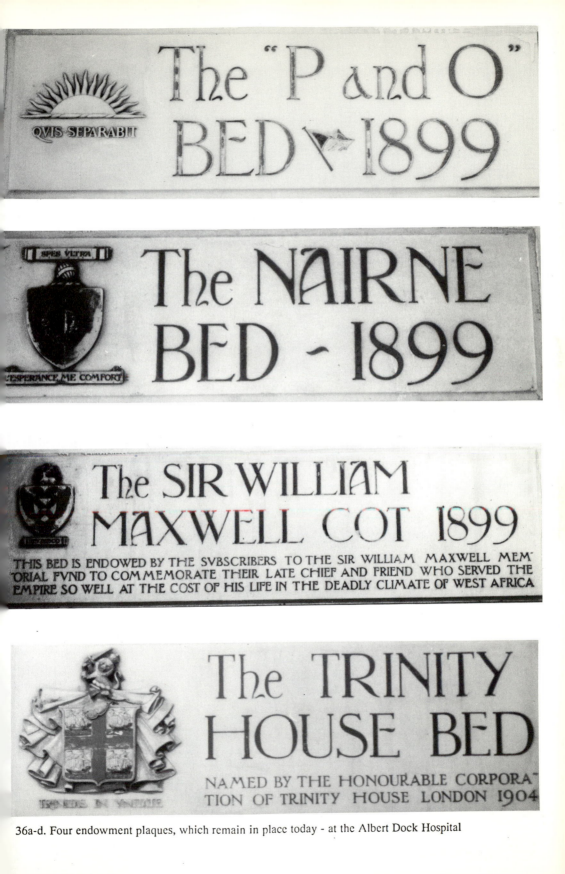

The "P and O" BED · 1899

QVIS·SEPARABIT

The NAIRNE BED - 1899

SPES VLTRA

ESPERANCE·ME·COMFORT

The SIR WILLIAM MAXWELL COT 1899

THIS BED IS ENDOWED BY THE SVBSCRIBERS TO THE SIR WILLIAM MAXWELL MEM-ORIAL FVND TO COMMEMORATE THEIR LATE CHIEF AND FRIEND WHO SERVED THE EMPIRE SO WELL AT THE COST OF HIS LIFE IN THE DEADLY CLIMATE OF WEST AFRICA

The TRINITY HOUSE BED

NAMED BY THE HONOURABLE CORPORA-TION OF TRINITY HOUSE LONDON 1904

36a-d. Four endowment plaques, which remain in place today - at the Albert Dock Hospital

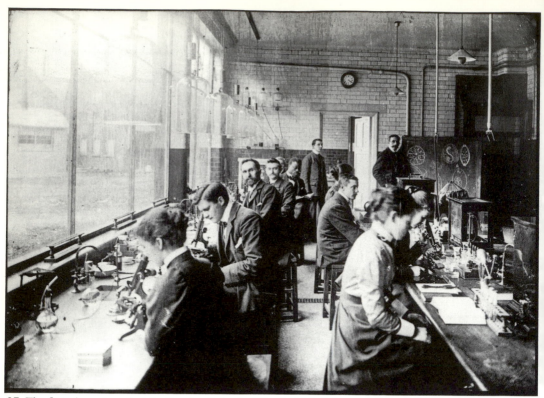

37. The first class at work at the London School of Tropical Medicine - 1899

38. Sir James Cantlie

39. Plaque commemorating Sir Patrick Manson at the LSHTM

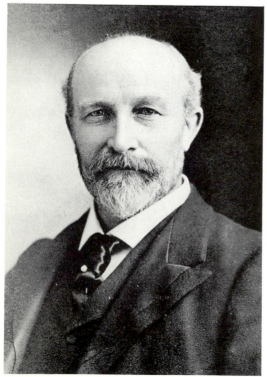

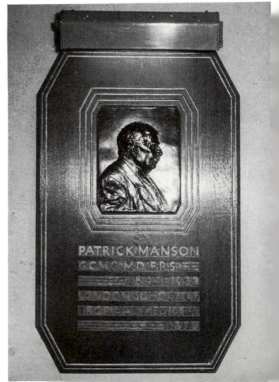

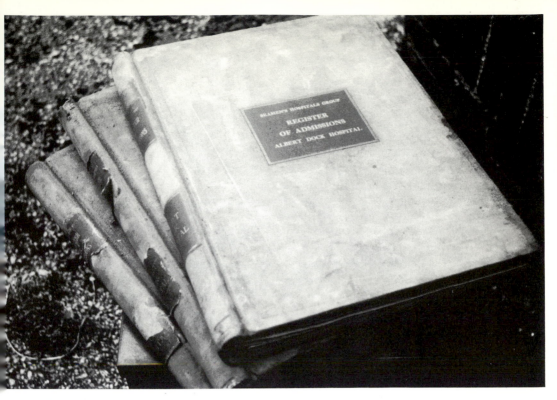

40. Admission books of the Albert Dock Hospital - in the early 20th century

41. The extension to the London School of Tropical Medicine opened in 1912 which consisted of laboratories and a student hostel

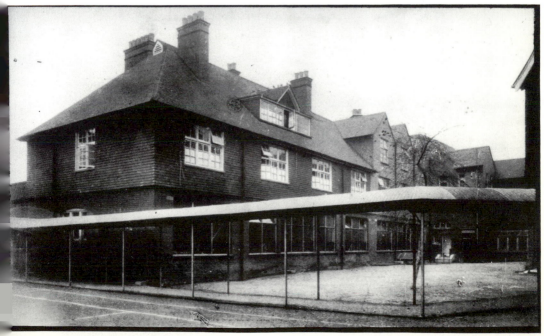

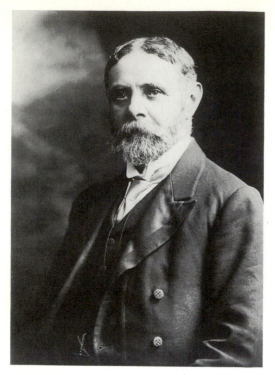

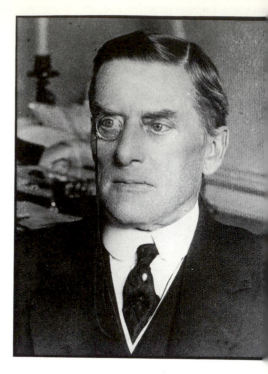

42. Dr Charles Wilberforce Daniels

44. Sir Austen Chamberlain MP

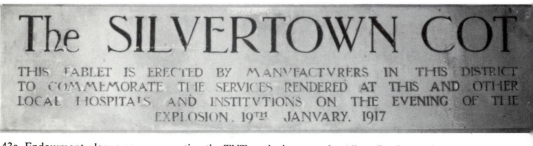

The SILVERTOWN COT

THIS TABLET IS ERECTED BY MANVFACTVRERS IN THIS DISTRICT
TO COMMEMORATE THE SERVICES RENDERED AT THIS AND OTHER
LOCAL HOSPITALS AND INSTITVTIONS ON THE EVENING OF THE
EXPLOSION. 19TH JANVARY. 1917

43a. Endowment plaque commemorating the TNT explosion near the Albert Dock Hospital in 1917

To perpetuate the memory of
MRS MAUDE ASHLEY
this bed is endowed by her father
SIR ERNEST CASSEL. PC. GCB. GCMG. GCVO.
1912

43b. Plaque commemorating Mrs Maude Ashley

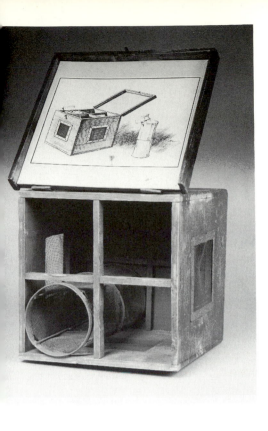

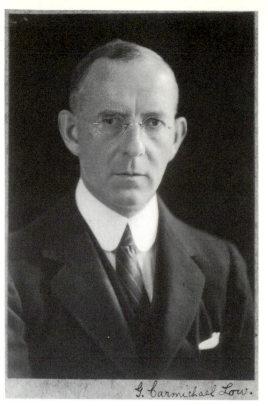

46. Dr George Carmichael Low

5a & b. Box used to convey mosquitoes from London to Rome - Campagna expedition 1900

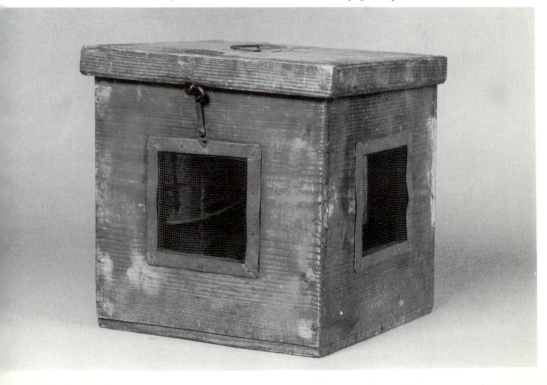

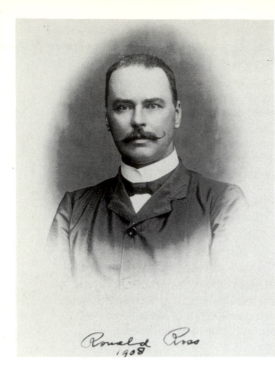

47. Major Ronald Ross in 1908

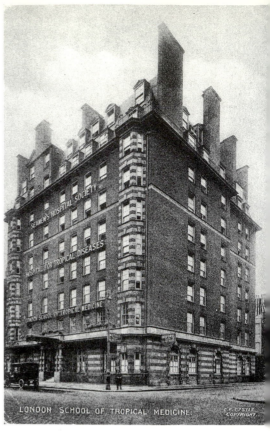

49. The Hospital for Tropical Diseases
and LSTM, Endsleigh Gardens - about 1920

48. Blue plaque at 18, Cavendish Square, W1

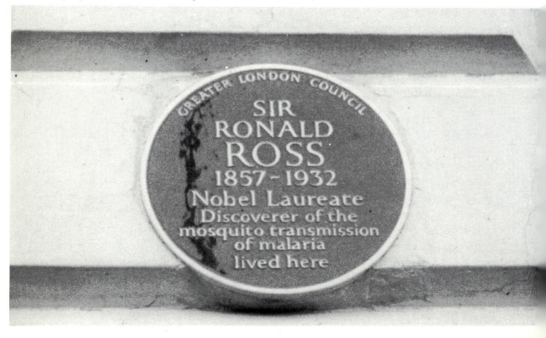

as a duty to be in any way associated with the school, a privilege because he could not think of any subject of scientific research and philanthropic enterprise which was more interesting, while it was a duty which we owed to the empire and from which we could not divest ourselves whatever our political opinions might be to see that all our possessions were rendered as healthy as possible. This duty had increased in recent years with the extension of our territory, with the increase of scientific knowledge, and with the awakening of our imperial conscience. We owed this duty to the vast population for which we had made ourselves responsible and owed it also to those of our own race who were daily risking health and life in order to uphold the honour and the interests of this country. Where the British flag was planted there must be established the British prosperity; we were unable, therefore, to stay where we began. Let them compare the position of Egypt as it was a quarter of a century ago with the Egypt of Lord Cromer and note the perhaps even more extraordinary advance in the condition of the Soudan and Nigeria. These miracles had been wrought by a handful of men, mostly very young, brought suddenly into the presence of great responsibilities, having to deal with crises of administration, of disease, of savage aggression, and with every problem of statesmanship. Science had given its martyrs recently in the persons of Myers and of Dutton, and owing to our ignorance of the conditions which had to be faced or our inability to deal with them, many others had left their health or their lives behind them in tropical climes. Our first duty was to do all in our power to reduce to the uttermost this blood tribute which we paid to the empire. To Sir Patrick Manson we owed the idea of a London tropical school and almost abreast of him came the promoters of the Liverpool School of Tropical Medicine. They in London felt no jealousy of the Liverpool school since there was room for all in that work, but they did envy them the liberality and energy of their citizens, who raised something like 40,000 by private subscription. Why could not London, the metropolis of the empire, the metropolis of the world of commerce, emulate more frequently the generosity of a provincial city? Mr. Chamberlain then referred to the work done by the London school and to the number of its students and appealed for the sum of £100,000 to repay the debt, to make proper provision for the teaching, and, above all, to subsidise research in tropical diseases of every kind.

The Times account[16] stressed 'our responsibility . . . for the great populations which policy, or accident, or destiny has brought under our control.' The importance of dealing with tropical disease was addressed, but it was considered, 'It may be that, as many now hold, the inhabitants of the temperate zones can never be more than migrants in tropical climates.' An increase in public funding was essential: 'This is another opening for the millionaires, and one which offers ample and speedy results to justify their liberality.'

In fact, Lyttelton on succeeding Chamberlain as Colonial Secretary, had written to all of the Colonial Governors seeking further financial support; these were not all in tropical climates however, and it is clearly recorded that the Governor of the Falkland Islands declined to contribute[17]. Under Lyttelton, these contributions were channelled not directly into the London School's funds but into a Tropical Diseases Research Fund (see below); this was a significant change for the funds were not earmarked for certain institutions, and were thus more widely available to departments of tropical medicine.

An overall statement of the finances during the first 12 years of the School's existence was compiled by Mr P J Michelli in early 1911[1]:

> The amount received in contributions during the first twelve years amounted to £39,597 of which:
> £3,550 was a Government Grant.
> £24,158 received in Students' Fees.
> £7,389 for special departments of Entomology, Helminthology and Protozoology.
> £1,300 for Scholarships and Prizes.
> £1,200 to create a Memorial Fund for research.
> £500 for investigation into some form of Tropical Disease
> £1,500 for Endowment Fund,
>
> | | |
> |---|---:|
> | making a total of | *£39,597* |
> | Special donations were as follows: | |
> | Tropical Colonial Contribution | |
> | (Through Sir Francis Lovell) (in 1910). | £836 |
> | Hon. Bomanji Petit | £6,600 |
> | Dr. Irvine Rowell (collection) | £2,000 |
> | Sir Wm. Treacher (collection) | £684 |
> | Sir John Craggs, M.V.O. | annually £50 |
> | Lord Sheffield 'Hon. Edward John Stanley Memorial Fund' | £1,000 |
> | Special contribution for Tropical Research | £500 |
> | E.W. Blessig, Garston Park, Godstone | £1,241 |
> | (i) Banquet at Hotel Cecil 1899 | |
> | (Mr. J. Chamberlain) | £12,000 |
> | (ii) Banquet at Hotel Cecil 1905 | |
> | (Mr. J. Chamberlain) | £11,000 |
> | | |
> | Grand Total | *£75,508* |

A financial support meeting in 1912 was reported as follows[18]:

> A meeting was held on Wednesday, Feb. 28th, at the Mansion House, by permission of Sir Thomas Crosby, M.D., the Lord Mayor of London, in support of the London School of Tropical Medicine, when Mr. Lewis Harcourt, the Secretary of State for the Colonies, delivered an impressive appeal for the public support of the school. He detailed the vast and

valuable work which had been done in our far-off dependencies to mitigate the ravages of tropical diseases, or to discover and eliminate their causes, and claimed on good grounds that the keepers of the national purse had not been niggardly in their contributions to the work. A few days later H.S.H. Prince Louis of Battenberg, taking the chair at the annual dinner of the London School of Clinical Medicine, supplied additional arguments for public digestion why the people of this country should endeavour to support, and support profusely, the grand medical work now being done throughout the borders of our vast Empire. The medical services, Naval, Military, and Colonial, are now collaborating with private workers and scientific missionaries from our universities and schools of tropical medicine in a manner that bears new fruit every day. The movement is the direct adjuvant to our rule as an Empire; for only by subjection of the inimical forces of disease can we as a nation come into full enjoyment of much territory that bears our name on the atlas, or discharge our duty as a superior race to those whom we have invited to depend upon us. Medical men have sacrificed their lives for this cause; the way for the public to make such sacrifices unnecessary is to facilitate the great object which medical men and sanitarians have in view, and support the multifarious movements now taking place to wipe out disease in our tropical possessions.

The overall state of funding of tropical research in Britain was well summarized in 1910[19]:

In no department of medicine have such signal advances been achieved of late years as in that of tropical medicine. Considering the comparatively small pecuniary encouragement which it has in the past received from the State for the purpose of scientific research, it is surprising to learn how much has been already accomplished. There are some signs that the Imperial and Colonial Governments are now more favourably disposed towards the efforts which are being made by the medical profession to prevent the ravages of tropical disease and to render some of our colonies more safely habitable. These remarks are prompted by the perusal of the recently issued annual report for 1909 of the Advisory Committee for the Tropical Diseases Research Fund. This committee was constituted in 1904, at which time the Imperial Government and various other bodies made themselves responsible for certain sums as annual contributions to the Research Fund for a period of five years. As that period terminated in 1909 the committee had to face the possibility of some at least of the contributors discontinuing their subscriptions. Fortunately, all the previous subscribers have agreed to renew their contributions for another period of five years, and there is also some prospect of further payments being received towards the fund from certain of the smaller British colonies which have not hitherto contributed. The total amount of revenue at the disposal of the Advisory Committee in 1909 was £3470, of which £1000 were contributed by the Imperial Government, £500 by the Government of India, £200 by the Rhodes trustees, and £1770 by various colonial Governments. The expenditure during the year amounted to £3333, of which £1383 were voted to the London School of Tropical Medicine, £1000 to the Liverpool School of Tropical Medicine, £750 to the University of London, and £200 to the University of Cambridge. Most of the money granted to these institutions was devoted to payment of the salaries of special professors or lecturers on tropical medicine, protozoology, parasitology, and economic entomology, also towards defraying part of the expenses of laboratories in which research work is carried out. It is obvious that much good is likely to follow this expenditure of money for special instruction in the various branches of tropical medicine to medical men about to proceed to our colonies and dependencies. In our opinion this wise expenditure is likely to bear good fruit in future years. No grant was made from the fund in 1909 towards the costs of the sleeping sickness investigations in Uganda for the reason that money for this purpose was forthcoming from other sources. Reference is made by the advisory Committee to the work of the Sleeping Sickness Bureau, which in its opinion has amply fulfilled the hopes which were expressed in the report for 1908 concerning it. The Australian Institute of Tropical Medicine, towards the establishment of which the committee in 1908 contributed £400, has now been definitely constituted and a director appointed. Adequate contributions for its future maintenance will be obtained in Australia; the Universities of Sydney and Melbourne are also interested in the matter. A small bacteriological laboratory under the charge of a skilled bacteriologist has been established in the island of St. Lucia, and the Advisory Committee hopes to include in its report next year some record of the work done in the new laboratory. The committee was consulted by the Secretary of State for the Colonies as to a proposal to enlarge the Medical Research Institute for West Africa at Lagos, and plans were ultimately passed for extension of the building at an estimated cost of £2350.

The committee has been greatly interested during 1909 in the question of malaria and its prevention. Appended to its report is a copy of a circular despatch which the Colonial Secretary addressed in March of last year to all the tropical colonies in which malaria is prevalent. Enclosed with the despatch was a reprint of a letter to the editor of the *Times*, by Professor W. Osler of Oxford University, on the subject of 'Malaria in Italy: a Lesson in Practical Hygiene.' Replies were invited from the various colonies as to the extent to which preventive measures against malaria had been carried out. The answers received show that on the whole a good deal had been done generally to combat the disease. Special attention was directed to the reply from Ceylon, containing as it did full and excellent statistics on the subject. Mention is also made that in Mauritius much had been done at a comparatively small outlay. In the colonies as elsewhere progress is hindered for want of funds and also by the attitude of many native races respecting measures for their own and others' benefit. An instance of this may be quoted from the report of Dr. D.M. Macrae, medical officer of the Bechuanaland Protectorate, who says that little can be done until the natives are educated up to some civilised ideas of disease and its prevention. At present they are largely in the hands of wizards and impostors, and notwithstanding a century of zealous missionary work among them and 25 years of administrative control the Bechuanas remain exactly where they were. Even the great medical missionary David Livingstone, who spent 13 years teaching them, was inclined to regard them as a "lost race". Hundreds of children and adults, says Dr. Macrae, have perished among the native population whose lives could certainly have been saved by the administration of quinine, yet though this drug is always within reach the natives somehow prefer to die rather than take any 'white medicine.' The committee append reports on the excellent work done at the Schools of Tropical Medicine in London and Liverpool; the report of the professor of protozoology at the University of London; an account of the work performed by the research student in entomology at the University of Cambridge and in the Quick Laboratory; a report on work done in the experimental treatment of trypanosomiasis under the supervision of a subcommittee of the Royal Society; and reports on the work at the several colonial laboratories, which have been sent in accordance with requests made by the Secretary of State for the Colonies. In these appendices are given the full details of the investigations carried out, and of the papers published in connexion with the grants made by, and under the supervision of, the committee.

Funding continued to be a major source of concern for all those involved in what was still regarded as a relatively new specialty. The overall importance of the discipline is however, reflected in a parliamentary discussion of the time[20]:

In the course of the debate on the report of the vote on account, Dr. HILLIER drew attention to the inadequacy of the Government contributions to the Tropical Diseases Research Fund. The report of the Advisory Committee for 1910 stated that the annual grant was insufficient, and that it was very important that the sums at the disposal of the committee should be very largely increased in view of the many questions which urgently required further research. The committee had noticed with interest the steps which had been taken to combat malaria in tropical colonies. The sum actually granted was only £1000, but there was probably no branch of human industry and scientific research which had brought a richer reward to the nation undertaking it and to mankind at large than the wonderful bacteriological researches of the great scientific men of the present generation. Let honourable Members look, for instance, at the very steadily decreasing rate in the deaths from malaria in India alone – a decrease which had gone on steadily since 1898 – the year in which the researches of Sir Patrick Manson and Major Ronald Ross established the true nature of that disease. It really behoved Parliament to deal more generously with the institutions in which distinguished men of science had given to the world these valuable results. This work was still being carried on. He wished to read to the House a few extracts from a letter from Major Ronald Ross of the Liverpool School of Tropical Medicine. "The amount at our disposal for tropical medicine," wrote Major Ross, "is £3245. Of that amount the Imperial Government contribute £1000 and the Government of India £500, and from the colonies we get £1745." He (Dr. Hillier), whilst he hoped the Chancellor of the Exchequer would see his way to increase this grant, would say that it equally devolved on the Government of India relatively to increase the paltry sum they were giving for this purpose. Major Ross continued: "Out of this total sum the London School received £1330 and the Liverpool School of Medicine £1000. The rest of the money goes partly to the University of London, and is distributed for a number of special researches. . . . We received £900 last year for the special researches. . . . This year we have only received about £250 for that purpose." Further on Major Ross wrote: "I am strongly of opinion that it would be a good sound national policy to increase the amount considerably to the school from the Treasury in order to enable the school to be properly consolidated. So long as we depend merely upon subscriptions, which may ultimately dry up to some extent, the organisation of the school cannot be completed. We have, in fact, to deal with the whole range of tropical medicine and sanitation, . . . also numerous investigations especially into practical public health sanitation. . . . The cause which we are dealing with is an Imperial matter. It is of consequence, not only to individual colonies, but to the whole of the British Empire, just as the navy and army are. . . . Our purpose concerns not only the health of the civil population in tropical countries, but also the naval and military forces there, and already our work has resulted in very considerable saving to the Government." He (Dr. Hillier) considered £1000 an inadequate contribution for the purposes of the research into tropical diseases. These researches could only be conducted with success by men provided with the necessary appliances and equipment. In aiding a cause of this sort the Government would be furthering the economic as well as the scientific and humanitarian interests of the whole nation.

Mr. J.A. PEASE (Chancellor of the Duchy), replying on behalf of the government, said: It is no discourtesy to the honourable Member that the Secretary of State for the Colonies is not here this afternoon. Another engagement accounts for his absence. The Government welcomes this subject being raised and the Colonial Office is anxious that more money should be spent in the direction which has been indicated by the honourable gentleman. The Secretary of State is sending representations to the Treasury and hopes that further moneys may be forthcoming. But I should like to remind the honourable gentleman that the amount of money which is devoted to this excellent humanitarian work is not limited to this particular vote. There is money devoted from India for exactly the same object, and my honourable friend the Under Secretary of State for India reminds me that recently a substantially increased sum has been given to this very object in India.

Mr. T.P. O'CONNOR spoke in appreciation of the work accomplished under the auspices of the Liverpool School of Tropical Medicine in Sierra Leone and other parts of the Empire.

Mr. LYELL thought that it was in the interests of true economy that adequate support should be given to the schools of tropical medicine in London and Liverpool. The work of these institutions would, he believed, go to reduce the invaliding of officers from tropical climates where the climatic conditions were bad.

But despite persistence on the part of Dr Hillier, the Chancellor of the Exchequer seems to have been unmoved[21]:

Dr. HILLIER asked the Chancellor of the Exchequer whether he proposed increasing the grant to tropical diseases investigation, and if so by what amount. – Mr. Hobhouse (Secretary to the Treasury) answered: The Treasury has recently sanctioned the appointment of a special commission under Sir D. Bruce, and including at the outset the services of Professor Newstead, to make further investigations into trypanosome diseases, the cost of which, amounting for this year alone to about £5000, will ultimately fall upon the Exchequer. In view of this large provision of money the Chancellor of the Exchequer does not see his way to increase the amount of the grants provided in the estimates for tropical diseases investigation, as Sir D. Bruce's commission will be carrying out this very work with great prospects of successful results.

And, a further report from Parliament early in 1912[22]:

The report of the Advisory Committee for the Tropical Diseases Research Fund for the year 1911 is now issued as a Parliamentary Blue-book. The Research Fund has now a revenue of £3345, of which £1000 is received from the Imperial Government. This sum did not quite meet the expenditure of the year, which amounted to £2795 6s 8d. It was allocated as follows: London School of Tropical Medicine, £1533 6s 8d., Liverpool School of Tropical Medicine, £1262; University of London, £750; and University of Cambridge, £250. The excess of expenditure over income was met by drawing on the accumulated balance of the Fund. Attention is called by the committee to the urgent necessity of further sums being placed at its disposal in view of the many important questions calling for further research. During the year the committee was consulted on various matters by the Secretary of State for the Colonies, including the appointment of an assistant in the research laboratory at Yaba and the selection of an officer to inquire into the diseases of vomiting sickness and peripheral neuritis which are prevalent in Jamaica. Returns in regard to mosquito-borne disease in various colonies and protectorates have been before the committee, but these are not yet complete. The report states, in conclusion, that the committee notes with pleasure the high standard of work which is being done in various colonial laboratories, and which shows the increased interest in research work which is being taken by the officers in charge. The committee is of opinion that the experiment of setting up these laboratories has fully justified itself, and that it deserves all possible encouragement.

The Lord Mayor of London presided over a large meeting of the London School of Tropical Medicine on 28 February 1912[23]; the principal speakers were: the Rt Hon Lewis Harcourt MP (Secretary of State for the Colonies), Lord Sheffield, Sir Patrick Manson, Mr Arthur Lampard, and Professor T Anderson Stuart (Professor of Physiology in the University of Sydney). In his appeal for further funding Mr Harcourt began:

> I come to appeal to you for additional assistance to the London School of Tropical Medicine. No one alas is better equipped than I by personal and official knowledge to assure you how worthy an object it is for your generous support. It is my painful duty to receive day by day as the ordinary and inevitable routine of my work telegrams from all our tropical possessions of sickness, danger, death, amongst the gallant band of men who throughout your Empire are laying the sure foundations of the Pax Britannica by their admirable administration of law, equity, justice, religion, medicine, civil rights, and good fellowship.
>
> But they carry their lives in their hands and too often lay them down as their last tribute to your service. They are exposed by the nature and locality of their labours not only to the familiar diseases of temperate climes but to the pestilences of the torrid zones – known too well by their results, but known too little in the domain of prophylaxis or of cure.
>
> Malaria, Blackwater Fever, Yellow Fever, Plague, Cholera, Leprosy, Sleeping Sickness, are all at hand and hungry to claim their toll.
>
> The most and the best that we can do for them is to give them specialised treatment when we can get them home, or to provide opportunities for specialised research which may hasten the discovery or perfection of curative methods.

The school needed a further £20,000 to put it on a sound financial footing. One of the primary needs was for more student accommodation (only 8 rooms were available); a further £10,000 was required for additional labora- tories and residential quarters for at least 20 more students. He continued:

> It may possibly be asked why if the services of this School have been so valuable to India and our Crown Colonies, why, if its extension is so

desirable, the Government, as representing the State does not itself find the necessary funds. The answer is twofold. First, it does find a large part of the money contributed nobly aided as I have said by private generosity and individual effort. Secondly, the State has no fund on which it can draw except the pockets of the people. *There is a curious popular misconception of the riches and resources of the State; it is regarded by many as a sort of anonymous millionaire with the bottomless purse of a Fortunatus* [my italics].

As a matter of fact the State is an incorporeal entity in a condition of chronic bankruptcy, and only saved from insolvency by frequent and legalized raids on the pockets of the tax-payer. It is only by the imposition of new or higher taxes that these demands for vicarious generosity can by any possibility be fulfilled.

It is on this ground, therefore, that I venture to ask this Company, and to ask through you my Lord Mayor, the general public to open their hearts and their purses in order to second and enlarge the not inconsiderable contributions of the State. I should not wish you to think that, even with the great and growing demands upon them, the keepers of the National purse have been niggardly in their practical assistance to this great work. I am happy to be permitted to announce that the Treasury are prepared to contribute a donation of £500 to the purposes for which we are appealing to-day – that is, a gift to this particular School and to this special object, and not to be treated as a precedent or the foundation of a claim for other, though similar demands.

If there are any amongst my audience whose lot it has been to try to tap the Treasury for public objects, they will, I am sure, afford me a mead of praise for my temerity and my success, and not omit their gratitude for the generosity of the gift. Indeed, in justice to the Treasury and in recollection of the old days spent there when I was still a gamekeeper and before I had turned poacher, I think I ought to tell you what in recent years they have given, at your expense, to the modern developments of Tropical Medicine.

The Treasury have contributed, and are contributing:

For the last five years, £1,000 per annum to the Sleeping Sickness Bureau.

For five years, £1,000 per annum to the Entomological Research Fund.

For three years, £5,000 per annum to Sir D. Bruce's Expedition to Nyassaland to enquire into Sleeping Sickness.

From 1904–1907, £500 per annum, and from 1908 onwards £1,000 per annum to the Tropical Diseases Research Fund.

Mr Harcourt's speech was in fact, seriously disturbed, as *The Times* reported[24]:

Several suffragists obtained admittance to a meeting held at the Mansion House yesterday, in support of the London School of Tropical Medicine, and interrupted Mr Lewis Harcourt at the commencement of his speech. They were removed by the police. [This 'scuffle' was then reported verbatim.]

Manson followed this with another 'state of the art' speech, in which he traced the origins of tropical medicine as a separate discipline:

Some thirty or forty years ago progress in medical science appeared to have come to a dead stop. There was elaboration of detail, speculation and theory in abundance; but for many years there had been no great discovery, no well-grounded enunciation of some general principle such as could lead to definite and marked advance along the whole line.

Then came [Louis] Pasteur [1822–95] and the thorough establishment on a firm basis of fact of the germ theory of disease. After Pasteur came our own Lister – whose recent death we deplore – and his beneficent work. [Robert] Koch [1843–1910], Paul Ehrlich [1854–1915], and a host of others carried the Pasteurian idea into the realm of general medicine, and in a few years almost the entire subject was revolutionised. The process is still in progress and gathering force.

For a considerable period Tropical Medicine, that is to say, that department of medicine which concerns itself with diseases peculiar to the tropics, or which are specially prevalent in the tropics and sub-tropics – and their name is legion – remained practically uninfluenced by the new ideas. The reason for this I need not dwell on, suffice it to say that such was the fact. Even when another distinguished Frenchman, Laveran, in the early eighties published his discovery of the long-sought-for germ of malaria, tropical medicine hardly stirred from its lethargy. It took over ten years to get Englishmen to accept and to recognise the importance of Laveran's discovery. At last we did recognise it, and when it was shown subsequently that the mosquito was the active agent in carrying and implanting this germ, and that the germs of other tropical diseases were spread in a similar way, the study of tropical disease received an impulse which it has never lost, and which in a few years has culminated in a series of discoveries such as hardly any other department of medicine can boast of, discoveries which already have borne abundant fruit in the saving of life and health, in making hitherto uninhabitable places habitable, in making otherwise almost impossible engineering feats possible, in lowering the cost of labour, in making unprofitable undertakings profitable.

In the eighties and nineties, just when the new era in tropical medicine was commencing, the British Empire was undergoing one of its periodical expansions – this time principally in Africa. Vast areas were being added to the Empire – Northern and Southern Nigeria, Uganda, British East Africa, Nyasaland, the huge territory included under the name Rhodesia, the Boer States, and, in a sense, the Egyptian Soudan. As a consequence of this expansion important problems in administration kept cropping up for our statesmen to grapple with; none more important than those entailed by the unhealthiness of many of the countries I have mentioned. Indeed, this matter of health was a very old problem in African administration, and one hitherto unsolved.

Tropical Africa, like so many tropical countries, though potentially rich is, under present conditions, a poor country. For this the unenterprising character of the native and the relatively scanty population may, in part, be responsible; but, undoubtedly, the main reason is the unhealthiness of the climate.

The European cannot, as a rule, live and thrive in Tropical Africa as he can in India and China, for example. Therefore, to induce the ordinary European to cast his lot there, even for a short time, he demands special advantages – more pay, less work, liberal furloughs; indeed, the latter are often necessary conditions of his being able to live there at all. And this was the most important problem our Government had to face in dealing with its new African possessions. It was an economic one; how to govern and exploit, or rather develop, a poor unhealthy country and at the same time to preserve its solvency. It seemed almost that some of the new African Colonies would follow in the steps of the older West African Colonies and become sleepy hollows and death traps.

After outlining Chamberlain's prescription for improving living conditions in the colonies, Manson went on:

To contend successfully with the unhealthiness, the nature and causes of African diseases and the means of preventing and treating them must first be ascertained, and, having ascertained these, the knowledge gained must be spread, and care taken that it be applied. And so, as, from circumstances I need not enlarge on, these things could not be done by the ordinary medical schools, he founded the London School of Tropical Medicine, and encouraged by every means in his power the sister establishment in Liverpool. In these schools tropical diseases are studied and taught as a speciality by men specially experienced in the subject, and through one or other of these schools every African Colonial Medical Officer has to pass.

Speaking of the enormous strides which had taken place in the understanding of the cause and management of these diseases he said:

As a result a man need no longer leave England for tropical Africa with the feeling that he is going to his grave. He knows now that he can protect himself from ills against which his predecessors were helpless. There is less sickness, less invaliding; better men are obtainable for the services and, throughout the countries concerned, altogether a far more hopeful feeling prevails. This happy state of matters is almost entirely attributable to Mr. Chamberlain's action in calling into existence the schools of tropical medicine, and from the encouragement they have received from his successors in office.

Having thanked the Treasury, the Colonies, India and the great 'Merchants of the City of London' for their support he continued:

> I would conclude what I have got to say with a personal reminiscence and a comparison. After eight years medical practice in China I returned to England in 1874. During my holiday, deeming it a great medical centre, I came to London, principally with the view of improving my knowledge of tropical disease. I was grievously disappointed. Nobody taught, or seemed to care very much about the subject. I learned very little. Again, after a further term of practice in China, I came to London on the same errand in 1883. Again I failed. Coming home for good in 1889 I found matters as regards tropical medicine very much as they were on my two previous visits – no teaching, no special opportunity for study, no guidance.

> Compare this with what London can offer to-day. Now-a-days, the out-going or the home-coming doctor has only to put himself and his portmanteau into a taxi-cab and drive to the Tropical School at the Albert Dock. There, besides being comfortably lodged and fed, he can learn all that is known about tropical disease, perfect himself in the appropriate laboratory technique, study actual cases of tropical disease in the wards of the hospital, and, if so minded, carry out original researches on the subject in laboratories placed at his disposal, and all this under expert guidance.

> Surely, such arrangements are in the public interest, and deserve encouragement and support?

Lord Sheffield followed with a further appeal for funds:

> Meeting as they did in the centre of commercial prosperity of the empire, he would like to say a few words to show why the great merchant princes of London should come forward and support this scheme. In Liverpool much had been done. He thought in Liverpool they had more money than the London School had. This was not because Liverpool had a greater tropical trade; but Liverpool had not such a universal trade as London had, and he felt that it had a more concentrated public spirit than was found in London, where people were bewildered by the multiplicity of exciting occupations, and did not concentrate themselves upon matters which elsewhere would be of local obligation and local pride. But London, with its vast commercial interests, might be asked to do something more for the school. It was not a school for Civil Servants: it was a school of true scientific character, the aim of which was to widen the basis of knowledge. It was invaluable, because it put in the very forefront that scientific research which was the only sound base of the healing art.

And, speaking of progress in research into tropical disease, Mr Lampard reminisced:

This increased rate of mortality is not confined to the native population as those of us who have lived in the East know only too well; and the saddest part of our knowledge is that much of this fearful waste of life – under better medical conditions – was preventible. Go into any Eastern Cemetery and it is appalling to find that the average age of the Europeans lying there does not much exceed 30.

Great progress has been made in Tropical Research since I first went to the East, and all honour is due to the men who – with inadequate resources – have carried it out. But it is time that the responsibilities of those residing in England was made known, for I am confident that when once realized generous support will be forthcoming.

When you realise that the population of the Empire is 425 millions, and that of these at least 370 millions live in tropical countries, the importance of the health of these people comes home to one.

Our import and export trade with these possessions amounts to some 500 millions per annum. Surely therefore, on business grounds alone it is our duty to prevent by all means the waste of life, for with the preservation of health and energy the future development of the East becomes possible, which will add immensely to the wealth and prosperity of the Empire as a whole.

I do not suggest, of course, that even medical science can entirely abolish the risks that are inevitable from the development of tropical countries. Nature seems to demand a price for converting tropical jungle into cultivated land for the use of man. The Uganda Railway, the Johore Railway, the Kelani Valley Railway in Ceylon, the Tea Industry, the Rubber Industry, all have had to pay the toll. But all progress is based upon sacrifice, which is exemplified by the loss of life in aviation and submarines. Some loss is inevitable, but a large percentage of the loss of life is preventible; and it is our clear duty to do all in our power to rectify this, and for this reason and upon these grounds I ask you to lend this movement your generous support.

And finally, a contribution about Australia:

Professor Anderson Stuart, in supporting the motion, said that he had lived in Australia for thirty years, and there they had a vast Northern portion of the continent which was entirely tropical. Its area was 300 million acres, but there were only 1,400 white inhabitants. All efforts to induce settlers of the British race to live there had failed, and now they were looking to tropical medicine to help the task. An Australian Institute of Tropical Medicine was now in working order at Townsville [see below]. There had been some private donations, but for the most part the Institute relied upon Government support and the help of the Universities. A request for an additional Government contribution of £4,000 a year had just been acceded to. He strongly recommended Government to that meeting as the best milch cow for the object they had at heart.

Meanwhile, to provide the badly needed extensions to the school, a £100,000 appeal had been launched. Progress with this was summarized at the Annual Dinner for 1913 which was held on 24 October at Prince's Restaurant[25]:

> Owing to the success of Mr. Chamberlain's appeal and the generous grant from the Board of Education the School has been able to make a considerable advance. The new buildings are now complete. The laboratory will be used for the first time next session, and the increased accommodation for resident students will be available. The new course in tropical sanitation and hygiene will also be inaugurated next session.
>
> Dr. F.M. Sandwith presided, and among the company present were Mr. Austen Chamberlain, M.P., Viscount Milner, Sir Patrick Manson, Mr. Perceval A. Nairne, Chairman of the Seamen's Hospital Society; Sir Charles Pardey Lukis, Sir J. West Ridgeway, Sir John Anderson, Surgeon-General Sir A. W. May, Sir W. Bennett, General the Hon. Sir Reginald Talbot, Sir J. Rose Bradford, Colonel Sir William Leishman, Sir Havelock Charles, Surgeon-General A. M. Branfoot, Sir F. Lovell, Mr. J. Cantlie, Dr. W. T. Prout, Mr. A. Aspinall, Sir R. Burnet, and Mr. P.J. Michelli, Secretary.
>
> During the evening the CHAIRMAN announced that, in response to a telegram which he had sent to Mr. Joseph Chamberlain, on behalf of those present, he had received the following reply: 'Thanks for your kind message. I wish you a pleasant dinner and I congratulate you on the progress made. – J. CHAMBERLAIN.'

> ### PROGRESS OF THE £100,000 SCHEME.
> The loyal toasts having been honoured.
>
> Mr. A. [later Sir Austen] [Plate 44] CHAMBERLAIN, in proposing the toast of "The London School of Tropical Medicine," said that he supposed it was entrusted to him because it had recently been his good fortune to be connected from the outside rather intimately with the fortunes of the School. He was glad of the opportunity which was afforded him of saying what had been done with the funds which had been collected. He accepted the invitation of Mr. Lewis Harcourt to take the chairmanship of the Committee to raise funds for the School for several reasons. The first reason, he need have no hesitation in saying, was a filial one – (cheers) – and it was on the ground of his father's connection with the School that Mr. Harcourt appealed to him. That was not the only reason. The study of tropical medicine had in the past twenty or twenty-five years made giant advances, and in the progress which it had made Englishmen had borne a distinguished and a leading part. (Cheers). As the possessors of the greatest tropical and sub-tropical Empire existing in the world Englishmen had a special obligation alike to the subject races, of whose well-being they were

the guardians, and to the young men of their own race who went out to other climes, carrying with them the honour of England, doing her work, spreading her civilisation, and increasing her reputation. England owed to them that at least she should do everything she could to minimise the risks they naturally had to run, and should show her appreciation of their work by striving to secure thorough research into the conditions of health and the cause of illness, to which their labours rendered them particularly exposed. It was a matter of national honour and national pride that in a movement so beneficial Englishmen should be encouraged to carry on the work and that England should stand in the forefront of the pioneers and of the new learning which was being acquired. They set out to obtain a sum of £100,000, and they had received the not inconsiderable sum of over £70,000. (Cheers.)

ALLOCATION OF THE FUND.

Acting on the advice of the committee of management of the School of Tropical Medicine and of the head of the Seamen's Hospital, they desired, in the first place, to make a not very large, but an absolutely necessary extension of the buildings of the school . . .

. . . The second object was to provide a fund for research. That they had been able to carry out by the kindness of Sir William Bennett in allocating to this purpose the legacy of £10,000 which the late Lord Wandsworth entrusted to his discretion. This object had been further served by strengthening the staff of the school. The third object of the Committee and the subscribers was to obtain a moderate endowment for the school, which should place it beyond immediate want and prevent it being always hampered by lack of funds. For that purpose there had been already allocated a sum which would produce an annual income to the school of about £1,400, and additional funds had been obtained which would allow of another £400 a year. The last of the objects was one of some delicacy. Men sometimes returned from the tropics suffering from tropical diseases, but with means insufficient to secure the attention of those with special knowledge of tropical medicine, which was confined to very few. They were anxious, therefore, to make some provision for cases of that kind, and owing to the help received from the authorities at the Seamen's Hospital they had been able to make arrangements for people of that class. A large measure of success which had attended the appeal would never have been obtained but for the hearty co-operation of numberless people. He had been moved by the response which had been made to the appeal from all quarters, and he was particularly touched by letters he had received from many tropical dependencies of the Crown, in which the writers sent their humble contributions. He wished to take that opportunity of asking the gratitude of the company and of recording his own in particular to the City Committee. Thanks to the London Chamber of Commerce, in the first instance, and to the City Committees formed under their auspices, in the second, the response from companies had exceeded his most sanguine expectations. It was unnecessary at that gathering for him to dwell upon the appreciation which was felt for the work of the school by those who most immediately benefited by it, and who were best able to judge of the results achieved. But he might give an instance showing how cordial was the response which was being made to the invitation issued to some of those tropical colonies by the Colonial Secretary for a contribution to their funds. When it was gently suggested by the Colonial Office to the Government of the Federated Malay States that in view of the importance of the School to them they might be willing to vote £500 of public money to the fund, a telegram was received in reply stating that in view of the importance of the work to them the unofficial members of the Council suggested that a grant of £5,000 should be made. Those who subscribed in this country need not, therefore, think that they subscribed to a work for an ungrateful few who could not appreciated what the School was doing. Great as had been the advance which tropical medicine had made in the last few years, he believed they had only scratched the soil so far, and that was a most hopeful and encouraging sign. The discoveries made were not final or conclusive; each opened up a new vista, and new possibilities, and they were changing the whole of our mental attitude towards the problems of tropical disease, health, settlement, and development. Diseases which were once thought to be the inevitable concomitant of that development were now seen to be preventable. (Cheers.)

The CHAIRMAN, in reply, referred to the great efforts of Mr. A. Chamberlain on behalf of the fund, and said that it was intended that one of the wards in the hospital should bear the name of the "Chamberlain Ward". (Cheers.) He was glad to be able to report that the School was in a fairly flourishing condition. They had the largest class of students they had ever had, and the greatest number of resident students.

PRESENTATION TO SIR P. MANSON.

Mr. JAMES CANTLIE and Dr. W.T. PROUT, in the name of the subscribers, presented to Sir Patrick Manson two portraits of himself, in recognition of his work in connection with the School.

Mr. A. CHAMBERLAIN, in unveiling the portraits, said that it was owing to the inspiration of Sir Patrick Manson that the London and Liverpool Schools of Tropical Medicine sprang into existence almost at the same moment. Sir Patrick's friends asked him to accept the portraits as a testimony to their gratitude to him for his help and of their affection for him. They wished to recognise the honour he had done his country and the great services he had rendered to mankind. (Cheers.)

Sir PATRICK MANSON having suitably acknowledged the gifts, the CHAIRMAN proposed the health of the guests, to which Sir JOHN ANDERSON replied. Viscount MILNER submitted the toast of "The Chairman," who acknowledged the compliment.

Fig 8.1 shows a cartoon in support of Chamberlain's appeal.

194

Manson had retired at the end of 1912 but was to continue taking an active interest in the School. He actually sailed to Ceylon in 1913 to join Dr P H Bahr (later Dr P H Manson-Bahr) who was engaged on his 'sprue project'; on a more permanent basis however, he moved to Ireland where fishing became a favourite hobby[1]. The Tropical Diseases Research Fund

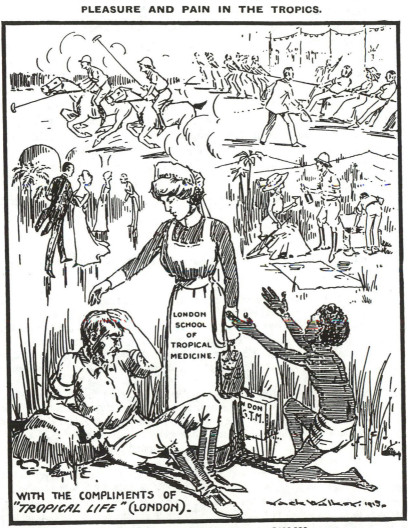

PLEASURE AND PAIN IN THE TROPICS.

LONDON SCHOOL OF TROPICAL MEDICINE.

DON S.T.M.

WITH THE COMPLIMENTS OF "TROPICAL LIFE" (LONDON).

Mr. AUSTEN CHAMBERLAIN's APPEAL for £100,000.

Fig 8.1: Cartoon in *Tropical Life* [July 1913: 135] supporting the appeal which had recently been launched by Mr A Chamberlain. The fact that donations were more likely to benefit the white man rather than the indigenous populations of the Empire is clearly emphasised. The caption reads as follows (see over):

remained an important source of income for the two schools and also others involved in researches into this area[26]:

> During 1913, as the annual report of the Advisory Committee shows, the expenditure of the Tropical Diseases Research Fund exceeded the revenue. The revenue was £3445 and the expenditure £3600. It appears that the excess of expenditure was met, as in the previous year, by drawing on the accumulated balance of the fund. The committee places upon record the importance of increasing the amount at its disposal, having regard to the large number of directions in which important research could be carried on if the means at its disposal could be permanently increased. The report notes how the grants to the London and Liverpool Schools of Tropical Medicine and to the Universities of London and Cambridge have been expended. It goes on to state that the committee were consulted on various matters during the year by the Secretary of State for the Colonies, including the important question of the measures to be taken to safeguard India and the eastern colonies against the danger of the introduction of yellow fever on the opening of the Panama Canal. Reports received from certain colonies and protectorates on anti-malarial measures are appended.

But in a detailed analysis of research work carried out in this increasingly important area, *The Lancet* clearly remained very dissatisfied with the low level of Government funding[27]:

> Since the Tropical Diseases Research Fund was established about ten years

---

We again appeal to all our readers to put aside a small percentage of their income during the past twelve months and remit it to Mr. Austen Chamberlain (9, Egerton Place, London, W.), in order to try and raise £25,000 out of the £100,000 needed for the work of the London School of Tropical Medicine in the Tropics, so that the lives and health of their families and friends, as well as of themselves, can be assured, and that, whilst they continue to grow rich and can make merry, others who are less fortunate shall not be forgotten.

If life in the Tropics to-day has become bearable and pleasant for Europeans, and if vast new areas can be utilized to-day which formerly were closed to "white" capital and enterprise, this is largely due to the Liverpool and London Schools of Tropical Medicine. Yet in spite of this, Mr. Austen Chamberlain's appeal to raise £100,000 to place the London School of Tropical Medicine on a sound basis, and extend its work, has only resulted so far in £63,000 being raised.

In the course of his lecture on "Medical Science and the Tropics," at the Royal Colonial Institute, on January 14th, Major Sir Ronald Ross, KCB, MD, FRS, told his audience: "Britain probably gives much less than £50,000 per annum throughout the British Empire for Medical Research which benefits 50,000,000 white people, not to mention hundreds of millions of coloured subjects. This sum divided amongst the white subjects only amounts to one-tenth of a Penny each per annum. We spend every day on public banquets many times more than this sum, but if the work of investigation is to continue it must be properly paid for by the country, and the Colonies ought to contribute more than they do. Those that go abroad are above the average, since they have the ambition to go and ability to prosper when they get there."

196

ago the advisory committee has effected a large amount of valuable work, but it is somewhat humiliating to a colonising nation like ours to find that the British Government does not give anything like adequate support to the scientific researches which have done so much already to reduce the excessive sickness and mortality rates recorded in many of our colonies and protectorates. The present income of the fund in unable to meet in a proper manner the pressing requirements of tropical research, the total receipts being only £3445, of which the British Government contributes £1000 and India £500, while the Dominion and Colonial Governments give £1945.

The Expenditure of the Fund.

The expenditure for 1913 amounted to £3600 – that is, £155 more than the income – the excess having to be met, as in some previous years, by drawing upon a balance accumulated in the past. It is obvious that something should be done to place the finances on a sounder basis. The committee strongly urge the extreme desirability of having the income increased in view of the many directions in which important researches might be instituted for the benefit of our tropical colonies and dependencies if only sufficient means were permanently available. In allocating the grants, and looking at the unsatisfactory position of the finances, it was carefully considered whether a reduction could be made in the amounts voted to the Schools of Tropical Medicine in London and Liverpool; but on certain representations being made it was decided to give £1200 to each of them, £750 to the University of London, and £450 to the University of Cambridge. The grant to the London School was expended in paying the salaries and maintaining the laboratories of the teachers and investigators of helminthology, protozoology, and entomology. The Liverpool School employed their grant to defray the cost of special researches in their laboratories on trypanosomiasis, general parasitology, helminthology, and entomology, as well as in carrying out some investigations on malaria. The sum given to the University of London was used as before in paying the salary of the professor of protozoology, and the grant to the University of Cambridge was employed partly to support a research studentship in medical entomology, partly in helping to pay the salary of an assistant in the Quick Laboratory and also that of a helminthologist, and partly in assisting to defray the general expenses of that laboratory. It is worth noting that the sum given to the University of Cambridge in 1913 was larger by £100 than in the previous year; in the opinion of the committee this increase was amply justified by the importance and extent of the research work carried on in the Quick Laboratory by Professor Nuttall and his assistants . . .

Teaching and courses at the LSTM at the Albert Dock

Fig 8.2 summarizes the position with respect to staff, lecturers and courses at the LSTM in 1906. Sir Francis Lovell had been appointed first *Dean*

LONDON SCHOOL OF TROPICAL MEDICINE
(UNIVERSITY OF LONDON),
Under the Auspices of His Majesty's Government.
CONNAUGHT ROAD, ALBERT DOCKS, E.
In connection with the Branch Hospital of the SEAMEN'S HOSPITAL SOCIETY.

THE SEAMEN'S HOSPITAL SOCIETY was established in the year 1821 and incorporated in 1833, and from time to time has been enlarged and extended. It now consists of the Dreadnought Hospital, Greenwich, to which is attached the London School of Clinical Medicine; the Royal Victoria and Albert Docks Hospital; the East and West India Docks Dispensary; and the Gravesend Dispensary.

Over 26,000 Patients treated annually. Of this number many are Cases of Tropical Disease.
The School buildings are situated within the grounds of the Royal Victoria and Albert Docks Hospital.

MEDICAL STAFF OF THE HOSPITAL AND LECTURERS IN THE TROPICAL SCHOOL.

Sir PATRICK MANSON, K.C.M.G., F.R.S., LL.D., M.D., F.R.C.P.	ARTHUR EVANS, Esq., M.S., M.D.(Lond.), F.R.C.S.	FLEMING MANT SANDWITH, Esq., M.D., F.R.C.P.
Professor R. TANNER HEWLETT, M.D., F.R.C.P.	L. VERNON CARGILL, Esq., F.R.C.S.	
ANDREW DUNCAN, Esq., M.D., F.R.C.S., M.R.C.P.	KENNETH W. GOADBY, Esq., D.P.H.(Camb.), M.R.C.S., L.R.C.P., L.D.S.R.C.S.	L. W. SAMBON, Esq., M.D.
JAS. CANTLIE, Esq., M.B., F.R.C.S.	Professor W. J. SIMPSON, M.D., F.R.C.P.	J. M. H. MACLEOD, Esq., M.D., M.R.C.P.
		E. TREACHER COLLINS, Esq., F.R.C.S.

DEAN—Sir F. LOVELL, C.M.G.
HELMINTHOLOGIST—R. T. LEIPER, Esq., M.B., Ch.B.
PROTOZOOLOGIST—C. M. WENYON, Esq., M.B., B.S., B.Sc.
SUPERINTENDENT AND MEDICAL TUTOR—C. W. DANIELS, Esq., M.B., M.R.C.S.

LECTURES AND DEMONSTRATIONS DAILY BY MEMBERS OF THE STAFF.

There are three Sessions yearly of three months each, viz., from October 1st to December 31st, from January 15th to April 14th, and from May 1st to July 31st inclusive. Women Graduates are received as Students.

Certificates are granted after Examination at the end of each Session, and the course is accepted by Cambridge University as Qualifying for Admission to their Examination for the Diploma in Tropical Medicine and Hygiene, and by London University as Study for the M.D. in Branch VI. (Tropical Medicine).

Fee for course £16 16s.; shorter periods by arrangement.

Students can be provided with Board and Residence, or partial Board, at the School, at moderate rates.

Medical men requiring posts in the Tropics may apply to the Tutor at the School, where a Register is kept.

A syllabus, with the general course of study, can be had on application to the undersigned, from whom further particulars may be obtained.

Students of the London School of Tropical Medicine, who join the London School of Clinical Medicine, will be allowed an abatement on their fees, and vice versa.

SEAMEN'S HOSPITAL, GREENWICH, S.E.   P. MICHELLI, C.M.G., Secretary.

Fig 8.2: Summary of the medical staff, lecturers, and courses at the LSTM in 1906. [Seamen's Hospital Society: The London School of Tropical Medicine. Opening of the 22nd session 8 October 1906].

of the school and remained in that position until his death in 1916. He collected large sums of money during travels in the Far East, and Malaya, which helped significantly with the funding in these early days (see above). The first Medical Tutor, Dr. D C Rees remained at the School for only one year (he resigned in April 1901)[1]; he was succeeded by Dr C W Daniels (seconded from the British Guiana government service)[28], and two years later Dr G C Low[29] became the third Tutor; Daniels returned to the position in 1907.

In 1905 Dr R T Leiper and Dr C M Wenyon joined the staff, and the departments of helminthology and protozoology were founded[30]. In 1906, the University agreed to the creation of a Chair of Protozoology (to be funded by the Rhodes Trustees – through the Colonial Office – and the Royal Society); E A Minchin, Professor of Zoology at University College was appointed. This proved to be a complex matter. In 1905, the Lister Institute of Preventive Medicine (at Chelsea) had joined the LSTM as a new member of the University's Faculty of Medicine; this Institute (which was far better equipped than the LSTM) decided that the new Professor should work there. The Colonial Office, which had assumed that he would be based at the LSTM, reluctantly acceded! After Minchin's unexpected death in 1915, the Chair remained unfilled until the LSHTM was founded (chapter 10). Shortly afterwards, Col A Alcock established a department of entomology[1].

In May 1910, Dr H B Newham succeeded Dr C W Daniels as Director

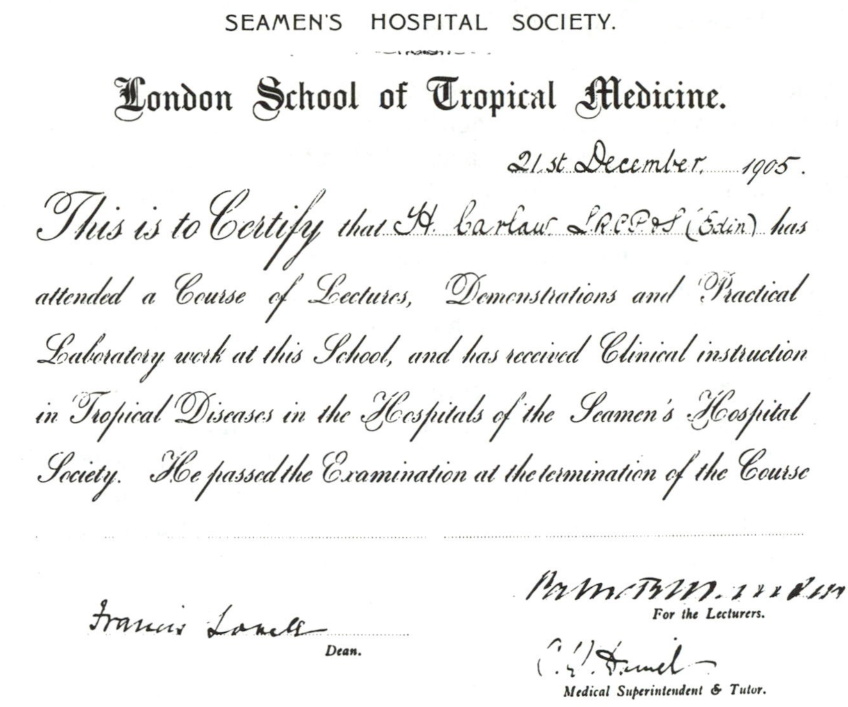

London School of Tropical Medicine.

21st December, 1905.

This is to Certify that H. Carlaw L.R.C.P.S. (Edin) has attended a Course of Lectures, Demonstrations and Practical Laboratory work at this School, and has received Clinical instruction in Tropical Diseases in the Hospitals of the Seamen's Hospital Society. He passed the Examination at the termination of the Course

Francis Lovell ....
Dean.

Pm.m.Bm. ... km.
For the Lecturers.

(......)
Medical Superintendent & Tutor.

Fig 8.3: Certificate awarded by the LSTM in 1905 which indicates satisfactory completion of the course and the passing of the examination. The signatories are Sir Patrick Manson, Sir Francis Lovell, and Dr CW Daniels.

of the School. In 1911 (the first issue appeared in December) the School began publication of its journal (*The Journal of the London School of Tropical Medicine*) – (7s 6d per annum), with Manson and Daniels as its Editors[31]; this survived for a mere 2 years (2 volumes) due to 'increasing competition'[1] – the last issue was dated November 1913.

Students in the early years came from America, India, Germany, west Africa and many other countries. Among the more distinguished foreign students were F Fülleborn (1866–1933) and Aldo Castellani (1877–1971)[1]. Fülleborn had previously joined the newly opened tropical school in Hamburg and came to England for one year in 1904.

A certificate from the early days of the LSTM is shown in fig 8.3. In 1903 Cambridge University recognised the school course and granted a Diploma in Tropical Medicine and Hygiene; Professor G H F Nuttall, FRS seems to have been largely responsible for this[1]. In 1911 the London conjoint board established a similar qualification; this was discontinued in 1915 but revived in 1920[1].

In 1913, the course was revised and enlarged (largely as a result of a report on the School by Sir Ronald Ross – see below); bacteriology was included under Dr Wedd, as was tropical hygiene. In 1913 also, the

199

International Congress of Medicine was held in London and the School was visited by the 'tropical section' of that organisation. Manson-Bahr recalled that it was there that 'Blanchard proclaimed Manson 'the Father of tropical medicine' and presented him with the fine bronze medallion which now graces the entrance hall of the School.' [This is presumably the plaque which is today on the wall of the LSHTM – chapter 7].

In 1916 Sir Frances Lovell died, and Sir Havelock Charles became Dean (he had previously been Head of the Medical Board at the India Office). The problem(s) of identity of 'the discipline tropical medicine' remained, and this was to some extent a result of the dilemma as to whether this 'colonial discipline' should be aimed primarily at patient care ('clinical medicine') or hygiene ('sanitation'). Was it fact essentially medicine or science? Were doctors or biologists what was really needed? Should the subject be centred on London, or based in the colonies themselves? Should it fall within the province of the Royal College of Physicians or the Royal Society?

Clinical research at the LSTM

The school was certainly not idle when it came to clinical research. An expedition to the Roman Campagna was organised to continue studies on human malaria[1]. As a result of two important pieces of clinical investigation the mosquito-man cycle in *Plasmodium* sp was established conclusively; it also engraved it on the public mind! Both were reported by Manson in 1900[3][2]. In the first, Drs. A Bignami and G Bastianelli with the help of Dr L Sambon transported (via the British Embassy in Rome) relays of malaria (*P vivax*)-infected mosquitos from Rome to London; they were sent in cylindrical cages (8 ¼ x 3 ½ inches) [the ventilated box (9 x 8 ½ x 8 ½ inches) in which these were dispatched is preserved in the library of the London School of Hygiene and Tropical Medicine – Plates 45a & b]. They were transported in the 'Embassy Bag' and arrived in London 48 hrs after leaving Rome. Here they were fed on the blood of Manson's elder son – P Thurburn Manson, who was a 23-year-old medical student at Guy's Hospital, London, and Mr George Warren – the Senior Laboratory Assistant. Both were non-immune. They both developed *P vivax* malaria (parasites were identified in blood films by Manson) with all of its clinical manifestations and were successfully treated with quinine. P T Manson did however suffer two relapses in 1901. In the second piece of clinical investigation, a wooden hut, which had been constructed in England, was shipped to the Roman Campagna and set up at a highly malarious area (the King of Italy's hunting ground near Ostia at the mouth of the Tiber). The hut had mosquito-netting in the doors and windows, and the beds were provided with mosquito-nets; 'not

200

a grain of quinine was taken'! Drs L W Sambon and G C Low (Plate 46), Signor Terzi (an artist) and their Italian servant (Silvestri) lived in the hut from dusk to dawn between early July and 21 September; they remained completely well, despite the fact that they went 'about the country quite freely' during day-time. During this time they were visited by Battista Grassi and King Umberto of Italy. Manson concluded his report[32]:

> These experiments, together with the work of Ross, Grassi, Celli, Bignami, Bastianelli, and other Italians, the recent observations on native malaria by Koch, and the representations of the Malaria Commission of the Royal Society and Colonial Office, plainly indicate that the practical solution of the malaria problem lies in:
> (i) Avoiding the neighbourhood of native houses – the perennial source of malaria parasites, (ii) the destruction, so far as practicable, of *Anopheles*' breeding pools, (iii) And principally: Protection from mosquito bite.

Dr C W Daniels went, on behalf of the Royal Society, to Calcutta to verify Ross' work on malaria. Dr G C Low demonstrated the emergence of larval filaria from the proboscis of the mosquito (the intermediate host); this was an important piece of work which virtually clinched the mosquito-man component, and hence the complete life-cycle of *Wuchereria bancrofti*. This he followed up with a series of research projects on the distribution of filariasis in the West Indies[1].

Manson's interest in trypanosomiasis continued. Between 1899–1905 a vast epidemic of this parasitosis occurred in the British Protectorate of Uganda[33]; estimates put the total mortality at a quarter of a million. Early observations of this epidemic were made by Dr (later Sir) Albert Cook and his brother Dr J H Cook – missionaries at the Mengo Hospital, Kampala[33], and pioneers of health care and training in Africa. The causative organism of West African 'trypanosome fever' was discovered by J E Dutton and J L Todd during the Liverpool School's 6th expedition (to The Gambia) in September 1901. Dr G C Low led a team sponsored by the Royal Society to Kisumu, Uganda in June 1902; the other members of the party were A Castellani and C Christy. The expedition proved something of a disaster because Christy did not accept Low's authority and apparently spent his time big-game hunting. However, Castellani discovered a 'fish-like' parasite (thought to be a streptococcus) in infected blood; the discovery was communicated by Low to Manson on 15 October 1902. The Uganda epidemic was extremely perplexing for the Colonial Office; clearly it seriously undermined the health of the indigenous population and there was even a fear that it might spread to the 'Jewel of the Crown' – India! It also captured the public's imagination. Incidentally, this disease also became a major preoccupation of the Belgian government (and remained so until 1960!); King Leopold II invited the Liverpool School to send an expedition (their 12th) to the Congo Free State to investigate the disease there. The team consisted of Dutton, Todd and Christy; they set off in September 1903. It has been argued that the enormous disruption of indigenous societies which was considered necessary to deal with these epidemics, actually made them a great deal worse[33].

Dr C W Daniels later studied blackwater fever in central Africa. In 1903, Low and Manson demonstrated *Leishmania* amastigotes (Leishman-Donovan bodies) in a patient from India who had died of Kala-azar at the Albert Dock hospital; this confirmed the observation of Leishman the previous year[34]; the work was published in 1904[35]. A second case was diagnosed in a London Missionary Society clergyman who had served in southern Sudan; he apparently made an uneventful recovery despite the lack of effective chemotherapy[1].

Dr R T Leiper visited the head waters of the Nile. In 1907 Dr C M Wenyon travelled to the Sudan, sailed up the White Nile in a floating laboratory, and studied parasites of man and animals; he later travelled to Baghdad, Aleppo and finally Malta (1913) in order to study leishmaniasis[1]. Beri-beri was investigated by Dr H E Durham and Dr P T Manson at Christmas Island. In 1908, A T Stanton who had been seconded to the Institute of Medical Research in Malaya demonstrated the role of polished rice in the aetiology of beri-beri. Dr L W Sambon travelled widely in Italy investigating pellagra. Dr W Simpson went to west Africa to carry out a plague survey for the Government in 1908[1]. Dr P H Bahr worked on dysentery and filariasis in Fiji (in 1910), and sprue in Ceylon (in 1912–13). Dr S Cochran investigated kala azar in China in 1912. Dr R T Leiper worked on the life-cycle of *Loa loa* in Nigeria and the Cameroons (also in 1912). H M Hanschell and S Coghill travelled to the Gold Coast (now Ghana) to report on yellow fever on behalf of the Colonial Office in 1913. Leiper and Surg-Cmmdr. Atkinson studied the life-cycle of *Schistosoma japonicum* in China. Col Alcock worked in Ireland on the breeding habits of *Chrysops* sp, with the intention of applying this knowledge to tropical species of the fly.

Sir Ronald Ross and the LSTM

Ross (Plate 47) was to play only a peripheral role in the development of the LSTM (see below). The eldest of 10 children, he was born in India on 13 May 1857 – his father was General Sir Campbell Ross, KCB of the 68th Bengal Native Infantry[36,37]. Aged 8 he was sent to Britain for schooling. In 1874 he entered St Bartholomew's Hospital Medical School and having qualified with the MRCS diploma in 1879 and the LMS in 1881, he returned (after a brief period as a ship's surgeon) to the Indian Medical Service (IMS). His seminal work which clinched the *Plasmodium* sp mosquito-man cycle was published in 1897[38–41] – Manson was his mentor throughout this period (chapter 4). At the time of the discovery, he wrote[36]:

I have found thy secret deeds
O million-murdering death.
I know this little thing
A million men will save.
O death, where is thy sting?
Thy victory, O grave?

The work resulted in an FRS in 1901, a Nobel Prize for Medicine in 1902 (the award was subsequently disputed – Grassi, Laveran and Manson's names being mentioned[42]) and a Knighthood (KCB) in 1911. Incidentally, this latter accolade was announced in the same Honours List in which Osler became a baronet. Between 1899 and 1912 he was Lecturer and then Professor of Tropical Medicine at the Liverpool School of Tropical Medicine. He then proceeded to London where he began medical practice; he lived at 18 Cavendish Square, W1. He became Physician for Tropical Diseases at King's College Hospital. Despite these extremely impressive credentials however, Ross was a most unusual character; those who knew him well described the hostility he generated professionally, the fact that he was 'quick to take offence and capable of magnifying a petty affair out of all proportions', and others considered him either 'chronically maladjusted' or 'a tortured man'[43].

One interesting facet of his life was an overwhelming financial ambition; he sought monetary reward for having solved the 'great malaria problem'. He contrasted his position with that of Louis Pasteur who had been awarded financially by the French Government[44]. He also compared this discovery with that of Jenner – who received £30,000 for developing smallpox vaccination (chapter 1) and petitioned Parliament for a financial reward for his discovery in November 1913; this never came and he became increasingly disgruntled[44]. The extent to which Austen Chamberlain was involved in this decision (Lloyd George seems to have been largely responsible) is not entirely clear, although he certainly seems to have been opposed to it and could well have been instrumental in blocking the claim. The lengths to which he went to seek financial reward have been clearly described[44]. He did in fact succeed in getting a great deal of support from many quarters and in some he was considered to have been very 'badly done by' for not being rewarded for this piece of research which had given so much potential benefit to mankind. Even the founding of the 'Ross Institute and Hospital for Tropical Diseases'[45] (see below) did not deter Ross from seeking further financial reward. In 1928

203

he offered his personal papers for sale[44]; his target was at least £2000; in October 1928 he sold them for exactly this amount to Lady Houston, DBE.* He incidentally dedicated his Memoirs to the people of Sweden – not of Britain!

Some other outrageous episodes in Ross' life were a series of libel actions which he took against various colleagues (including Grassi) – and not least Manson – his former mentor[43]. It is important to stress the fact that Manson's paper[41] ('Surgeon-Major Ronald Ross's recent investigations on the mosquito-malaria theory') which had been published in the British Medical Journal in 1898, was very largely responsible for giving Ross priority for his seminal discovery, bringing it to the profession's attention, and it probably paved the way for Ross's Nobel Prize[46]. This astonishing legal affair took place in 1912–13, and it centered on the appointment of Ross' successor at the Liverpool School of Tropical Medicine. Dr (later Sir) William Prout applied for the post and asked Manson for a letter of recommendation[43]. Manson's testimonial was sent to the Secretary of the School (Mr A H Milne) immediately before he departed on a journey to Ceylon (with his son-in-law – Dr P H Manson-Bahr):

13 November 1912

Dear Mr. Milne,

I have just heard that Dr. Prout has applied for the Professorship of Tropical Medicine in your School, vacated by Sir R. Ross. I sincerely hope that his appointment may be successful, for it would, if I may use the expression, *make good a defect in your system of teaching* [my italics] which I have long been anxious, in the interests of tropical medicine, to see remedied. A teacher of tropical medicine to be considered efficient should be *not only a scientific man, but one having had extensive experience in tropical practice* [my italics]. Dr. Prout is such a man, and I know of no other in Liverpool with a similar record. Moreover, he is a good speaker, and by his academic and subsequent career both in research and practice, has shown himself to be a man of talent.

I have known him for many years, and entertain a high opinion of his personal character.

Yours sincerely,
PATRICK MANSON.

On 18 November Prout wrote to Ross from Leopoldville that he had

---

* The larger part of the Ross Archive (c20,000 items) is now deposited in the Library of the London School of Hygiene and Tropical Medicine; another collection (about 12,000 documents) is maintained as the Ross collection at the Library of the Royal College of Physicians and Surgeons of Glasgow.

visited Manson who had given him a "splendid" testimonial, and 'I should be very pleased if you could send such a testimonial supporting my candidature . . .'

On becoming aware of Manson's letter, Ross and seven senior colleagues wrote to Milne expressing 'very serious objection to the insinuation in [Manson's] testimonial regarding the teaching at the School' and requesting that the letter be withdrawn immediately. Milne complied and notified the selection committee members of the objection.

The following day Ross' solicitors wrote to Manson ('c/o Postmaster, Colombo') stating that 'It appears to Sir Ronald Ross that [Manson's testimonial] letter contains a serious reflection on him in his capacity of Teacher of Tropical Medicine, and also in his capacity as Practitioner in that subject.' The libel was 'especially injurious' because Ross planned to begin practice in London, and 'The letter most distinctly implies that he has not had sufficient experience in tropical practice.' The solicitors' letter to Manson, also indicated that the staff of the Tropical School resented the insinuation and asked for the testimonial's withdrawal. Finally: 'We shall be glad to receive a full apology from you by mail, or in the event of your deciding to contest the matter, please let us have a reference to your London Solicitors.' Ross replied to Prout's Leopoldville letter, saying that '. . . an unfortunate event has occurred. The letter which Sir Patrick Manson wrote in support of your candidature has been declared by my lawyers to be libellous . . . The lawyer says that anyone circulating the letter will be concerned in the libel, so that I advise you to tear it up at once! All the same I have . . . strongly recommend[ed] that you should be given a paid appointment with the School and hope that this will be given.' The rest of the letter is informal and cheerful, ending, 'We are all looking after your interests here in spite of the libel.' In effect, Ross seems to have derailed Prout's candidacy well before any of the academic or legal issues could come to a head.

In a letter to his solicitor, Ross expressed concern that some of the copies of the objectionable testimonial were missing, and that 'It is a very serious matter altogether, more especially that it opens up an old wound that everyone had hoped was healed years ago.' A Milne, the School's Secretary and Ross's personal friend, wrote to Ross to apologize and to dissociate himself from Manson's remarks. Ross accepted Milne's apology on behalf of himself and his protesting colleagues, but added that he was 'obliged to take [legal] steps which will reopen, much against my own will, an old trouble which we all hoped had been healed long ago; and I fear the matter is not likely to be closed for years to come.' In a letter explaining to the Acting Chairman of the School the history of the affair, and how serious he found it, Ross asked the School to dissociate itself from the libel, and to underwrite his legal expenses. There was no reply. In response to a note from the solicitor saying he had received no word from Manson, Ross replied (from his new residence in Cavendish Square): 'I fancy that Manson got the letter but has taken up a position of masterly inactivity.' Ross, (surprisingly) waited until Manson returned from abroad. 'After all,' said Ross, 'he is pretty old and may have written the testimonial in a great hurry without appreciating what he said.'

In mid-March, Ross's solicitors received a cablegram from Ceylon: 'Letter just received Manson away will communicate – Lady Manson,' and on 7 April Ross's solicitor received a handwritten letter from Manson, still in Ceylon. The letter (which is not in Manson's own hand) reads:

Messrs Batesons Wurr and Wimshurst
Liverpool

18th March 1913

Sirs,
Your letter of 7th Dec ult. I received only two days ago, and now take the earliest opportunity to reply.

I confess I do not understand it how wherein the libel on Sir Ronald Ross to which you refer lies. I have no copy of my letter of 13th Nov. 1912 to the Secretary of the Liverpool School of Tropical Medicine to guide me. But of this I am quite sure that in writing it I had no intention of reflecting in any way on Sir Ronald Ross' capacity as a Teacher of Tropical Medicine, nor on the Liverpool School of Tropical Medicine. Indeed I do not think I mentioned Sir Ronald's name. If however such reflection can be read into my letter I sincerely regret having written it and apologise for my carelessness. I may mention that the letter was written in great haste and while I was busy preparing to leave England for the East.

Yrs. faithfully,
PATRICK MANSON

Back in London, Manson received a copy of his original testimonial from Bateson, and in a covering note said he regretted that 'Sir Ronald Ross and the Liverpool School of Tropical Medicine have interpreted [the testimonial] in a way I never contemplated.'

Considering Manson's expressions of regret, Bateson felt that nothing was to be gained by further correspondence unless Ross wished to pursue legal action, a course Bateson advised against. Since Ross had received an 'ample apology', and Milne had recalled and destroyed all the copies of the libellous letter, 'I think if I were in your place,' Bateson advised, 'I should be content to let the matter rest where it is.' Ross told Bateson that he was anxious to pursue the libel but he thought that Manson or the School should pay his legal expenses. Bateson, who may have begun to lose patience with Ross's persistent niggling, offered to inquire about payment for his fees, 'but if I do not succeed I am perfectly willing to write them off.' Bateson soon secured Manson's permission to circulate his letter of apology at the Liverpool School, and also his agreement to pay legal costs. In due course, Manson's letter of apology was sent to the original recipients of the disputed testimonial, Manson paid Ross's solicitor £4.4/–, and Ross the balance of £1.1/–. These transactions formally closed the Ross-Manson libel episode![43]

In December 1912 Ross wrote to the Chairman of the Liverpool School, Sir William Lever (later Lord Leverhulme), expressing a preference for J W W Stephens as his successor; he was duly appointed to Ross' former Chair in February 1913[43]. Ross then proceeded to support Prout for a lectureship in tropical medicine on the grounds that since Stephens had no clinical experience in the tropics Prout's appointment would redress this; Prout soon received an appointment, but as Lecturer on Tropical Sanitation!

According to Manson-Bahr in his overview of the 'malaria saga'[46]: 'from 1913 onwards till Manson's death nine years later the relations between the two formerly congenial and mutually helpful collaborators became increasingly strained so that it is better to draw a veil over what actually transpired.' It should be recalled that they had first met in 1894 when Ross had first approached Manson for advice on the investigation of tropical diseases; he had offered direction and encouragement throughout Ross' days in India, and pulled strings at the India Office in London to prevent postings which would have interrupted Ross' work[42]. Other factors too were involved in the increasingly sour relationships between Ross and Manson. Ross' decision in 1898 to write on the *practical* applications of his research, both took him out of the realm of scientific and medical debate and put him into direct confrontation with the colonial administration. He got nowhere with the Colonial Office but he and other members of the Liverpool School found an ally in the Governor of Nigeria – Sir William MacGregor (chapter 2) – who was sympathetic to the 'sanitary' approach. Ross also distorted the facts in some of Manson's writing and concluded (in typically paranoid fashion) that he was siding with Grassi (malaria) and Dutton (trypanosomiasis) regarding priority in discovery[42]. Despite all of this, Ross had a few good words to say of Manson after he died in 1922[47].

In 1923, the 25th anniversary of Ross' malaria discovery, he persuaded a group of distinguished individuals to launch an appeal to establish the Ross Institute and Hospital for Tropical Diseases[45,48]. This was founded in his honour and opened at Putney Heath, London SW15; Ross became the Director-in-Chief. But it never really succeeded. It was plagued by poor finances throughout, and of course there simply were not enough 'tropical cases' in London to warrant another tropical hospital[49]. After

Ross died on 16 September 1932 the institute was incorporated into the then London School of Hygiene and Tropical Medicine (chapter 10)[50].

A blue plaque has recently been placed on the house in Cavendish Square, London, W1 where Ross lived following his removal from Liverpool (Plate 48).

Ross' inspection of the LSTM in 1912

In July 1912, Ross was invited to inspect the LSTM on behalf of the Board of Education; a satisfactory report was required before the courses could be officially recognised. The basic course was of 3-months duration; those who completed it could sit an examination and obtain a certificate; some also took the Cambridge University Diploma in Tropical Medicine and Hygiene. There was also a 3-month advanced course on medical zoology; this consisted of: arthropodology (entomology), helminthology and medical protozoology. An outline of what was involved can be found in the following letter (*Ross Archive*):

BOARD OF EDUCATION,
WHITEHALL, LONDON, S.W.
31st May, 1912

Sir,

The Board of Education are about to recognise the London School of Tropical Medicine (Royal Albert Dock) with a view to the payment of grant under their 'Statement of Grants available for Technological and Professional work in Universities', a copy of which is enclosed for your information. Before finally granting recognition, however, the Board have informed the authorities of the School that expert inspection will be necessary, and I am directed to write and ask you whether you would be prepared to assist the Board by visiting the School and making the necessary inspection. If, as the Board hope, you are in a position to place your services at their disposal, I should be glad to hear from you on what dates before the close of the current term it would be convenient for you to conduct the inspection.

The Board are in a position to offer you a fee of £4.4. a day during the period of your employment, and they anticipate that you will find it necessary to spend at least two days in work connected with the inspection and the preparation of your report. The fee for your services would consequently be £8.8. together with first-class railway fare and necessary travelling expenses, and a subsistence allowance of £1.1. for each night spent away from home.

On hearing from you that you are able to undertake this work copies of certain forms to be used in connection with the inspection would be sent to you, together with the necessary preliminary information of an administrative kind.

I should be happy to discuss the question with you if you cared to come and see me when you are next in London should this be in the near future.

I am, Sir,
Your obedient Servant,
F. FRANK HEATH [*sic*]

Major Sir Ronald Ross, KCB, FRS &c.,
The University,
Liverpool.

and the final arrangements for the visit:

WHITEHALL
LONDON, S.W.
26th June, 1912.

Dear Sir Ronald,
    Our visit to the London School of Tropical Medicine at Albert Dock is for next Wednesday, July 3rd. If it will suit your convenience we will leave Fenchurch Street Station at 11.21 a.m. If, however, you would greatly prefer 10.50 a.m. I think I could be at the Station at that time. Will you kindly let me know what would suit you best?

Yours very truly,
GEORGE NEWMAN

Major Sir Ronald Ross, KCB,
The University,
Liverpool.

Ross' subsequent report contained an accurate and comprehensive description of the state of the School, and in almost all of his account he is agreeably disposed to the facilities and syllabus. But his major reservation concerned the lack of a satisfactory course on 'sanitation':

It may be asked whether the ordinary diplomas of public health given in this country would not cover the field of tropical sanitation. I have had much experience in this line and can emphatically state that those diplomas will not nearly cover that field. Tropical sanitation is quite distinct from the sanitation of civilised temperate countries. The methods of water supply, food supply, sewage disposal, government, statistics, and the special diseases, are quite different in the two cases. I myself possess a diploma of public health and am therefore fully qualified to judge.
The proposed course of tropical sanitation should, I think only be allowed to follow a previous course in tropical medicine. This would be owing to the fact that a grounding in the study of tropical parasitology and disease is absolutely necessary before we can come to a study of the methods of prevention. It may be asked whether the course of tropical sanitation

should not be affiliated rather to courses of instruction of public health than to a course of tropical medicine. On the whole I think not. There are only two or three institutions where tropical sanitation can be taught, and these institutions are precisely those which are engaged in teaching tropical medicine. The bodies which now issue diplomas of public health would not possess the necessary staff of [sic] and sanitation together in the space of a single term of three months.

My remarks regarding the small amount of pay given to the lecturers, apply very strongly to the remuneration of the lecturer on tropical sanitation. The sanitary lecturer is on a different footing from the medical lecturers, because sanitary work does not necessarily connect itself with medical practice. Hence I consider that the pay, including examination fees of the sanitary lecturer, namely only £39. 18. 0. per annum is quite inadequate. Only six guineas are given for the lectures on Port Hygiene. The Lecturer on Epidemiology receive £31. 10. 0, but this is probably because his lectures include matter of importance in other lines. Besides these sums, only a few pounds are spent on the additional demonstrations. Professor [of Hygiene] Simpson is not provided with a special assistant.

I think therefore that the best way in which any grant which may be allotted by the Board can be spent would be in the line of establishing a special three months course for the adequate teaching of tropical hygiene and sanitation. I may add in confidence that this matter is already under consideration by this school, and that I have suggested it to the Colonial Office. Such a course would be very much welcomed by all Government officers who propose to take up the sanitary side in their careers in the tropics. At present medical men are often appointed to sanitary posts without having had any previous training in tropical sanitation whatever — not even training in general public health. This is a very serious situation, because such medical officers are to teach tropical public health. This point may however be open to future discussion and a means might be found by which a course of tropical sanitation could in some way be affiliated to both the proposed courses referred to. Another difficulty however lies in the fact that a diploma of public health already requires six months training, and that Government medical officers in the tropics could not be spared for this six months in addition to a three months for tropical medicine and another three months for tropical sanitation.

If a course of tropical sanitation is inaugurated at the London School, the following funds would be required.

(a) I think that the Lecturer on the subject should be given a salary which will demand first class men to take up the work.

(b) He should also be given the services of an assistant of a rather senior grade, to teach different kinds of analyses, inspections, statistical science, and to collect and keep on hand all the vast information on sanitary matters which is contained in the innumerable official reports. But the principal part of his work will be to teach water bacteriology and other branches of public health microscopy and many items which it is unnecessary to mention here.

(c) Room should be found for a suitable sanitary museum, which should be under the lecturer and his assistant.

(d) Many of the teachers in other lines will be required to give some lectures in connection with the course of tropical sanitation, because this subject actually overlaps tropical medicine on many points, for example entomology is perhaps the leading feature of tropical sanitation. Personally I think that such teachers will require additional fees.

The establishment of the proposed course would be very beneficial to the course of tropical medicine, because it would help to lighten the load on the latter. For instance it would relieve much of the higher entomology in addition to the public health lectures. This would give time for a complete teaching of tropical medicine and parasitology.

In conclusion I should like to remark that the whole medical curriculum would be very greatly benefited by a little more instruction on tropical medicine than is now given. At present men are supposed to be qualified without possessing any real knowledge of the subject, and the result is that they are employed on board ships and in factories, plantations and on expeditions in the tropics, although they really possess neither experience or training in the elementary details of tropical medicine. It may be argued that this is a very serious matter and should be corrected. I cannot see why teaching bodies cannot arrange to give more instruction on tropical medicine than they do now. There are numerous retired and well qualified medical officers available for such posts. Manchester gives a special course of lectures under Dr. Stephens of this School, and other bodies could do the same.

The report seems to have been more or less satisfactory from the point of view of the LSTM, and it was gratefully received by the Board of Education:

> Board of Education,
> WHITEHALL, LONDON S.W.
> 23rd July 1912.

London School of Tropical Medicine (University of London)
  U.I. 232/12.
Sir,
    With reference to your letter of the 18th instant, I am directed to express the thanks of the Board of Education for the full report received on the London School of Tropical Medicine.

Drafts for £13. 5. 1 are being forwarded to you in payment of the account submitted, the slight difference in the amount from that of £13.14.10 being due to the deduction of income tax on the £8. 8. 0 fee.

> I am, Sir,
> Your obedient Servant,

H FRANK HEATH [*sic*]

Sir Ronald Ross
The University
Liverpool.

Thus, Ross felt that the basic course was sufficiently long but that the amount of time allocated to hygiene was insufficient – and that this subject should be taught as a separate 3-month course. As a result of this inspection (and subsequent satisfactory report)[51] the School was recognised by the Board.

The Liverpool School of Tropical Medicine and other newly established schools

Progress of the Liverpool school during the early years of the twentieth century has been documented[52]. Between its foundation in 1899 (chapter 7) and 1914, 32 scientific expeditions to the tropics took place; details of these have been preserved[52]. In 1907 the *Annals of Tropical Medicine and Parasitology* (which still flourishes) was founded by the staff of the school.

When the Great War began in 1914, teaching (summarized below) had been in full swing for 15 years[53]:

Two full courses are given annually, beginning in January and September. An advanced practical course of one month is also given in June, and it is designed to meet the convenience of practitioners at home on leave; those who attend it are excused the first month of the other course. Three times a year special courses on entomology are given for officers in the West African Medical Service and others. A certificate of satisfactory attendance is given; this is independent of the diploma granted by the University. Special research work at the laboratories of the school and at Runcorn research laboratories (16 miles from Liverpool). Full particulars can be obtained from the Secretary, 10B Exchange Buildings, Liverpool.

The success of the two British schools did not go unnoticed in Europe. Schools were founded at Hamburg (1901), and later at Amsterdam (1910) and Antwerp (1931). France also established schools at Paris, Bordeaux and Marseilles. Basel later followed suit. Further afield, Australia, the northern part of which had significant tropical health problems, also elected to have its own school[54]:

The Bishop of North Queensland, Dr. Frodsham, is making arrangements with the Schools of Tropical Medicine at London and Liverpool to send out to Australia a trained man to initiate the work of an institute which it is proposed to establish with a laboratory at Townsville, the principal city in Northern Queensland. If the institution can be started the general management will be undertaken by the three Australian Universities having medical schools, Sydney, Melbourne, and Adelaide. The Federal Government of Australia has agreed to subsidise the work at the rate of £450 per annum and the Government of Queensland will give £250; thus the institute will start with an assured annual income of £700, a sum which it is hoped will be increased by private subscriptions.

And two years later (1910) the following report appeared in *The Lancet*[55]:

The Queensland Institute of Tropical Medicine was practically inaugurated at Townsville on Jan. 4th. The new director, Dr. A. Breinl, was entertained at dinner by Dr. Frodsham, Anglican Bishop of North Queensland, who was the originator of the scheme. Dr. Breinl, in the course of a speech, stated he had promises of aid from the Australian Universities and Commonwealth and States Governments. He dwelt on the necessity of solving the question of making tropical regions habitable both from humanitarian and commercial standpoints.

India too, joined the list of countries with a tropical medical school of its own[56]:

In connexion with the proposal to establish a Pasteur Institute in Assam, public interest has been quickened in the more important question of a School of Tropical Medicine for India. The subcommittee of local medical men which reported on the proposed institute urged that original research into such diseases as kala-azar, blackwater fever, &c., could be carried out with great advantage in Assam. But if India is to have its tropical school, and it certainly should have, something more must be done than the creation of an annexe to the small Pasteur Institute at Haflong. The time has come when the Government should move in the matter and no longer entirely rely upon the London and Liverpool schools for post-graduate instruction for medical officers. In no country is the necessity for a tropical school of medicine more urgent than it is in India, and the endowment of such an institution should no longer be delayed. Calcutta would seem to be the place indicated, and the school should be founded in connexion with the Medical College where the opportunities for clinical study are unrivalled. The Government of India is being appealed to constantly for more grants for sanitation, the prevention of malaria, &c., but if there are spare funds available some portion of them could well be diverted to the scientific school, for which there is now so clear a demand. The question is one which claims immediate attention, and this it will doubtless receive at the hands of the responsible medical authorities.

Commenting on the proposal for a new School of Tropical Medicine at

Calcutta, Dr Andrew Balfour put forward an alternative but nevertheless novel scheme for an even more useful institution[57]:

> ... a marine floating laboratory [similar to one used by a Wellcome expedition on the Nile] would be of the utmost service. Every year I am inundated by appeals for material for teaching purposes from England, Scotland, Ireland, the United States, and various parts of the continent. It is noteworthy that amongst the institutions which apply are the two great English Schools of Tropical Medicine at London and Liverpool, and it is evident that even the latter school, despite its numerous and valuable research expeditions, cannot obtain all it requires for the instruction of its students; hence I believe the difficulty might be solved by the provision of a well-equipped laboratory on board a vessel of from 800 to 1000 tons burthen. Such a ship would be able to visit any portion of the globe, could ascend large navigable rivers, and would be the means of bringing back a store of most valuable material both for museum and teaching purposes. . . .
>
> If properly approached I believe those in charge of such institutions would be glad to assist in every possible way, and they might be repaid by demonstrations of new technique and interesting specimens. These institutions are often in cities on or near the sea, as, for example, Calcutta, Bombay or Madras, Cairo, Alexandria or Leopoldville, Hong-Kong, Rio de Janeiro, Manila, and so on. It is on the littorals of tropical countries that dengue, yellow fever, and other important diseases occur, and in the event of epidemics the infected places might be speedily visited and perhaps materially aided and benefited, while at all times the collection of specimens bearing on tropical medicine would form a most important duty. Specimens could be brought back in good condition, diseases studies on the spot, and parasites, especially blood parasites, observed in a living state. It will be at once apparent that such a laboratory ship could be utilised for the study of zoology, especially economic entomology, botany, geology, and hygiene, all subjects more or less intimately connected with tropical medicine. . . .
>
> There is a vast deal in environment, in tropical conditions, a vast deal to note both as regards symptoms and treatment. Think how tropical hygiene might be studied by those fortunate enough to travel in such a vessel. The ordinary medical man at home, however he may read and re-read the excellent manuals on tropical sanitation which now exist, has, I am convinced, but a vague idea of the conditions which obtain in tropical countries and the problems to be faced. . . .
>
> That our English Schools of Tropical Medicine have accomplished a great deal I would be the last to deny. They have been a boon to mankind, but if, under the control of the Colonial Office, a marine floating laboratory was affiliated to these schools their usefulness would be increased four, ten, a hundred-fold. Apart from anything else, what a link such a laboratory would be in binding together the Mother country and her colonies in humanitarian bonds, in establishing relations between schools at home

and their *alumni* working in the dark places of the earth! The thought is a fascinating one, but it is chilled by the bogey of expense. Still money is found, rightly and readily found, for polar expeditions. Valuable though these may be, can they for a moment compare, as regards benefit to mankind, with repeated expeditions of the kind outlined? Emphatically no. Even in their scientific aspect I do not believe they can serve so useful a function. It is the beginning of a new reign [King George V had succeeded to the British throne]. Is it too much to expect that some of our wealthy philanthropists may mark the occasion by the gift of such an institution? Its value is not to be reckoned in money, but in health and energy and human lives and the spread of knowledge, and the forging of yet another link between Britain and her children.

I am Sir, yours faithfully,
ANDREW BALFOUR.

Wellcome Tropical Research Laboratories, Gordon Memorial College, Khartoum, June 2nd, 1910.

This suggestion seems to have survived in the minds of some, and nine years later *The Lancet* recorded[58]:

... Dr. Louis Sambon, in a lecture delivered before the Royal Society of Medicine on June 14th [1919], by arrangement with the West India Committee [developed] the theme of bringing students periodically into the tropics by means of a floating school. The islands of the Lesser Antilles, which he had recently visited, were ravaged each by its particular breed of epidemic, and nothing would co-ordinate the isolated efforts of medical officers on these lonely isles so thoroughly as a regular circulation of expert advice and help. He advocated a development on international lines, having already received encouragement from the French and Italian Governments. The idea thus timely set forth was not allowed to drop and came up for discussion at a private meeting held under the chairmanship of Sir Humphry Rolleston on Thursday, July 10th, at the same place. Here Dr. Balfour set out the views summarised above, adding the further claim of a floating laboratory as a link between the Dominions and the Mother Country. Sir David Bruce and Dr. G.C. Low, among others, doubted the feasibility of the floating school as a substantial agent of research, the latter pointing out that sleeping sickness and kala-azar at all events could not be studied on the littoral. The extended establishment of local shore laboratories appealed to the majority of those present for the purpose of actual research work, neither nostalgia nor rolling and pitching apparatus being specially conducive to the desirable mental detachment. Sir Thomas [later Lord] Horder voiced the general consensus in finding the floating school an attractive idea for teaching purposes, adding that finance should not be an impediment if the ruling authorities were satisfied of the practicable character of the proposal. A committee was appointed, with Dr. Balfour as chairman, and Dr. Low, Dr. R.T. Leiper, and Dr.

Sambon as secretaries, to inquire into the question in all its aspects. We are inclined to agree with Dr. Balfour, who has from first to last been the moving spirit in the proposal, that the cost of such a floating school might reasonably be regarded by Parliament and public in the same light as polar expeditions. The adventures and prizes are much the same, the gain, indeed presumably much greater: the difference consists chiefly in the substitution of pith helmets and mosquito nets for fur caps and moccasins. Within a generation, if ankylostomiasis and pellagra are not then extinct, we doubt not that the floating school will be a routine method of education and preventive study.

Despite these words of advice, by 1915 progress had been made in establishing this school (on land) close to the Calcutta Medical College[59]:

Good progress is being made with the scheme for the establishment of a school of tropical medicine in Calcutta, with which the name of Sir Leonard Rogers, IMS, is so honourably associated. An excellent site has been secured close to the Calcutta Medical College, and the buildings are now going up. The first subscription list shows that Rs.1¾ lakhs have already been obtained and another half lakh is practically secured.

And in 1928, the role of Sir Leonard Rogers in this enterprising venture was duly acknowledged by *The Lancet*[60]:

The annual report for 1927 of this school [THE CALCUTTA SCHOOL OF TROPICAL MEDICINE] records under appropriate headings the manifold activities in teaching and investigation of the now great school established by Sir Leonard Rogers [1868–1962]. Although under the Government of Bengal, the school in reality serves the whole of India, and students attend it from every province. The chief work of its staff is research in the special diseases of the country, and their published contributions give some indication of the zeal and ability with which it has been carried on. In judging their results, however, it is necessary to remember the influence they have in stimulating and maintaining all over India a new appreciation of the value of Western medicine.

The Society of Tropical Medicine and Hygiene

Another significant development during the 'Albert Dock days' was the foundation of the (later Royal) Society of Tropical Medicine and Hygiene. The initial inspiration seems to have come from Mr (later Sir) James Cantlie[61,62], although Dr G C Low was from the outset extremely enthusiastic about the idea; Manson (who was to become the first President) was 'at first a little doubtful about the idea, thinking that the time was not yet ripe[1].' In 1907 the Lancet announced the formation of the society[63].

216

The Society of Tropical Medicine and Hygiene was formed on Jan. 4th of this year at a meeting held at the Colonial Office for the purpose of the study and discussion of diseases met with in tropical countries. The second meeting of the society will be held on Friday, March 15th, at 5.30 p.m., at the Royal College of Physicians of London, to consider the rules drawn up by a sub-committee for the constitution of the society and the regulation of its work. So much has been done in recent years to advance the knowledge of the diseases of warm climates that there must be ample food for discussion and study in this branch of medicine, and the meetings of the society should prove interesting not only to medical men with tropical experience but to every medical man engaged in the practice of medicine wherever his lot may be cast.

This rapidly became a flourishing organisation which acted as an excellent venue for the discussion of any problem relating to clinical medicine and 'sanitation' in relation to the tropics. *The Transactions of the [Royal] Society of Tropical Medicine and Hygiene* has been published since the foundation of the Society. An account of the early days has been provided by Dr G C Low, one of the founders[64]. Low also gave an account of the early days of 'tropical medicine' in his Presidential address to the Royal Society of Tropical Medicine and Hygiene in 1929[65].

9

Removal to central London

True democracy does not consist in the dismemberment and disintegration of the Empire, but rather in the knitting together of kindred races for similar objectives.

Joseph Chamberlain (1836–1914)

In July 1917, the Dean of the LSTM – Sir Havelock Charles (1858–1934) – suggested to the Committee of the Seamen's Hospital Society that the time was ripe for removal to a new site[1]; the idea was formally accepted at the first meeting of the committee for 1919[2]. The Endsleigh Palace Hotel, 23 Gordon Street, Euston, had already been identified as a suitable building.* There was some pressure from another bidder, but by May 1919, the SHS helped by some financial assistance from the British Red Cross (who made a grant of £100,000 to the SHS and also endowed some beds) and the Order of St John of Jerusalem, bought the building for £70,000[3-5]. *The Lancet* informed its readers in May 1919[6]:

> A hospital devoted solely to the treatment of patients suffering from tropical diseases will be opened shortly by the Seamen's Hospital Society in the Endsleigh Palace Hotel near Euston-square. The building has been used during the last four years as a hospital for wounded officers and was recently acquired through the aid of the British Red Cross. It is understood that the clinical material will be available for post-graduate instruction in connexion with the London School of Tropical Medicine. The new hospital will be within easy reach of University College Medical School, Middlesex Hospital, the School of Medicine for Women, Charing Cross Hospital, and Bedford College, and should prove a useful accession to the claims of Bloomsbury to become the future home of the University of London.

And by October of the same year[7]:

---

* This building, although severely damaged during the second world war (1939–45) remains extant and now houses the Student Union of University College London (UCL), together with the Departments of Physics and Mathematics of that college.

218

The London School of Tropical Medicine will within the next few months remove from its abode at the Albert Dock Hospital to a permanent home in what was the Endsleigh Palace Hotel, close to Euston Station. The journey from Fenchurch-street Station to the docks was described by Dr. Andrew Balfour at the annual school dinner on Oct. 16th, in the words used by one Scottish divine of another, as "short, dark, and dirty," and whatever reason there may have been at the time of its foundation for placing the school at the point of disembarkation of its patients, in these days of motor ambulances and quick road transport that reason no longer exists. It cannot fail to be of great advantage to the school to be located in the neighbourhood of one of the largest medical teaching centres in London, and the gain will doubtless be mutual. Of clinical material there can be no lack. The return of our citizen army from many tropical regions, bearing with them not only wounds but the protozoal fauna of the parts from which they came, will ensure that, and as Professor J. L. Todd of McGill has recently pointed out to Canadian doctors [Todd J L. *Canad Med Ass J* 1919; 9: 709–716]; they must be prepared to meet with "Uncanadian diseases." We understand, too, that the India Office is to avail itself of the services of the school for the observation and treatment of its employees of whatever grade. Staff and salaries will have to be reconsidered in the new and palatial surroundings. It is hardly to be expected that the numbers of students will remain limited to those as yet taking the course, who are for the most part entering the Colonial Medical Service. An intensive three months' training in tropical medicine is likely to become the equipment of every ambitious medical student, and the school now has on its register a number of members of allied or associated nations on their way back from the European turmoil. We may gratefully remember Mr. Joseph Chamberlain's keen intuition, to which the school owes its inception, and congratulate Sir Patrick Manson on seeing this fruit of his long toil.

Progress was rapid and by January 1920 *The Lancet* was able to report[8]:

It is expected that the new hospital for tropical diseases . . . will be ready for patients this month. Roughly speaking, 58 to 60 beds will be available. One floor will be devoted to private patients, including cases from the India Office and Colonial Office, and for them small private single- or double-bedded rooms have been set aside. On another floor general cases will be dealt with, and here there will be two roomy wards, with a few single rooms in addition for special cases. The old tropical hospital at the Albert Docks, a branch of the Seamen's Hospital at Greenwich, is to be utilised as a source of supply for the new hospital, cases being transferred from there as required by ambulance. The physicians will be Dr. C.W. Daniels and Dr. George C. Low, both old superintendents of the London School of Tropical Medicine and both widely known for their researches and work on tropical medicine. As assistant physician Dr. P. Manson-Bahr has recently been appointed. Such a hospital should prove a great boon to a large class of sufferers from the tropics, because here they can be properly housed, have every attention, and, what is most important, be treated by expert consultant physicians with special knowledge of their diseases.

Running in connexion with the hospital will be the London School of Tropical Medicine under the care of Dr. H.B. Newham as director. Students will thus have the advantage of studying the cases at first hand and will also be trained in the scientific methods required for their diagnosis and treatment. It is expected that there will be a wealth of clinical material available and valuable research work will, we have no doubt, accrue from its study. The easy accessibility of the new building will be one of its chief assets.

For a relatively short period therefore the hospital and school would continue to be housed in the same building – but with the enormous advantage of being situated in the centre of the metropolis.

Manson-Bahr[9] reflected: 'at the close of 1919 the move to London was carried out. No longer, then, were the dismal and boisterous Connaught Road and the dingy Albert Dock to remain the centre of the world of tropical medicine.' . . . 'the buildings in which it had been born were to be handed back to their original owners – the Dock Authorities.' He also recalled[9]: There were nine storeys; the lower four were used by the School and the upper five by the Hospital; there were two public wards of 'fair size' and numerous smaller ones for 2–4 beds, and there was one floor mainly for single rooms for private cases. The surgical block was at the top of the building, and the X-ray Department was somehow or other wedged into the basement! The ground floor was fully occupied by a lecture room, library, board room, refectory and offices. The remaining space accommodated the various departments of the school, the museum, and the Tropical Diseases Bureau. Plate 49 shows the newly opened Hospital and School at Endsleigh Gardens in 1920.

The first student course to be held there began on 2 February 1920, and the first patient was admitted by Sir James Cantlie on 9 February[10]. The new School and Hospital were formally opened by HRH the Duke of York (later King George VI) on 11 November 1920[11]. Few contemporary reports of the Endsleigh Gardens building at this time seem to have survived. Manson-Bahr[9] however later recorded a series of reminiscences: 'During this period the clinical side reached its acme.' 'An outpatient department had been established by Dr W E Cooke.' 'The bed-state was increased to seventy-five and these were filled!' Of the 'lecture room on the ground floor which replaced the dining hall of the erstwhile hotel' he recalled: 'It was dingy, dusty and noisy where it impinged upon Gordon Street and with the bustle of the traffic outside at times it was difficult to make oneself heard, and when the lantern was in use, it was inky blackness, so that the class found it convenient on these occasions, to

The Seamen's Hospital Society accepts in THE HOSPITAL FOR TROPICAL DISEASES Paying Patients of either sex suffering from diseases peculiar to the tropics.

It is a voluntary hospital, and voluntary contributions alone enable the Society to afford treatment and maintenance at the charges set forth below, or to make special arrangements in certain cases.

Patients from H.M. Colonial Office are charged according to the agreement existing between that Office and the Seamen's Hospital Society.

A similar agreement exists with H.M. Foreign Office in respect of Consular Officers, Commercial Diplomatic Officers and H.M. Trade Commissioners and their established Chief Clerks in the Dominions and Colonies.

The same terms are also extended to the staffs of certain commercial firms in consideration of the latter's annual subscription.

The India Office and the High Commissioner for India arrange for the special tropical treatment in accordance with their conditions of service, upon receipt of a recommendation from the India Medical Board, which, in all cases, should be obtained before attending at the Hospital.

The Ministry of Pensions arrange to grant treatment to suitable cases in receipt of a disability pension.

WARD ACCOMMODATION.

The accommodation available is of the following nature :

(A) Rooms with two beds.

(B) Private wards with more than two beds.

There is suitable accommodation for women and children. In the case of very young children the full charges are not made, and it is sometimes possible to arrange for the mother or nurse to occupy the same room as the child.

COST.

MAINTENANCE.	CONSULTANT'S FEE. (at least two visits weekly)	WEEKLY TOTAL.
A. 15s. per day	£1 11 6 per visit	£8 8 0
B. 12s. „ „	£1 1 0 „ „	£6 6 0

The following charges may also be incurred :—

RADIOLOGIST.	PATHOLOGICAL TESTS.
A. £3 3 0 per examination	£1 10 0 (minimum fee)
B. £1 1 0 „ „	£1 1 0 „ „

(For repeated or bio-chemical tests the total fee shall not exceed £5 5 0).

MASSEUSE.   10/6 per visit or according to circumstances. 2/6 per exposure for artificial sunlight.

Operation fees are made by arrangement.

Anæsthetist's fee 10 per cent. of Surgeon's fee in addition.

Dental or other special treatment by arrangement.

Consultations with other Physicians or Surgeons incur an additional fee.

"Maintenance and Treatment" includes attendance by a Resident Medical Officer, all board, nursing, medicine, necessary stimulants and surgical dressings. Special nurses are an extra charge.

PAYMENT.

All financial arrangements must be made with the Resident Secretary, who is authorised to make all necessary enquiries, and who will give every consideration to special cases.

For the convenience of patients, their whole account (Hospital services and Consultant's fees) is rendered, and is payable weekly.

The Visiting Hours are from 2 to 4.30 p.m. daily.

Fig 9.1: Centre pages of a pamphlet entitled: 'Facilities for Paying Patients' to the Hospital; this was issued sometime between 1920 and 1930.

lapse into deep slumber.' [The plaque of Manson which was placed on the wall of this theatre (Plate 50) is now at the Albert Dock Hospital]. 'There were certain aspects of the Endsleigh Gardens building which remained impressed on one's mind. It was dark, awkward and inconvenient, with multitudes of doors and narrow passages.' 'Everyone then agreed that the Endsleigh Gardens building was not satisfactory as a hospital, though it had been cleverly adapted, having been primarily designed as a residential hotel.' However 'though there were grumbles, a fine spirit prevailed in those days and the patients acknowledged that they were well served, both by the medical and nursing staffs.' 'The laboratory was of a high order under Dr Hamilton Fairley ... Director of Pathology, and all possible steps were taken to ensure that the correct diagnosis should be arrived at and appropriate treatment determined.' 'The patients came from many sources – from the Colonial Office, the India Office and other government departments, from many tropical and commercial companies, notably those associated with W. Africa, while for teaching material it was always possible to rely on seamen, European, Indian and Chinese, from the Dock Hospitals under the management of the Seamen's Hospital Society.' Fig 9.1 gives a list of charges for paying patients at this time.

Plate 51 shows the staff of the HTD in 1930. Manson-Bahr[9] also considered that: 'For the members of the staff who were attached to the [SHS] institutions to visit those hospitals was a laborious duty, but it was

221

one which was faithfully fulfilled, though it entailed frequent journeys to the East End, and these hospitals lay far away.'

Research into tropical disease

Interest in research into tropical disease was never greater than during this period (1920–39). However, it is clear that the overall orientation of the discipline was moving increasingly away from the clinical (bed-side) approach, towards prevention and (hopefully) eradication! Thus the Tropical Disease Prevention Committee was set up in 1920[12]:

> . . . While much has already been done in the patient investigation of tropical diseases [claimed *The Lancet*], it would be idle to deny that we are still ignorant of the exact causes and mode of spread of many of them, or that there is still a vast field of investigation open before the problem of their successful control can hope to be solved. Great territories, not a few of them forming part of the British Empire, are still ravaged by leprosy, yaws, beri-beri, pellagra, plague, blackwater fever, bilharziasis, hookworm disease, filariasis, and other loathsome diseases; and in many cases the loss of man-power entailed by their prevalence is so great as to form a serious barrier to the progress of the State or the success of great commercial undertakings therein.
>
> . . . there is no organisation like the Rockefeller Foundation, in this country whose aim is solely or even principally that of the eradication of tropical diseases.
>
> . . . The Committee rightly aims high. It is hoped to raise immediately a sum of £100,000, and it is proposed to begin work by undertaking a thorough medical survey of the Lesser Antilles. The advantages offered by small islands, as compared with vast continental areas, for such a survey are obvious. But the work is not to be confined to purely scientific research; it is hoped that the Committee will be able to apply, with the co-operation of local authorities, practical preventive measures, and for this purpose the Island of Barbados is suggested as a suitable field for an active campaign against ankylostomiasis, filariasis, pellagra and leprosy.
>
> . . . It will be among the objects of the Committee, we gather, to render impossible in future such ruthless slaughter of innocent individuals, to make universally known the lessons already learnt as to the methods of preventing many preventable diseases, and to widen the field of applied hygiene in tropical countries by research into the natural history of other diseases. These aims are as truly humanitarian as scientific, and as commercially promising – to descend once more to the levels of self-interest – as either. They cannot, we think, fail to appeal, and we gladly and warmly commend them, to the support of administrators in all tropical and subtropical countries, of the leaders of commerce in regions where disease is still a formidable obstacle to the full development of trade

and labour, and, indeed, of all who are in any way interested in the future welfare of the earth's warmer zones.

The future study of tropical disease, and the important role which London should to be playing formed the main theme of a Presidential address to the Section of Tropical Diseases and Parasitology of the Royal Society of Medicine in 1921[13]:

> ... Sir Leonard Rogers pointed out that the research work done at the Calcutta Medical College, where he had been professor of pathology, and at the large hospital of 600 beds affiliated, had led to vast public benefit by the prevention of disease, as well as to the promotion of the spirit of research. He described the methods employed to make intelligent appeal to the Home and Indian Governments and to wealthy individuals for money to equip and support this work. Large contributions for the upkeep of the institutions, he said, had come from Indian rajahs and Indian merchants, while subsidies for scientific research had been received from English men and business firms as well, to mention two names, from Sir David Yule and Sir Dorab Tata, of Bombay. He proposed that London, the wealthiest city in the world, having before it the examples of Calcutta and Bombay abroad and Liverpool at home, and the stimulating actions of philanthropists like Mr. H.S. Wellcome and the late Sir Alfred Jones, should endow the London School of Tropical Medicine, so that research laboratories in British tropical countries could be founded in connexion with the school. He believed that the support of the Colonial Office would be forthcoming for such a movement, and suggested that the start should be made by obtaining annual contributions towards the support of research workers to proceed to certain British colonies. He considered that the colonial authorities should supply laboratories wherein the researches should be carried on, these being adjacent to the largest available hospital. The men to do the initial work should, he pointed out, be selected by a strong organising committee, and it was particularly important that their early choice should fall on the right man, as the first five years of work would be critical. This plan, he said, would eventually ensure that all important British tropical possessions would obtain permanent laboratories and the services of scientific workers whose efforts could be supplemented, in accordance with urgent or special need, by temporary workers sent out from the London School ...

The increasing emphasis on sanitation and hygiene is also clear from the increase in publications in this area. The Tropical Diseases Bureau (which had been set up as the *Sleeping Sickness Bureau* in 1908, and had altered its name in 1912), had now moved into the new School/Hospital; it began publication of 'Sanitation Supplements' to the *Tropical Diseases Bulletin*[14]. [Incidentally, the Tropical Diseases

Library – which was formed by amalgamating the LSTM library with the collection of periodicals belonging to the Tropical Diseases Bureau was founded soon after the removal to Endsleigh-gardens, in February 1921[15].]

An update on the research activities of school and hospital was provided by *The Lancet* for 1923[16]:

> ... Since the removal three years ago [to the Endsleigh Gardens building] the 56 beds have been filled with examples of interesting and rare diseases from all parts of the British Empire. In association with the hospital itself, a laboratory has been specially fitted up for clinical investigations and clinical research, and the activities of the helminthological, protozoological, and pathological departments of the School testify to the value of the co-operation between the wards, the research laboratories, the lecture theatres, and the bureau from which is issued the *Tropical Diseases Bulletin*.
>
> Among the results of practical importance derived from the association may be mentioned a new theory and treatment of sprue by Dr. H.H. Scott, now a member of the School and himself a former sufferer from this terrible scourge, as also the discovery of Weil's disease in London and the treatment of trypanosomiasis by Bayer "205." The staff of the hospital counts among its numbers a distinguished physician who has been appointed in order to originate and conduct research in clinical medicine. Certain tropical diseases, sprue among them, are probably more profitably investigated in London than in the tropics. It has, however, been fully recognised that the really great advances are to be obtained by special researches in the tropics themselves. This can be done in two ways: by training workers for positions in the laboratories now established in most of the British tropical possessions or by the despatch, from time to time, of special investigators most fitted to conduct an intensive research for a limited length of time on some special problem.
>
> During the last 23 years the School has despatched no less than 21 of these expeditions and, as the publications of the School will show, they have been fruitful in many ways. The researches of C.M. Wenyon in protozoology and R.T. Leiper in helminthic disease are known to all. At the present moment two of the staff are actively engaged in research in the tropics. Dr. J.G. Thomson, for the second time, is investigating blackwater fever in Rhodesia, and Dr. H.B. Newham the prevalence of undiagnosed fevers in British Honduras, while at the end of the present year Dr. P.A. Buxton, accompanied by assistants, is proceeding to Samoa with the co-operation of the New Zealand Government, with the object especially of devising methods for the prevention of filariasis. Dr. Cecil Cook, the recently appointed Wandsworth scholar, will investigate the aetiology of ulcerating granuloma in New Guinea, where this intractable and loathsome disease is rampant.
>
> This active prosecution of research in the tropics has been made possible

owing to the endowment by Lord Milner of a magnificent research fund with an income of over £2,600 a year. The helminthological department also expends over £1,000 a year in special research facilities, and Prof. Leiper has constantly attached to him three or more research students, their activity being reflected in the publication of the bi-monthly periodical the *Journal of Helminthology*. The publications of the School as a whole include the production of the *Journal of the London School of Tropical Medicine* as well as the *Research Memoir* series, of which four volumes have already appeared and others are in course of preparation.

The London School thus provides ample and generous opportunities for laboratory and clinical research, the popularity of which is reflected in the increasing attendance at the post-graduate classes. Still greater opportunities are assured to the School in association with the scheme for an Imperial Institute of Hygiene.

Another organisation which had tropical research as one of its major thrusts was the Wellcome Bureau of Scientific Research, which was situated next to the LSTM – at 26, Endsleigh Gardens[17]. But in addition to research, it had a large teaching and research museum devoted to tropical medicine and hygiene; this proved to be of enormous value to the LSTM. Museums modelled on this one had by then been established in Calcutta, Zanzibar and Dar-es-Salaam[17]. The Medical Research Council (in conjunction with the Colonial Office also decided (in 1936) to support tropical research[18-21], and a committee (the forerunner of the 'Tropical Medicine Research Board') was set up; this consisted of: Prof J C G Ledingham, FRS (chairman), Prof A J Clark, FRS, Dr N Hamilton Fairley, Prof W W Jameson, Dr Edward Mellanby, FRS, Miss Muriel Robertson, DSc, Sir Leonard Rogers, FRS, Dr H Harold Scott, Sir Thomas Stanton, Dr C M Wenyon, FRS, Prof Warrington Yorke, FRS, and Mr. A Landsborough Thomson, DSc (secretary). In addition to providing both junior and senior fellowships, some permanent and pensionable appointments were also established: 'while the exact terms of service are still undecided, . . . they will be not less favourable than those which apply to other Government appointments at home or overseas for men of similar professional standing'[20,21].

Qualifications for the practice of tropical medicine

The increasingly complex system of diplomas in tropical medicine was addressed by *The Lancet* in 1923[22]:

Although a qualification in tropical medicine has not been made registrable by statute, a diploma is regarded as indispensable for appointments in the Colonial Medical Service and similar positions abroad. Systematic instruction for these diplomas is given at the Incorporated Liverpool School of Tropical Medicine (founded in 1898), and at the London School of Tropical Medicine, 5, Endsleigh-gardens, London N.W.1 (founded in 1899), which is a school of the University of London in the Faculty of Medicine.

University of Cambridge. – Two Examinations in Tropical Medicine and Hygiene are conducted yearly by the State Medicine Syndicate of the University of Cambridge. The examinations are held in Cambridge early in August and at the end of December. Each examination will extend over four days.

Any person whose name is on the Medical Register is admissible as a candidate to the examination provided

(I.) that a period of not less than 12 months has elapsed between his attainment of a registrable qualification and his admission to the examination;

(II.) that he produce evidence, satisfactory to the Syndicate, that he has diligently studied Pathology (including parasitology and bacteriology) in relation to Tropical Diseases, Clinical Medicine, and Surgery at a Hospital for Tropical Diseases, and Hygiene and Methods of Sanitation applicable to Tropical Climates. As evidence of study and attainments a candidate may present to the Syndicate (1) any dissertation, memoir, or other record of work carried out by himself on a subject connected with Tropical Medicine or Hygiene; (2) any Certificate or Diploma in Public Health or Sanitary Science he may have obtained from a recognised Examining Body. Such evidence will be considered by the Syndicate in determining whether he is qualified for admission to the examination and by the examiners in determining whether, if admitted, he shall be included in the list of successful candidates.

The examination will be partly in writing, partly oral, and partly practical and clinical (the clinical part will be conducted at a hospital for tropical diseases, at which cases will be submitted for diagnosis and comment), and will have reference to the nature, incidence, prevention, and treatment of the epidemic and other diseases prevalent in tropical countries. Every candidate who passes the examination to the satisfaction of the examiners will receive from the University a diploma (D.T.M.&H.) testifying to his knowledge and skill in tropical medicine and hygiene.

The fee for the examination is £9 9s., and applications should be addressed to Dr. Graham-Smith, Medical Schools, Cambridge.

University of London. – The MD degree may be taken in tropical medicine at an examination held twice annually, for which a thesis may be submitted.

University of Liverpool. – The University grants a Diploma in Tropical Medicine. At the end of each full course an examination is held by the University for its Diploma of Tropical Medicine (DTM), which is open only to those who have been through the course of instruction of the school. The subjects of examination are (a) Tropical Pathology, Parasitology and Entomology; (b) Tropical and Applied Bacteriology;

(c) Tropical Hygiene and Sanitation; (d) Tropical Medicine, including Aetiology, Symptoms, Diagnosis, and Treatment of Tropical Diseases. The advanced course consists entirely of Practical and Clinical Laboratory Work, given at the laboratory at the University. The fee for the full course of instruction is £21, with an extra charge of 10s. 6d. for the use of a microscope if required. Applications should be made to the Dean of the Medical Faculty, University of Liverpool. Two University Fellowships of £100 a year each are open to students of the school, amongst others. Accommodation for research work is to be had at the University Laboratory. The Mary Kingsley Medal is awarded by the school for distinguished work in connexion with Tropical Medicine.

Conjoint Board RCP Lond, RCS Eng. – The diploma of D.T.M. & H. Eng. is awarded on the results of an examination held thrice yearly in January, April, and July. Candidates must possess a registrable qualification, and produce evidence of having attended (1) practical instruction in pathology, protozoology, helminthology, entomology, bacteriology, and hygiene in relation to tropical medicine in a recognised institution during not less than three months, (2) clinical practice of a recognised hospital for the same period. Conditions of study may be modified in the case of candidates of special experience. Fee for admission to the examination, £9 9s., 14 days' notice of entry to the Secretary, Examination Hall, Queen-square, London, WC1.

A medical career in the tropics

Unquestionably, *research* into tropical diseases dominated much thought at this time. However, a suitable training and career structure were clearly important and this was emphasised by Balfour in a lecture to the International Continuation Course of the League of Nations in 1927[23]. Balfour also addressed the subject of the possibilities for women in medical service abroad, in an address to the students of the London (Royal Free Hospital) School of Medicine on 1 October 1928[24]. The work open to them (he concluded) could be summarized as follows: (i) the Women's Medical Service for India; (ii) mission hospitals; (iii) private practice; (iv) public health work; and in addition there were 'a few other openings, including research posts.' He seemed however, to have undoubted reservations about the role of women in the latter! What to do if one had a tropical qualification and wished to work in the tropics was later addressed (in 1937) by R T Leiper, Professor of Helminthology in the University of London[25]:

It is natural, and indeed inevitable, that most medical graduates should seek to make their future careers in this country; either in general practice or in whole-time medical service under the State in one form or another. If I may use a motoring simile they take the broad trunk road and they have

227

their security. But while its surface is smooth it is becoming increasingly crowded, the pace is slower, and the journey more monotonous and exasperating. There are, however, secondary roads and by-paths which, leading to the same destination, enable one to make a quieter journey and enjoy a wider horizon. As it has been my lot to make my own professional life's journey along one of these by-paths of medicine, I should like to tell you something about it. Although in recent years it has become a good secondary road, it has increased, rather than lost, its original attraction; for the road has become smoother and the prospects widened. This is the road which runs through the tropics.

It is necessary first to stress the fact that nowadays overseas work is no hazardous adventure. The amenities of life in the tropics have greatly improved. Indeed medical science has transformed them during the last quarter of a century. "White man's grave" is an almost forgotten epithet for West Africa. . . .

The type of Englishman acceptable to-day in our sphere of life in the tropics is the good all-round man with a sound body, a sound mind, and a good record – a good mixer of the social, not the alcoholic type. For persons with poor nervous outfits, the tropical climate and environment are particularly unsuited.

In this survey of career prospects, Leiper identified 5 main categories of medical service in the tropics:

(i) The Indian Medical Service,
(ii) the Colonial Medical Service,
(iii) independent private practice,
(iv) subsidised private practice,
and (v) medical service with big commercial and industrial corporations – which we may call the Unofficial Medical Service.

And he concluded with a few reflections on everyday life in the tropics:

So much then for the professional aspects. But what of life in these tropical lands?

Strangely enough, it is the fear of heat and not of disease which is often the chief deterrent from a tropical career. Yet I personally know of no one who has left the tropics on that account. The summer heat of London can be more trying than that of Central Africa, where dress and mode of living are more suitably adjusted to climatic conditions.

Even in small communities games and amusements are organised, and there is far more frequent and general participation in them than at home; for there is a pressing sense of need to compensate for enforced banishment and the severance of home ties. Usually there are tennis and golf and in many places cricket, football, hockey, polo, and racing. The club, with its rooms for billiards, cards, and dancing, is the chief social centre. Dinner provides more frequent occasions for the exchange of hospitality than here. Wireless brings news and music; open-air cinemas are springing up in many places. If there is abundant rain or where water is available, a garden can be made as deeply satisfying as at home. In many districts there are opportunities for sport and in some for big game shooting. In all these social activities the doctor shares as fully as the other members of the community. He has few night calls and work ceases early, for the afternoons are hot and night falls suddenly at, or soon after, six o'clock.

But if these English pastimes become the sole relaxation they are merely anodynes. There are many serious interests with which to fill leisure hours. All around are strange and fascinating subjects for study: local dialects, customs and legends, native medical lore, bird watching for European migrants, and other aspects of fauna and flora. Perhaps more fascinating than these: native psychology, and the effects of the impact of European civilisation upon it, with all its unplombable potentialities. If in the past there had been better understanding of native motives, many errors, involving heavy loss of European and native life, misunderstanding, and bitterness could have been avoided . . .

Health hazards of the tropics

During the 1920s the health problems facing the expatriate in the tropics still received a great deal of attention, and a few solutions were to hand; certainly much was being written on this topic. In 1924, *The Lancet* carried a first leader 'The curse of the tropics'[26]; the main thrust of this account related to the British Empire Exhibition held at Wembley that year. While extolling the fascination of the tropics to several groups of individuals, some of the potential disadvantages were brought to the fore.

> . . . Altogether tropical medicine is an amazing business, and most of it has been crowded into the last 30 years. But it would be a mistake to view the exhibits at Wembley merely in the light of an historical pageant. The burden of which we have spoken still exists, doubtless infinitely lighter than of yore, but for all that pressing heavily on many of our tropical possessions. Blessed in many respects the tropics have their disabilities. From the European stand-point the climate is trying, exhausting, sometimes almost unbearable, there is often an acute sense of isolation; the surroundings are frequently irritating, monotony may make for melancholy, the molehill with marvellous celerity becomes the mountain. Yet, excepting possibly climate in some of its aspects, all these trials and troubles sink into insignificance compared with the presence of disease. Disease is the true curse of the tropics: it militates against their conquest by man and has in the past defeated him time and again. In the old records it is strange to read how men groped in darkness, attributing tropical maladies, as, for example, malaria and yellow fever, to all kinds of causes – miasmata from marshes, effluvia from decomposing material,

atmospheric disturbances, and even to celestial displays like comets. It is, moreover, pitiful to note how, when someone more enterprising or enlightened than his fellows, a SUSRUTU, a RUSH, a NOTT, a BLAIR, a BEAUPERTHUY, a FINLAY, or a KING, advanced a theory which we now know approached the truth, little or no notice was taken of his hypothesis, and when it was not actually ridiculed it was soon relegated to the limbo of forgotten things.

These men were in advance of their times, and it was not until new conceptions on protozoology and entomology had been evolved, and the microscope and the laboratory had begun to take a serious part in the fray, that any real progress was forthcoming. Once, however, LAVERAN and MANSON had led the way, the path in respect of malaria was open for ROSS to commence his brilliant and unforgettable researches; open in one sense, but beset with difficulties and obstacles in another, for he, like others before and after him, was the victim of official stupidity and neglect. The Italians played their great part, and the mystery of malaria transmission was solved. As a direct result the Americans grappled with the problem of yellow fever, and with the loss of some valuable lives wrested the secret which "Yellow Jack" had for so long managed to conceal. But the Americans went farther. They realised and appreciated the great opportunity vouchsafed to them, and, fired by that idealism which so often spells success, they set out to obliterate the disease altogether. What is more, they have well-nigh succeeded, and the burden of yellow fever has been almost lifted from the New World. Yet on the African West Coast the disease still lingers and flares out at intervals, while apathy and a false economy tolerate the presence of its mosquito vector. At the same time it may be admitted that the problem on the eastern side of the Atlantic is in some respects different to that upon the western, so that an equitable comparison cannot easily be drawn. Meanwhile malaria still remains the second or third great killing disease of the world, dysentery slays outright or makes miserable wrecks of men and women, cholera sweeps away the unwary, plague claims its victims in thousands and hampers commerce, ankylostomiasis saps the energy of native labour, leprosy makes pariahs and outcasts of hapless sufferers, and sleeping sickness, far from asleep, takes toll of the African negro. Yet in every instance we know the why and the wherefore of these maladies, and to a very large extent could and should extend our mastery over them. In many cases a great deal has been accomplished – how much no one can say who has not made a study of the past with its truly appalling records, who has not read of veritable armies of men disappearing as the result of epidemics, of thousands of young and promising lives cut short on the threshold of the tropics, of the crippled beings, a mere remnant of those who had sallied forth, returning from India and elsewhere with ruined constitutions, a burden to themselves and to their country. The wonder is that any survived, and that acquired immunity can be such a potent force as it has proved itself to be. It would, however, be a bad business if we had still to rely upon acquired immunity;

and, though it will continue to play its part, its beneficent action must be reinforced by measures based on a sound knowledge of tropical pathology. In certain directions there is good cause for especial satisfaction. New light has been thrown upon plague by NORMAN WHITE; leprosy, thanks to SIR LEONARD ROGERS, is to be attacked upon a scale never hitherto attempted, the parasites of ankylostomiasis and sleeping sickness are being countered by new and surprisingly effective remedies, leishmaniasis is controlled by tartar emetic, yaws has been conquered by the organic arsenicals and bismuth, and schistosomiasis has yielded to antimony and emetine.

So far so good, but in other directions the outlook is somewhat depressing. Malaria in many places still defies us, largely because we do not take it seriously and spend enough upon its suppression; dysentery in its chronic form remains an enigma as far as treatment goes; the epidemiology of cholera eludes us, while in many hygienic directions our tropical possessions lag behind the times and pay a corresponding penalty. Let us then welcome the Tropical Health Section at Wembley. It should excite interest and create enthusiasm. Not only does it furnish information regarding the cause, nature, and treatment of many tropical diseases, but it shows, by models and otherwise, how we have learned to safeguard the public health in those lands beyond the sea. In this all-important and humanitarian work men of our race and lineage have played a notable and a noble part, and it is fitting that in the great display of the Empire's resources there should be emphasised those disease factors which exercise a malign influence upon those resources and their exploitation. We welcome this record – a fascinating record – of what has been accomplished by the combined efforts of the clinician, the laboratory worker, and the hygienist.

A detailed description of the exhibition 'Health in the tropics' was provided in two subsequent articles[27,28]. But most interest undoubtedly still lay not in the health of the indigenous populations, but in that of the 'white man'. One example is the following letter entitled 'White men and work in the tropics'[29]:

To the Editor of THE LANCET.

SIR, – In the *Archiv für Schiffs- und Tropen-Hygiene* (vol. xxvii., 5, p. 177) [*sic*] Dr. H. W. Knipping, of the Physiological Institute of the University of Hamburg, discusses the heat regulation of the human body in the tropics, inquiring whether white workmen, who suffer more often from heat-stroke than do natives, have greater difficulty than these others in adjusting themselves to tropical conditions. He shows that after numerous investigations by many men, there has been found no material difference in the heat-regulating mechanisms of these two classes, though coloured men have probably more sweat glands and larger cutaneous capillaries. The great reducer of temperature is perspiration, but that does not help as it might unless there is a sufficient current of dry enough air to evaporate the sweat secreted. As an example of the absolutely worst place in which to work in the tropics he takes a boiler-room (furnace-room, stokehold) in the Red Sea, and observes that there, with a temperature of 49° C. (120° F.) and a relative humidity of 88 per cent., men drank, in a four hours' watch, 5 litres, and that 2 ½ litres were to be evaporated through lungs and skin. Probably this means that 2 ½ litres of urine were passed, but that is not directly stated. To evaporate this 2 ½ litres, 1343 calories are claimed as necessary, and 300–400 cubic metres (10,000–14,000 cub. ft.) of air at this humidity to carry this vapour away. There was not enough air supplied, so the men's temperature rose; sometimes he found it as high as 38.8° C. (101.8° F.). Even here it was not men in good health who took care of themselves who got heat-stroke. Coloured firemen escape because they do not work so hard; they do rarely more than half a white man's task. Their modest demands on life are satisfied with less exertion. The white man trying to work in the tropics as he could and did in the temperate zone exposes himself to a great risk. Dr. Knipping reaches the conclusion that, for any climate, the maximum safe output of work is a function of the drying power of the air, in relation to the temperature of the atmosphere and its rate of movement.

A very important question in reference to colonisation is raised by this communication.

I am, Sir, yours faithfully,
R.N.

Physiological acclimatisation to heat remained a topical subject for some years[30]. But adaptation in a wider sense was addressed later that year[31]:

In presenting the play "White Cargo," which is now being performed in London, the author, Leon Gordon, states that he has made no conscious effort to create or eliminate sensationalism, but has attempted to portray the struggle for development in a country which steadily defies the encroaching civilisation, and where the reaction of an ever-shining sun breeds inevitable rot – a rot which penetrates not only the vegetation and inanimate objects, but the minds and hearts of the white men who attempt to conquer it. The symptoms of mental and physical decadence produced by residence in a hot and malarious district are, indeed, well reproduced. Acclimatisation in such an isolated and unhealthy area may mean simply mental and physical deterioration. A treatise, published recently by a French author, reaches a similar conclusion as regards physique and morale in the tropical French colonies. He states that sojourners in the French tropics compare unfavourably with those in the British tropics, the chief reason being the lack of active exercise in the former. The Britisher plays games regularly all the year round, whereas the French colonist leads a uniform sedentary life. Possibly the Britisher is nearer to true acclimatisation thereby.

Perhaps in its most exact meaning acclimatisation is the process of becoming accustomed to a new climate and its conditions, with maintenance of full physical and mental vigour. The main difficulties in the way of acclimatisation in the tropics are evil influences of climate per se, parasites, unhygienic conditions, altered habits of life, altered social states, sedentary routine, over-indulgence in food, and last but not least, alcohol. Many have seen the tableaux in the Tropical Health section housed in the pavilion of His Majesty's Government at Wembley. These demonstrate how, by human effort intelligently directed, the "white man's grave" of 25 years ago has become a centre of health and prosperity. Indeed, there exist some tropical cities from which all the opposing influences enumerated, with the exception of climate, have been eradicated, at least in so far as some white men are concerned. Having reached this advanced state of sanitary and moral excellence, are we in a position to say that these white men have become fully acclimatised in the sense defined above? Judging from the evidence reviewed recently by such authorities as Prof. van Eijkman and Dr. Andrew Balfour, the answer must be No. In spite of our success in stamping out malarial and such-like parasites, and in introducing all kinds of outdoor and indoor exercise and other healthy recreation, there still remains the depressing effect on the nervous system with its states of exhaustion and psychical irritability, for which the only cure is a prolonged vacation in a temperate clime. Possibly we are now just beginning to see clearly these effects on the efficiency and nervous mechanisms of the white man, because formerly such symptoms were masked by concomitant tropical disease due to known bacteria and parasites. Very probably these nervous effects are due to continuous heat, although we must not forget the possibility of an unknown bacterial or parasitical agent. At present it would appear that brain-work, with its more sedentary and indoor conditions, leads sooner to nervous symptoms than an outdoor occupation such as planting. It is only by a clear understanding of the present position that we shall make any real advance towards maintaining our fellow countrymen in the tropics in the full mental and physical vigour to which they have been accustomed at home, and which alone spells content to the white man.

The condition 'tropical neurasthenia' was given in-depth attention at a meeting held at the Royal Society of Medicine in 1933[32]; this prompted an annotation[33]:

Most of the speakers in [this] discussion . . . had lived in the tropics, but most of them are now living in London. The verdict of men on the spot might have been less favourable to a tropical life, and in face of breakdown they might be disposed to lay more emphasis on faults of environment and less on faults of personality. For example, in the December issue of the *Malayan Medical Journal* Mr. Kenneth Black, professor of surgery at Singapore, writes with envious enthusiasm of the benefits of a temperate climate. Times, as he says, may change, and in another 1000 years the belt of optimum climate may have shifted to Egypt and Mesopotamia. Meanwhile, however, Europeans who leave England for the tropics must expect a physical and mental deterioration which occurs independently of the onslaughts of disease, and is observed even in countries, such as Malaya, where the incidence of tropical infections among Europeans in comparatively low. Evidence of such deterioration was collected by Dr. G. H. Garlick, who, in reporting on the Colonial Survey Station making a topographical survey of Johore, stated that the graph showing the area surveyed per white man per month rose steeply at the beginning, as the man became accustomed to his work, maintained a steady level until he had been working for two and a half years, and then showed an equally steady decline until he was relieved at the end of his third year. Mental deterioration cannot be demonstrated so neatly, but it is significant that out of the total number of European government officials sent home on sick leave from the Dutch East Indies, the numbers suffering from neuroses and psychoses during the past 12 years have averaged just over 50 per cent. Prof. Black falls into line with speakers at the Royal Society of Medicine when he wonders how far this high incidence of nervous disorder is due to lack of training for self-control. Missionaries rarely get 'nerves,' he says, and he goes on to quote a medical authority experienced in examining people from the tropics who said that he never found neuroses in those who were really keen on their work. At the same time he urges that in Malaya three years should be the maximum tour of service for white people if they wish to keep their efficiency, mental equilibrium, and alertness. The editor of the *Malayan Medical Journal* remarks in comment that 'the pendulum of lay opinion appears to be swinging from the former unjust extreme of referring to certain tropical countries as deathtraps to the other no less erroneous extreme of now regarding the same parts as health resorts.'

Diet too, was the source of a great deal of interest[34]:

During his long service in the Navy Sir P. W. Bassett-Smith had constantly to deal with the practical application of dietetic principles and the fruits of his experience are manifest in an address which has now been reprinted. Just as in civil life the ultimate result of a deficient dietary is to produce civil disobedience and political unrest, so, in former times, bad rations fomented open mutiny in the Navy, as in the reign of George III. In the tropics the maintenance of a balance between the intake and output of heat should be the main consideration underlying the dietary, so that the ration supplied to naval ratings in the Persian Gulf has to be based upon a different scale from that supplied in more temperate climes. The value of protein in the dietary should depend largely upon the amount and kind of amino-acids which it contains, two only of which – tryptophane and lysine – appear to be indispensable for life. The greater the similarity of the protein supplied to the tissues, the higher is its value; hence the biological protein value of meat and milk is three to four times as great as that of maize. In the tropics people tend to rely more particularly upon one kind of food – e.g., rice, maize, bananas, manioc, figs, or dates – for the maintenance of life, and this very dependence on one particular product tends to produce, in times of scarcity, malnutrition and susceptibility to disease. The lecturer showed how the dietaries of the several navies when compared showed considerable variations, those of the United States giving the highest caloric value, the French and Japanese showing much lower fat values than those of the British and Americans, more in conformity with tropical conditions. Tropical heat has a depressing action upon many physiological processes, lessening the respiration rate, and with it the absorption of oxygen and the excretion of carbonic acid, resulting in retention within the body of CO_2 with production of glycosuria and acidosis. In addition to the basic supply of protein, fats, carbohydrates, and salts, accessory food substances – the vitamins – or "food hormones" are essential to health. Sir P. W. Bassett-Smith concluded by directing attention to the experiments on guinea-pigs which showed that animals fed on a diet rich in vitamins, such as marmite, exhibited an enhanced resistance to tuberculous infection as compared with a control series fed on a normal dietary.

And practical advice was given on details of a correct diet whilst living in the tropics[35]:

. . . taking food also raises temperature, especially protein food; fats and carbohydrates exert less effect, and can be stored if taken in excess of immediate requirement. Proteins break up into amino-acids which, circulating in the blood, stimulate the tissues to increased metabolism, so raising the temperature of the body; this is their specific dynamic action. Since they cannot be stored, any excess taken in must be at once further broken down, whereby temperature is still further raised. Dr. Kipping [sic] [the author cited in reference 29] concludes that in the tropics, proteins should be taken only sparingly during the hotter part of the day, the main protein meal being arranged to occur in the cooler evening. Where fruits are plentiful, the need for vitamins is supplied. Protein is more of a difficulty; 100 g., according to Voit, are required daily, but to get that from rice, for example, would compel the eating of five pounds daily, with a total caloric value of 5400, or about double what is required. The protein must not be supplied from a single source, as the right proportions of cystin, tyrosin, tryptophane, and the like, do not exist in every food. As to cellulose, Dr. Kipping holds strongly that there must be in the food some element, bulky, unabsorbable, and yet unirritating, to increase the mass of the intestinal contents and, by assisting peristalsis, to prevent constipation. This cellulose is easily obtained from fruits, salads and bread made from coarse flour. After this evening protein meal, the office-worker can be quiet in a long chair, not further raising by muscular activity his temperature, already slightly raised by digestion. In Java, Dr. Kipping tells us, doctors not vegetarians in principle took to living exclusively on vegetable food.

CHRONIC DYSENTERY AND COLITIS.

(Low Starch, Low residue diet).

Diet for one month during convalescence after leaving Hospital.

The following articles of diet are <u>not permitted</u>.

Potatoes.
Cheese.
White Bread.
Fats : meat-fat, bacon-fat.
Rich sauces.
Rich cakes.
Pastry.
Pickles.
All shell-fish.
Coarse fruit and vegetables, *i.e.*, turnips, carrots and cabbage.

Commoner articles of diet <u>permitted</u>.

Milk.
Eggs.
White fish—haddock, plaice, sole, cod and whiting. (If the fish is fried remove outer skin.)
Chicken, roast or boiled.
Game, rabbit, pigeon.
Grilled liver and kidneys.
Lean beef, mutton, ham, tripe and sweetbreads—for lunch only.
Toast, rusks, brown bread.
Jams, jellies, plain marmalade.
Plain milk puddings (with the exception of rice pudding), milk jellies, junket and custard.
Stewed fruit, apples and pears. Baked apples.
Grapes, orange juice, grape-fruit juice, bananas.

Beverages.

No alcohol (including beer and stout), for one month. Lemonade, ginger beer, etc., permitted.
Tea and coffee.

General Instructions.

Avoid over-exertion and over-fatigue. Dress warmly, change clothes immediately if damp or wet. No cold baths, or outdoor bathing allowed.
Live as simply as possible.

H.T.D./B.

Fig 9.2: A diet-sheet for a patient suffering from 'chronic dysentery' (whilst undergoing treatment at the HTD) - in 1925.

He puts forward himself the following scheme for food for a tropical day – Breakfast: tea or coffee, bread, butter, jam, pineapple or banana fritters, fruit. At midday: rice (not too much) with vegetables, salads, a little fish, fowl, or egg; all to be nicely cooked, but taken in small quantity. In the evening comes the main meat meal. The moral of Dr. Kipping's articles may be put briefly: Self-denial at lunch will keep you cooler through the afternoon.

Incidentally, it was not only in the tropics that a correct diet was considered important. Fig 9.2 shows a diet sheet used at the HTD, for a patient suffering from 'chronic dysentery'. An overview of the problems and hazards of living in the tropics was well summarized[36]:

The experiences of one who has not only travelled widely in the tropics but has worked there as an active investigator of local diseases can hardly fail to be of interest. Dr. [Alfred] Torrance [*Tracking Down the Enemies of Man*. London: Alfred A Knopf. 1929. Pp. 319. 7s. 6d.] describes his African and Asian journeys and supplies maps to show the routes taken. In Africa, he passed from Angola to Mombassa in the middle south, and in the middle north, from Kenya to Gambia; while in Asia he sampled Burma, Annam, Siam, Malay States, Sumatra, and Borneo. His book is addressed rather to the laity than to the medical profession, and he deserves congratulation on the simplicity and freedom from technicalities of his accounts of tropical diseases such as malaria, yellow fever, trypanosomiasis, relapsing fever, dengue, and cholera. He gives the history of the curative measures adopted for each at different times. These medical details are interwoven with tales of big game, native dances and other adventures, some of which are exciting enough. Those who like swatting flies will appreciate his notes on "man-handling the mosquito." The first chapter, in defence of the big jungle beasts, points the moral that, dangerous as these may be, they are no more dangerous than the insect perils that beset all travellers in the tropics. A useful table of the more important tropical forces, their transmitter, geographical distribution, and diagnosis completes a book which those meditating a sojourn in the tropics might well read before they start.

However, the health of the indigenous inhabitants of the Colonial Empire did not completely escape attention[37]:

The material betterment of the conditions of native races is the aim which inspired Prof. Blacklock to write an essay on the house and village in the tropics. [*An Empire Problem: The House and Village in the Tropics*. D.B. Blacklock, M.D., Professor of Parasitology, Liverpool School of Tropical Medicine, the University of Liverpool. The University Press of Liverpool. London: Hodder and Stoughton, Ltd. 1932. Pp. 100. 3s. 6d.] He is anxious to create and maintain public interest in the development

237

of the tropics, and suggests that an annual exhibition in London, where the existing village defects of various tropical countries could be fully demonstrated on the model of the Ideal Home Exhibition, would be a useful method of propaganda. In this book he does not deal only with housing, but discusses the growth of tropical medicine, the staffing of hospitals and medical services in the tropics, and the relation of tropical medicine to trade.

A section is devoted to a consideration of the native house and its attendant parasites, the jigger, the flea, the Tumbu fly, the Congo floor maggot, and various species of tick and bed-bug. The parasites which infest the roof (rats, ants, and other insects) are also considered, and the water-supply, which may convey cholera, typhoid, both forms of dysentery, ankylostomiasis, bilharziasis, or the Guinea worm.

This useful little work closes with a popular account of malaria, elephantiasis, sleeping sickness, and other filarial diseases. An entertaining chapter concerns the skin of the native child who, from the hour of its birth upwards, is subjected to a perpetual series of injuries and pin-pricks of every kind; this is an aspect of medicine to which too little attention has so far been paid. It would be interesting to pursue this study on psychological lines; such questions as the effect of the darkness of the tropical village, and of the impossibility of obtaining mental relaxation during the long hours of the night, are worth consideration. It is small wonder that the African often becomes a prey to the native magician. Those who intend to live in tropical Africa will do well to read this book, and even old-established residents there will find in it a fresh point of view.

An interesting concept which formed the basis of a Chadwick lecture by Professor Blacklock as recently as 1935 was that certain houses in rural areas of the tropics encourage disease, eg malaria houses, blackwater-fever houses, yellow-fever houses, and others which gave rise to relapsing-fever, plague, typhus and kala-azar[38]. Of Kala-azar, he wrote:

. . . Dodds Price and [Sir Leonard] Rogers (1914) said:
'The facts collected having established that the infection clung to the houses or their sites, this sufficed to enable us to evolve a simple plan of dealing effectually with the epidemic which was ravaging the Nowgong district and ruining its chief industry.' Coolies in new lines, only 400 yards from the old ones, had remained free from kala-azar for 16 years, whereas of 50 coolies of the same batch who had lived in the old infected lines for want of room in the new ones, no fewer than 16 per cent. were already dead of kala-azar, while others were suffering from the disease. Rogers (1905) records how some native peoples realised the infectiousness of kala-azar, and mentions an effective sanitary measure adopted by the Garos; they isolated cases of kala-azar in their huts, rendered them

comatose with drink, and then burnt the hut and patient together. Dodds Price (1902), commenting on his nine years' supervision of kala-azar in Assam, said that segregation of the sick was of the utmost importance, and where coolie lines were badly infected they must be burnt and abandoned at all cost; and that the results he obtained by adopting these measures were gratifying in the extreme.

He concluded:

... Although much evidence of association with the house has accumulated since Dodds Price's time, it is not yet possible to assign accurately the reasons for this connexion, owing to the fact that the method of transmission is still in doubt. We are therefore unable to convict either the method of construction or the material, or the site, or even the habits of the inmates as being the predominant factors against which preventive measures should be directed. The discovery of the value of segregation of the healthy might equally well incriminate faulty structure or material, some peculiarity in the site, or in the habits of the inmates – including in this last item over-crowding and close contact with infected cases.

The emergent London School of Hygiene and Tropical Medicine (LSHTM)

The origin and early years of the LSHTM are the subject of chapter 10. On 1 August 1924 the LSTM in effect became merged into the new institution[39]. Some of the background is to be found in the proceedings of a presentation ceremony (of a rose bowl) for Dr Andrew Balfour (Plate 52), who had been appointed Director of this new institution, in 1926; in his speech, Professor R T Hewlett had this to say[40]:

... Some of us of the old London School of Tropical Medicine, so successful in the past under the aegis of the Seamen's Hospital Society, to whom a warm tribute ought to be paid for their wisdom and foresight in undertaking so desirable, though at the same time so great, a venture, some of us of the old Tropical School may feel some regret at its disappearance as a separate entity, for believe me under the inspiration and leadership of Sir Patrick Manson we throve wonderfully and were a very happy family. But all of us, I think, agree that the incorporation of the Tropical School in the new School of Hygiene was a right and proper step, and we in particular, members of the old Tropical School, welcome your appointment as Director because we believe that the great Mansonian tradition will be worthily maintained in your hands as regards the tropical side of the School's activities.

As regards other activities of the School, in your hands, too, we may rest assured that they will be in equally safe keeping. The physical side of health training certainly will, for have you not won, if not spurs, at least many hacks and bruises on university and international football fields? You have experience of public health administration, you have travelled widely and have a broad outlook on health problems, you are a research worker and know the importance of a live school combining teaching with research. When I look at the list of decorations and degrees you have acquired, of the prizes you have won, of the appointments you have held, of the campaigns in which you have taken part, and of the committees upon which you have served, I begin to ask myself: Has Scotland produced only *one* Admiral Crichton?

Moreover, by your silver speech and ready pen you do much for the School. Was not the last named (your ready pen) partially trained in the realm of romantic fiction? We may be sure you will not be "Cashiered," may we hope that your course may be a smooth one, not determined 'By Stroke of Sword' nor recourse 'To Arms,' and that in your present post you have in some degree entered into 'The Golden Kingdom'. . .

And so the permanent separation of the School (of Hygiene) and Hospital had begun, a development which was perhaps to benefit the new school, but did very little for the *clinical* discipline! Although this is what in fact happened, it was not the outcome which many envisaged at the time[41]. The Education Committee of the Board of Management of the LSHTM set up, in 1925, a Hospital Sub-committee to look into 'the future needs of the School in regard to Hospital provision'. At the first meeting on 23 September 1925, Sir James Michelli pointed out that the SHS Hospital was being maintained in large part to provide adequate facilities for the School until other arrangements were made. As a result of this, the Sub-Committee decided to prepare an outline of accommodation required for a new hospital, and in 1926, it recommended that the committee should remain in being to advise a committee which the Minister of Health was expected to set up[41]. On 28 July, 1926, a meeting of the Board of Management was held with Sir Cooper Perry in the chair; the minutes state that:

> After careful consideration of the powers of the Board under the Charter, and while recognising that it was not the Board's ultimate intention itself to erect a hospital, it was decided on grounds of urgency to authorise the Finance Committee (or during the vacation the Chairman of the Finance Committee) – (a) To instruct Mr. Walford to negotiate on behalf of the School with the Bedford Office for the purchase of one of the alternative Malet Street sites which had been the subject of correspondence (the one to the south with a frontage to Keppel Street being preferred) – and (b) to pay the necessary deposit subject to an adequate term being granted for the completion of the purchase.

There is no specific mention as to where the money would come from, either for the erection or indeed the maintenance of the hospital, but it was expected that the Minister of Health's Committee would enquire from the Rockefeller Trustees and others as to the possibility of raising funds[41]. Apparently the sum offered to the trustees of the Bedford Estate was not accepted and it was decided at a further Board Meeting not to increase the offer unless the Bedford Office should receive a better offer and consider parting with the site, whereupon 'the Treasurer should use his discretion in making an increased offer'.

When the Board of Management met on 24 November, 1926, Sir Alfred Mond, who was in the chair, said that 'as a matter of business he deprecated the locking up of funds, which might be required at short notice for building contracts, in a site which might not prove readily saleable.' He said further that he thought it premature for the Board to purchase a site before the Minister of Health's Committee had even begun to consider the question and moved that the negotiations for the purchase of the Malet Street site should be stopped: this motion was carried[41].

In their fourth Annual Report to the Court of Governors for 1927–28 the Board of Management recalled that the Committee appointed by the Minister to study 'the hospital question' came into being because the SHS had declared their intention of closing the hospital in Endsleigh Gardens. It was then mentioned in the Report that the Society had now informed the Minister that they were no longer going to close down the hospital at Endsleigh Gardens. As a result of this the Minister decided that the time was inappropriate for adopting the recommendations of the Committee which he had appointed[41].

The withdrawal of their application for a hospital site in Bloomsbury was made to the University after the Board of Management meeting held on 13 June, 1928; this was a sad day for *clinical* tropical medicine!

10

The London School of Hygiene and Tropical Medicine, and the Ross Institute and Hospital for Tropical Diseases

In 1922, the Rockefeller Foundation promised financial support towards a new School of Hygiene; the establishment of such an institution had been recommended in the 'Athlone Report'[1,2] which resulted from the deliberations of the Post-Graduate Medical Education Committee – chaired by the Earl of Athlone (1874–1957) – set up by the Minister of Health, Dr Addison, in 1921. The committee's brief was to 'investigate the needs of medical practitioners and other graduates for further education in medicine in London, and to submit proposals for a practicable scheme for meeting them.' The other members of the committee were: Sir George Newman (the first Chief Medical Officer), Sir Walter Fletcher (first Secretary of the Medical Research Committee), Sir Herbert Read, Sir John Rose Bradford, Sir Wilmot Herringham, and Sir Cooper Perry. In fact, the proposals contained in the Athlone Report were principally concerned with the setting up of an Institute of State Medicine which would be attached to the University of London (whose sole functions for 65 years had been to examine and award degrees[2]); tropical medicine was barely mentioned[1]. The Institute was to unify the various courses in *public health* under one roof; forensic medicine, toxicology, industrial medicine and medical ethics should all be subjects of postgraduate courses[3]. This Institute would fulfil part of the Committee's overall recommendations for the development of postgraduate medical education in London in general.

The Rockefeller Foundation (whose motto is 'the wellbeing of mankind throughout the world') was a great philanthropic organisation in health promotion; this was largely a consequence of concern for education in the southern United States and the deleterious effect of ancylostomiasis (hookworm disease) on childrens' learning ability[2]. In August 1913, the

Secretaries of State for India and for the Colonies dined with Wickliffe Rose (who was in charge of the Rockefellers' anti-hookworm campaigns in the American south, and was the Administrative Secretary of the Rockefeller Foundation's International Health Board); this had been arranged by the US Ambassador in London. In addition to establishing a School of Hygiene and Public Health at John Hopkins University, part of Rose's remit was to 'organise the English-Colonies hookworm service'. [Exactly how the 'Colonists' viewed this altruistic endeavour is not recorded.]

Manson-Bahr has summarized this and subsequent events[1]: in 1913 'the Rockefeller Foundation was grappling with its 'hookworm campaign', the target being the total eradication of this disease, which it was felt would improve labour conditions and hence efficiency in tropical populations'. [This was in his view, an indirect catalyst for the foundation of the LSHTM.] The representative of the Rockefeller Foundation, Rose, was in correspondence with the Colonial Office, and was referred to Dr (later Sir) Arthur Bagshawe, Director of the Tropical Diseases Bureau. However, the matter was left in abeyance during the war years (1914–18)[1]. By 1919 Rose had established firm links with R T Leiper (Professor of Helminthology at the LSTM)[2]. Details of subsequent non-productive negotiations and the complex political machinations of Rose and the senior administrators in London have been summarised[2]. In 1921 Leiper (now the 'go-between') (Plate 53) was engaged in some research on filariasis in British Guiana; whilst there he became acquainted with the Athlone Report, and having read it proceeded to New York where he again met Rose to furnish him with more facts. Shortly afterwards Rose made a 3-week visit to London as the representative of the Rockefeller Foundation; here he met the executive members of the Athlone Committee – including Sir George Newman – and offered $2 million [approximately £450,000] to the Ministry of Health to establish an Institute of State Health as part of a new School which must include Hygiene[1]. In fact the letter Rose and G H Vincent (president of the Foundation) drafted on 8 February 1922 for Sir Alfred Mond (Minister of Health) to present to the Cabinet stated: 'the Trustees have no doubt that such a school . . . would also become a centre of world-wide influence in the encouragement of research and the training of public health personnel . . . The functions of the school would be primarily educational, but . . . its scope would be the maintenance of health and the prevention of disease in their widest application, not only in temperate but tropical climates.' Therefore, the distinction between foreign and domestic objectives had become obscured[2]. The resultant institution would later become the London School of Hygiene and Tropical Medicine (LSHTM)[4]. Leiper and Wickliffe Rose thus became, in effect, the founders of the LSHTM.

[It is of interest that, in 1921, the LSTM had approached the SHS for a grant (capital = £2,170; annual = £1,200) to teach *tropical hygiene* – as recommended by Ross in 1912 (chapter 8) – but this had been rejected on the grounds of expense[5].] We are told that Manson, by then ageing in years, gave the scheme his blessing[1], although it is known that he had fought to keep his school independent[2]. Initially there was a good deal of doubt as to the scope of the services which the new School would provide; the *British Medical Journal*'s reporter considered[6]:

> It is intended that it shall be an imperial institute, prepared to receive post-graduate students in hygiene, not only from Great Britain, the Dominions and Colonies, and India, but from foreign countries also. It will therefore be necessary to provide class-rooms, lecture theatres, and research laboratories. To fulfil these conditions it will probably be considered desirable, when planning the building, to make provision for some 300 postgraduates. . . . London already possesses some of the elements of an Institute of Hygiene, and it is intended that the new institute shall be formed, in part at least, by entering into arrangements with existing institutions. Thus it is hoped that the London School of Tropical Medicine and Hygiene will become the Tropical Section of the Imperial Institute of Hygiene, and that the schools now giving courses for the diploma of Public Health will pool their resources within the new institute. It is intended, also, that the Lister Institute of Preventive Medicine shall be brought into intimate relation with the scheme, and it is hoped that it will undertake to provide facilities for teaching and research in certain departments.

The writer continued:

> the provision now to be made through the munificence of the Rockefeller Foundation is concerned with only one part of post-graduate instruction, which in London is greatly in need of better organization and larger resources. The words of Sir Clifford Allbutt seem appropriate to be recalled: 'A post-graduate scheme consisting of desultory side-shows will not continue to draw serious visitors. The visitor wants not cut flowers but a nursery garden. If students are to come to study medicine in England . . . there must be something large and creative for them to come to.' We can only express the hope that the country may before long be fortunate enough to witness the realization of the aspirations in this respect to which the Athlone Committee gave form if not substance.

On 18 October 1922, the Senate of the University of London ratified a 3-way agreement. The government would ask Parliament to grant £25,000 annually towards the expenses of the School, and the School would become semi-autonomous with its own Board of Management and Court of Governors; it would be recognised as a part of the Faculties of

Science and of Medicine of the University; it would 'negotiate with the SHS with a view to the union of the LSTM, and to make arrangements at their discretion for action in co-operation with other cognate institutions'[2].

On 6 November 1923, Dr Andrew Balfour was appointed Director of the new School (chapter 9) by Mr. Joynson Hicks, the Minister of Health. Also, Sir Havelock Charles succeeded Lovell as Dean. There were to be two foundation departments devoted to public health; Major Greenwood (of the Lister Institute) became Professor of Epidemiology and Vital Statistics, and W W C Topley became Professor of Bacteriology and Immunology[2]. While the new building was under construction – on a site previously intended for a national theatre[6,7] – the new departments were given temporary accommodation in various University buildings in the Bloomsbury area. In fact, the Royal Shakespeare Company very nearly had its home on this site, rather than at Stratford-on-Avon; the London Shakespeare League had begun fund raising to establish an 'adequate Shakespeare Memorial' on the site as early as 1904, and the Shakespeare Memorial Committee had acquired the site from the Duke of Bedford's estates in February 1914. However, it was sold in 1922 to Rose by Sir Carl Meyer, representing the Shakespeare Memorial Committee, for £52,000[7]. Rose wrote to Vincent that the site was preferable to Endsleigh Gardens, because it 'is also much more quiet – no freight traffic, no buses'[2]! The origin of the LSHTM actually dates back to 1 April 1924 when it was given a Royal Charter (of Incorporation); however, the physical (geographical) division between the School and the clinical facilities was not to take place until 1929 – when the new building at Keppel Street was completed. In 1924 the management of the LSTM was relinquished by the SHS, and it came under the sway of an interim Executive Committee. The administrative offices for the new school were opened in Malet Street in June 1924[1]. The origins of the LSHTM are summarized in *The Lancet* for 1925[8]:

> It was on August 1st, 1924, that the London School of Tropical Medicine became merged in the new London School of Hygiene and Tropical Medicine. At a meeting of the court of governors on Oct. 22nd some account was given of the present position and prospects of the school. The site for the new building is near the British Museum and has frontages on Keppel-street, Gower-street, and Malet-street. It was bought by the Ministry of Health in 1923 for £52,610, and it is hoped that on the plans of the architect, Mr. P. Morley Horder, the new home of the school will be ready for occupation in 1928. One cause of anxiety to the governors has been removed by the generous action of the trustees of the Rockefeller Foundation, who have amended their original undertaking, to provide a sum of $2,000,000 by promising to pay £460,830, which is the value in sterling of the money offered in 1922. By this the Rockefeller Foundation

has cancelled the loss due to the gradual rise in the cost of sterling which threatened the school with a diminution in the value of the gift of more than £50,000 if conversion had been made at the rate of exchange now established. Concurrently with the task of preparing for the building, the Education Committee and the Director have given considerable thought to the general educational organisation, and the Board has recognised the necessity for taking early steps to secure the services of prospective heads of divisions in order particularly to have their advice and assistance before the details of accommodation in the new building and of its equipment are finally settled. A grant has been made by the University Grants Committee for this purpose, and in order to supplement in some essential respects the teaching for the Diploma in Public Health, which is now given at University College, Middlesex Hospital, and at the Royal Institute of Public Health. Arrangements will also be made for the equipment and organisation of the museum, which will play an important part in the educational work of the school. The Director, Dr. Andrew Balfour, has issued a report on the work of the Tropical Division for the year 1924–25. The number of students was 227, which was a record, and on the research side there have been important developments. A field station has been established in Southern Rhodesia, in pursuance of the view that available research funds should be applied primarily to setting up field stations, though expeditionary work may be undertaken in exceptional circumstances. Four research studentships in London have been arranged, and the general courses in tropical medicine and hygiene will in future be spread over 20 weeks instead of 13, and much more time will be given to clinical demonstrations and to the teaching of tropical hygiene. There is no doubt that this will equip students far more fully for their work abroad, and that the already excellent reputation of the school will be enhanced.

Future direction, and courses at the new LSHTM were also summarized in *The Lancet* in 1925[9]:

> The munificent Rockefeller gift . . . does not come to full fruition until the London School of Hygiene and Tropical Medicine is both built and equipped. This will not be for another two years or so, although the decision will shortly be taken regarding the five excellent series of competitive plans submitted to the Advisory Committee.
>
> . . . The diploma course in tropical medicine has been extended by the addition of lectures on biochemistry, by giving much more attention to tropical hygiene and by the introduction of tutorial weeks. Two courses of study, each lasting five months, now occupy the academic year; one course begins in October and terminates in February, the other in March terminating in July. More clinical demonstrations will be given in the wards and opportunity offered for the study of minor forms of tropical disease at the Albert Dock Hospital and on ships adjacent thereto. Research is to be put in the forefront of the programme and a number of studentships

have been instituted, carrying an income of £250 per annum. Holders of these research studentships will give help as demonstrators in the diploma courses, but will have a large part of their time free for independent research. The demand at present for skilled workers in protozoology and entomology by Colonial Governments is greater than the supply. That these Governments are themselves awakening to the value of research was indicated in recent replies . . . by Mr. Amery in the House of Commons, although the proportion of expenditure on this head to the total cost of medical and sanitary services is as yet conspicuously small. The London School is now proposing to utilise overseas laboratories on a concerted basis rather than to continue the policy of research by expedition, as has been the practice in the past. Within the last few days a proposal has been made to develop the Natural History Museum at Nairobi into a centre for tropical research as a memorial to the late Sir Robert Coryndon, and a Rockefeller gift of £44,000 to the Singapore College of Medicine has been announced for the endowment of chairs of bacteriology and biochemistry. The aims of the London School are typified in its new seal [Plate 54] . . . The design, executed by Mr. Allan Wyon, owes its inspiration to a coin of ancient Sicily, where with little doubt the allusion is to the deliverance of the city of Selinus from a pestilence caused by the stagnation of the waters of the river. Apollo and Artemis are proceeding slowly in their chariot, Artemis driving while her brother, the sun-god, discharges arrows from his bow. The arrows are the healing rays of the sun, which drive away the malaria mists; and Artemis is beside him as the goddess who eases the pains of women labouring with child. The palm tree and the snake have been added to the Sicilian design.

The arrangements here described concern the teaching of tropical medicine for its special diploma, rather than the more general work on public health teaching which will be taken over by the school when completed. The requirements of public health students are being met in London at present at University College, King's College, Middlesex Hospital Medical School, and the Royal Institute of Public Health, with a special course on sanitary law and administration at St. Bartholomew's Hospital Medical School. It is proposed to develop the teaching of applied physics, physiology, and principles of hygiene, for which at present facilities simply do not exist, and public health students will also attend a course in parasitology to be given at 23, Endsleigh-gardens by Colonel A. Alcock, Prof. R.T. Leiper, and Dr. J.G. Thomson. At the same time opportunity will be taken of collecting a graphic museum of public health, something on the lines of the Ministry of Health exhibit now showing at Wembley [chapter 9], which will not be allowed to be disbanded when the Exhibition closes.

Detailed descriptions of the structure of the new building and the 'scope of the institute' were spelled out on the occasion of the laying of the foundation stone (Plate 55) in 1926[10]:

. . . In 1925, after a limited competition, Mr. P. Morley Horder and Mr. Verner O. Rees were appointed the architects of the new building, the foundation-stone of which was laid by the Minister of Health [Mr Neville Chamberlain (Plate 56)]* on Wednesday, July 7th, 1926. . . .

In the construction of the building certain requirements had to be met which, together with the extent and form of the site and the funds available, determined the architectural form which the school is to assume.

Provision had to be made for teaching hygiene in all its branches, for instruction in tropical medicine, and for research work in both these subjects, and in any of the ancillary sciences. The balance had to be maintained equally between teaching and research. Both have received sympathetic consideration. As a result, it was finally decided to provide for research one-sixth of the total space available for instructional purposes. This is a liberal allowance when it is remembered that the space devoted to teaching includes a big lecture theatre, numerous roomy classrooms and general laboratories, together with the library, a very large museum on two floors, tutorial rooms, and other accommodation. The number of students which the school is intended to accommodate is 250. Of these, it is considered that 100 will be engaged upon the study of tropical medicine, a figure based on the present attendance at the course given in the tropical division at Endsleigh-gardens, where there has of late been an average of nearly 70 per session. The remaining figure, 150, representing students studying for diplomas or degrees in public health, has intentionally been placed very much on the safe side. At present there are only about 45 students attending courses in London for the diploma in public health, but it is noteworthy that a recovery has taken place from the marked fall in numbers which followed the introduction of the new regulations of the General Medical Council, and there can be no doubt that this increase will continue, although it may be many years before there are as many as 150 aspirants for a public health qualification.

. . .[The building] will front south upon Keppel-street, and it is hoped that at least the frontage, which contains the main entrance, will be of Portland stone. This Keppel-street elevation will be enriched by a wide fringe composed of wreaths and of the names of some of the great pioneers in hygiene and in tropical medicine. Finality has not yet been reached as regards these names. Over the main entrance there will be a large panel on which the handsome and interesting seal of the school will be engraved. The general shape of the building is that of a letter H, with the Keppel-street front closing the southern end of the H, and the crossbar dividing the enclosed space into two nearly equal courts, one of which, the

---

* (Arthur) Neville Chamberlain PC, LLD, DCL, FRS (1869–1940) (later to become Prime-Minister – 1937–1940) was a son of Joseph Chamberlain and his second wife, and therefore half-brother of Sir Austen Chamberlain. He was MP for Birmingham (Ladywood and Edgbaston Divs.), and Minister of Health (1923, 1924–29, and August–November 1931).

northern, is not encroached upon, while the other, the southern, is partly occupied by the lecture theatre. This arrangement provides a building singularly well ventilated by natural means and well lighted, while it will be easy to find one's way about it, especially in view of the manner in which the different sections are grouped.

The provisional scheme of studies provides for six main divisions – namely, those of applied physics, physiology and principles of hygiene; chemistry and biochemistry; immunology and bacteriology; medical zoology, including parasitology and comparative pathology; epidemiology and statistics; and, finally the principles and practice of preventive medicine, general sanitation and administration. This grouping has been retained but, in addition, there has been recognition of the fact that the clinical pathology of exotic diseases forms a most important part of tropical medicine and, accordingly, as will be seen, a special laboratory has been devoted to the joint needs of this subject and of certain branches of tropical hygiene with which, of course, tropical pathology is intimately associated.

It has been decided, subject to satisfactory estimates of cost, to warm the building by the panel system of heating. This is a modification of the old Roman hypocaust method and has many advantages, while its disadvantages and difficulties can, it is believed, now be discounted.

Progress on the building was seriously delayed in 1926 by a dispute in the coal industry. Plate 57 shows the building under construction in 1927.

Opening of the LSHTM

Further details of the structure and functions of the school were provided when the new building was completed in 1929[11]:

> The great new building opened in London this week is something more than the Institute of State Medicine envisaged by the Athlone Committee of 1921. It will be an international, as well as a national, centre of public health, and its definition of preventive medicine will cover the needs not of this country alone, but of the whole inhabited world.
>
> So wide a view of its functions is justified partly by its constitution, and partly by the way it has come into being. On the one hand, union of the new school of Hygiene with the old School of Tropical Medicine gives it a large basis and historical continuity, whilst on the other, it has an international status from the first, because it is built with American money for the benefit of the world at large, and not of Englishmen alone. London has many advantages as the site of such an institution, but its chief claim to outside assistance for public health work lies in this country's past record rather than its present needs. The Rockefeller Foundation's grant . . . to build a new school is doubtless made in the lively expectation that this branch of English medicine is still capable of contributing something important and individual to the progress of mankind.

It will be remembered, however, that the grant was conditional on financial support from the British Government, and that the capital sum available was not to be used for running the School. Thus, from the time of its opening, the new building, though the gift of American citizens, will be a national concern, in which we hope to take a national pride. Moreover, thanks to the generous terms of the grant, the design and construction has been left to those who will control the fortunes of the School – notably, Dr. Andrew Balfour (the Director) and the heads of the various divisions.

. . . The walls of Portland stone confer an air of permanence desirable in public buildings, and the work has been carried out with imagination as well as restraint. Thus the roving eye is at once edified by a frieze bearing the names of twenty-one pioneers of public health, and entertained by gilded insects on the balconies – surely the first official appearance of the louse as a decorative emblem?

The pioneers whose names are commemorated in the frieze are as follows:–

H.M. Biggs (1859–1925), Edwin Chadwick (1800–90), William Farr (1807–83), J.P. Frank (1745–1821), W.C. Gorgas (1854–1920), Edward Jenner (1749–1823), Robert Koch (1843–1910), C.L.A. Laveran (1845–1922), William Leishman (1865–1926), T.R. Lewis (1841–86), James Lind (1716–94), Joseph Lister (1827–1912), Patrick Manson (1844–1922), E.A. Parkes (1819–76), Louis Pasteur (1822–95), Max von Pettenkofer (1818–1901), John Pringle (1707–83), Walter Reed (1851–1902), Lemuel Shattuck (1793–1859), John Simon (1816–1904), and Thomas Sydenham (1624–89).

. . . a certain amount of information about [the organisation of the School, and its connexion with special institutions and branches of the public health service] can be gained from the list of the principal members of the staff. . . . There is, however, one aspect of the work to which special attention may be drawn. In the words of Prof. Jameson 'it is earnestly desired that the School should become a centre to which all those interested in public health may look for assistance and advice. Members of the public health service will have a common-room placed at their disposal, and will be welcomed at all times – not only at the lectures given by the staff of the School, but also at the series of special afternoon lectures to be delivered by recognised experts on special public problems. We have no greater need at the present time,' he says, 'than for some sort of centre where our own public health workers can meet those from other lands, and discuss how best the experience of both may be made of service to the world at large. In this respect the London School of Hygiene and Tropical Medicine may be expected to play a not unimportant part' . . .

In July 1929 the new building was opened; *The Lancet* reported[12]:

The new building of the London School of Hygiene and Tropical Medicine [Plate 58] was formally opened on Thursday, July 18th, by H.R.H. the Prince of Wales.

... The proceedings commenced with the reception of the Prince of Wales at the main, or Keppel-street entrance, by Lord Melchett, Chairman of the Board of Management, Sir Holburt Waring, Chairman of the Court of Governors, and Sir Gregory Foster, Vice-Chancellor of the University of London. The Director of the School, Dr. Andrew Balfour, was presented to his Royal Highness, as were the architects of the building, Mr. Morley Horder and Mr. Verner O. Rees, who offered the Prince of Wales the key to the building.

... In the beautiful library a large and representative group of visitors were assembled to hear an address of welcome to the Prince, offered by Lord Melchett. The speaker pointed out that those responsible for the management of the School had embarked upon an enterprise made possible only by the benefaction of the trustees of the Rockefeller Foundation, which had realised that the claims of London as a centre for the teaching of hygiene and tropical medicine were unparalleled, and that assistance to provide the building of a central institute was therefore urgent. Lord Melchett reminded the audience that when three years ago the foundation-stone of the building in which they stood was laid by Mr. Neville Chamberlain, then Minister of Health, the American flag was flying side by side with the Union Jack above their heads, and the same was occurring to-day as a fitting reminder of their debt to American generosity. The absence from the ceremony of any representative of the Rockefeller Foundation was, he said, characteristic of the self-effacing policy of that establishment, while the Ambassador of the United States unfortunately had another engagement which could not be cancelled. Lord Melchett continued:– 'The gift of the Foundation followed immediately upon, even if it was not the direct consequence of, the recommendations of a committee which met in 1921 under the presidency of a distinguished relative of your Royal Highness, the Earl of Athlone. The committee found the arrangements for teaching for the Diploma of Public Health in London scattered and inadequate. The great post-graduate teaching centre which the Athlone Committee visualised as a necessity at once became possible by the fact that the trustees of the Rockefeller Foundation offered the munificent gift of $2,000,000 for carrying out the project which the Athlone Committee recommended. In this way it became possible that hygiene and public health should have a university institution of its own. And when further in the course of our deliberations the Seamen's Hospital Society expressed their willingness that the old School of Tropical Medicine should become merged in the institution, we felt indeed that these great twin subjects of hygiene and tropical medicine had at last their long-sought opportunity, and that a new epoch in the history of medicine and related sciences, and in hygiene, was about to be opened. Mr. Chamberlain at the foundation-stone laying, reminded us of the distinguished part which his father, Mr. Joseph Chamberlain, had played in founding, at the instance of Sir Patrick Manson, the School for the study of diseases of the tropics, and it is a pleasure again to recall this fact. We shall continue to be indebted to the Seamen's Hospital Society for clinical and pathological facilities for the study of these diseases, now that we have entered into our new home.' The speaker went on to point out that to-day the presence at their gathering of Mr. Chamberlain, the ex-Minister, and Mr. A. Greenwood, the present Minister of Health, was evidence that the School which, in union with the University of London, would be partly maintained by Parliamentary grants, and be open to all nations, would be in a position where party politics played no share, a position that was necessary for the establishment of the laws of health. It was, he concluded, the future duty of the British public and British Government to see that the School was adequately maintained.

... The Prince replied to the address of welcome by formally declaring the building open in the following words:–

'You have right to be proud of the magnificent building in which we are, and if the museums [Plate 59] and theatre and laboratories make good the promise of this library, you are to be congratulated upon a building that will be a notable addition to the homes of learning in London. While the part played by America has been described to you, the duty lies on both the British Government and the British people to see that this School is worthily endowed and maintained. The building is a sign that post-graduate education in medicine is about to come into its own. The establishment and endowment of this centre of teaching in preventive medicine is a signal example of the bond between the two great English-speaking races of the world. The chairman has rightly said that there are no territorial frontiers in hygiene [Plate 60]. The instruction in the class rooms and laboratories of this building will be conveyed by medical practitioners of every nationality to the far corners of the earth. This research will find its results wherever man lives and moves and has his being.'

'Three periods in medical science are stamped definitely, each with its own characteristics. The first, from 1870 to 1900, was a period of sanitary reform. The next period was marked by growing concern for the protection of the individual, which had been the basis of recent legislation, as evidenced by maternity and child welfare, the treatment of tuberculosis and National Health Insurance. *We stand now in the early days of an era of preventive medicine in which the progress made in sanitation and care of the individual will be developed, and fresh research will lead to the solution of problems not yet solved and to the prevention of much ill-health* [my italics]. The establishment of this school is of special importance to the British Empire, and it has undertaken great responsibilities. In my travels I have learned personally the appalling loss of life and effort due to tropical diseases, and I realised the great need for research in tropical medicine and hygiene. In the cause of hygiene generally the school will help and develop the growing work that has already been done. For these reasons I believe that the establishment of this school provides a great opportunity for this country and for the whole world.'

'If its work is properly conceived and carried out, there should follow a special development and interest, and a quickening of the public conscience, which will lead to a steady decrease in preventible diseases, suffering and death. By its work in this connection the school will be judged.'

. . . A fanfare of trumpets sounded by the Coldstream Guards followed, when an address of thanks was presented by Sir Holburt Waring. Sir Holburt pointed out that throughout the erection of the building, and in every stage of its rise, the notion of a workshop had been kept clearly in view all the time. He said that the London School of Hygiene and Tropical Medicine was intended to be a centre of Imperial effort, and alluded to the pertinent fact that already the Court of Governors, as part of a policy of future development, had taken over from the Government of Southern Rhodesia the research station there. It would, he knew, be the policy of the School to establish a chain of such research stations throughout the Empire as adequate funds were forthcoming, and to send out expeditions from time to time to the tropics. As Chairman of the building committee he recalled that at the conception it had been decided that the first condition laid down for competing architects should be 'Let there be Light,' and in the employment of half a million sterling real concern he believed and hoped had been shown to make the expenditure wide and judicious. The Director of the School, the professors, and the departmental heads had throughout been consulted in the construction of their laboratories and workshops, and it had not been found necessary, thanks to the generous measure of the Rockefeller gift, to refuse a single request for any piece of essential equipment. He associated the Director, professors, and staff with the governors and the board of management in thanking His Royal Highness for the encouragement and inspiration of his presence.

Sir Gregory Foster, also, in thanking the Prince, said that the new School would rank as a part of the University of the metropolis – the University of the capital city of the Empire – and that its work would be organised, not for London, and not even for the Empire, but for the world. In alluding to the many great men who had been educated at the University of London, and who had gone forth to make the world a better and happier place, he said he would mention one name only, that of Lord Lister, who was a graduate of the University of London, and received his education in London. The Vice-Chancellor described in humorous terms the curiosity that had been aroused in the neighbourhood by the new building, the reason for whose existence the local public had not yet grasped, while he was certain that the new School would increase the tradition of magnificent service in the cause of humanity which the University of London possessed, by sending back students, who had arrived from all parts of the world to be taught, as missionaries of health.

His Royal Highness then visited the museum, the laboratories, and the lecture theatre, and before leaving the building met the workmen employed in its construction who were having their mid-day meal in a tent adjoining the premises. Here the health of the Royal visitor was drunk in beer with musical honours.

A large number of those who were invited to be present at the opening ceremony remained to luncheon as the guests of Lord Melchett, and afterwards, under the supervision of the Director, professors and members of the staff were shown around the building, and were present at cinematograph displays in the lecture theatre.

Continuation of funding for the 'clinical' discipline

Despite Government assurances, there seems to have been a great deal of confusion about the method(s) for continuous funding of *clinical* tropical medicine. The future of voluntary hospitals was the subject of a speech by Mr Neville Chamberlain (Minister of Health) in Coventry in 1926 – reported in a leading article in *The Times*[13]. In it he referred to the Endsleigh Gardens building owned by SHS: '[the LSTM was] until recently a self-supporting body' but 'the old voluntary London School has now disappeared, and become merged in the new School, in accordance with the terms of the American benefaction.' Maintenance of the new school had he said been guaranteed by the State after the Rockefeller School was built. Meanwhile he had appointed a committee to investigate 'the alleged need for 'more permanent hospital facilities' for the Rockefeller School'. . . . 'This may or may not mean that the Government is contemplating the opening of a new hospital for tropical diseases to serve the needs of the Rockefeller School, the responsibility for maintaining which has already devolved on the taxpayer.' The leader writer supported a continuation of the role of the SHS, which thanks to its 'close relationship to the great shipping companies and to the fact that it owns the Dreadnought Hospital at Greenwich, the Albert Dock Hospital, and the Tilbury Hospital, it virtually commands the whole of the available clinical material'; he suggested that the 'SHS . . . appeal to the Empire for help to extend the accommodation. That, in the long run, is likely to prove a wiser course than the suggested intervention of the Ministry of Health – or of one of the bodies working in close association with it'. The writer went on to add: 'as has been amply proved in connexion with the general hospitals, the voluntary system is by far the best system of hospital administration which it is possible to devise.' The Chairman of the Board of Management of the LSHTM (Sir Alfred Mond) replied the following day in a letter (which referred to this leading article)[14]:

> . . . there is an underlying suggestion that Mr Neville Chamberlain, in his attitude towards voluntary hospitals, is treading the path followed by Socialist predecessors. . . . we remain a School of London University [he continued]; we have taken over the endowments of the old school, and we

look, and shall continue to look, for the splendid support from Colonial and commercial quarters

. . . I know of no reason for the statement in your article that the old 'voluntary' school has now disappeared.

Regarding hospital accommodation, his view was that:

. . . 'the present facilities on the spot, . . . cannot (so we have been assured by [the SHS]) be regarded as permanent, and that a hospital for tropical diseases in close proximity to the school is essential [a concept which has not incidentally materialised to this day!]. It can safely be said' he went on 'that the board of management of this school has no intention of submitting proposals for 'a Government-owned, or subsidized, hospital for tropical diseases'.'

The Lancet succinctly summarized the uncertainties regarding the financial situation facing both School and Hospital (as well as the *future* of the hospital) in December of that year[15]:

The question of the hospital at Endsleigh-gardens is still in abeyance, the Seamen's Hospital Society having announced its intention to maintain it for a limited period only, and the Minister of Health has appointed a committee, of which Sir Alfred Mond is chairman, to report on how the necessary clinical and pathological facilities can afterwards be secured to the School. The arrangements for financing the work of the School are incomplete and representations were made to H.M. Treasury as long ago as 1925 that the commitment of £25,000 a year entered into by the Government when the Rockefeller gift was accepted, would fall far short of the requirements for the staffing and upkeep when the School is fully established in the new building. The suggestion has been made that additional funds might be raised, in support of the Tropical Division of the School, from Colonial Government and commercial sources, so as to ease the burden on the Imperial Exchequer. The board is at present exploring this possibility.

In 1936 the school's position in relation to the Colonial Office was strengthened by the setting up of the Colonial Research Committee, at the Colonial Office (chapter 9) – on which several members of the staff were included.

The new School becomes established

The first annual report from the LSHTM in its new building indicated the general lines along which it was developing[16]:

. . . A division of public health has been inaugurated under the directorship of Prof. W.W. Jameson [shortly to become Dean of the School]. It has been staffed on special lines, and its members represent various aspects of public health life and activity. A scheme of study in public health, framed on novel lines, has been drawn up. It is hoped that the scheme will succeed in coordinating the different branches of study into a combined and logical exposition of the whole subject of the public health. A new course has also been drawn up for tropical medicine and hygiene. One feature of the new arrangement in this subject is that the summer course ends before the beginning of July – a 'stale' month, and one much occupied with congresses and meetings. The division of epidemiology and vital statistics has moved into the School from the National Institute of Medical Research. The study of experimental epidemics is being continued in conjunction with the division of bacteriology and immunology. An interesting feature of the School's work is the informal instruction given for short periods to medical officers proceeding abroad and the liaison work with other nations. Dr. Andrew Robertson has left the department of protozoology to work with the United Fruit Company of New York, in Tela, Spanish Honduras, and the School has been visited by teachers of tropical medicine from Berlin, Hamburg and Shanghai. A system of library services has been organised to supply information on any branch of the School's work to members of the staff and outside inquirers. The library has been expanding very rapidly, as has also the museum, which contains many interesting exhibits supplied by commercial firms. Research work, as always, plays an important part in the year's activities, and investigators have contributed from all over the world. The appendix gives a list of about a hundred original papers published during the year. One group of research is financed mainly from the Milner Research Fund, and another through the Ministry of Agriculture. Meanwhile the teaching work has continued with success. During the year, 166 students attended courses; they came from the Colonial and Indian Medical Services, the Royal Army Medical Corps, other Government services and missions, and they went to every part of the world, the majority to Africa and India.

The full programme of activities is not yet in operation, and the Governors look forward to an early expansion of the department of biochemistry, the section of applied physiology and the work of the School in relation to industrial hygiene.

The annual report for the following year again recorded steady progress[17]; developments in bacteriology, biochemistry, chemistry applied to hygiene, entomology, helminthology, and protozoology were outlined; agricultural parasites were under study at the Institute of Agricultural Parasitology at St Albans. The following remarks are of more general interest[17]:

The public health division has been particularly concerned to provide courses of instruction for public health students, and this end has been forwarded by arranging for a series of lectures to be delivered by recognised experts. Cooperation on the part of various Government departments, local authorities, and medical officers of health has made it possible for students to visit places of public health interest. A collection of plans and specifications is being collected with the aid of the public health service which will make it possible for the division to act, in time, as a clearing station for the public health data which accumulate from year to year. Already increasing numbers of persons are applying to the school for information and assistance, and many visitors are sent to the division by the League of Nations and the Rockefeller Foundation. *Thanks to the Seamen's Hospital Society an adequate supply of clinical material has been available for teaching purposes at the Hospital for Tropical Diseases, and experiments are being made to prepare clinical cinematograph films, of which one on beri-beri has already been completed* [my italics]. The museum of the school is still incomplete but includes sections on water-supplies, sewage disposal, contagious diseases, milk production, and tropical medicine. The library is growing steadily, and the use of a medical library is demonstrated to the students at the beginning of every tropical course.

The financial position, though satisfactory at the moment, calls for the backing of a large endowment; but, as the annual report points out, *anything in the nature of a hospital appeal would be unlikely to excite widespread sympathy. It is not generally appreciated that the familiar assertion that prevention is better than cure is a grotesque understatement* [my italics]. An increased income may ultimately be secured from the colonial Governments, and when Sir Andrew Balfour's health permits he will visit the colonies to make the necessary appeal on behalf of the school.

A year later, a modification to the tropical medicine course – making it shorter – was introduced[18]:

> ... The five-months' course of intensive study hitherto in force, followed by examinations first for the certificate issued by the school and then for the Diploma of Tropical Medicine of the Conjoint Board, has been found to impose an undue strain upon candidates. Many of the colonial governments have found it difficult to release their medical officers for a sufficiently long period to enable them to combine what is in effect six months' study-leave with a much needed holiday in this country. Further, the requirements of the colonial service are so urgent that a demand has arisen for a short course of instruction for recruits about to proceed overseas. After consultation with the Colonial Office and the Conjoint Board, it has been decided to divide the course of study into two parts: a three-months' course of clinical and laboratory instruction and a two-months' course in tropical hygiene. Each course can be taken independently, and the Conjoint Board is arranging for an examination to follow closely upon each course of study. The internal school examinations will be discontinued, and

students will be encouraged to sit for the diploma examination. Application has been made to the University of London for recognition of the revised course. The new three-months' course includes clinical tropical medicine, applied pathology, medical zoology, and elementary bacteriology; the two-months' course includes instruction in the relation to tropical hygiene of bacteriology, medical zoology, anthropology, and vital and medical statistics. In order to meet the requirements of the modified course, *the school has established a new division of clinical tropical medicine which can call on the combined resources of the Seamen's Hospital Society* [my italics]. The innovation will undoubtedly fill a need, and the facilities offered should make it easy for many more medical men and women to learn or revise the ground-work of tropical medicine, pathology, and hygiene.

Clinical tropical medicine was therefore recognised (presumably because it was regarded as a necessity for teaching) by the LSHTM! This was a significant development. The report for 1931 was overshadowed by the death of Balfour[19]:

The seventh annual report of the London School of Hygiene could have no other opening than a mention of its great loss in the death of its Director, Sir Andrew Balfour. His passing has signalised a certain change in the management of the School, which is now a school of the University of London, but one which has imperial and international responsibilities of a more direct kind and in greater degree than are usually found in university schools. The board of management felt that the School should have regard for university tradition and university standards, and the post left vacant has not therefore been filled by the appointment of another director, but the duties have been entrusted to a member of the professorial staff acting as dean. Prof. W.W. Jameson was appointed dean for five years from May, 1931. His first report shows the immense amount of work carried out in the School. There are now six departments, some of them with subdivisions: public health; bacteriology and immunology; biochemistry, with chemistry as applied to hygiene; epidemiology and vital statistics; *clinical tropical medicine* [my italics]; and medical zoology, with helminthology, protozoology, and entomology, while the Institute of Agricultural Parasitology at the St. Albans farm forms another department in close touch with the work of the School. Almost a separate division, though at present included under public health, is the department of medical industrial psychology and applied physiology, which is enabling the School to play a large part in the revolution that is taking place in psychological training. The students have given an excellent account of themselves in examinations, and a list of their countries and destinations emphasises once again the cosmopolitan field influenced by the School. *An agreement has been made with the Seamen's Hospital Society whereby members of the medical staff of the Hospital for Tropical Diseases form the staff of the new division of clinical tropical medicine at the School. This places the valuable clinical resources of the Society at the disposal of the students* [my italics]. Through the special programmes of instruction and study tours, the whole health organisation of Great Britain is laid open by the School for the information of students from overseas, and the dean's report shows throughout that the conception of the School as a great centre of teaching and research is being realised.

So great an international service naturally involves a large budget. When at least £10,000 per annum must depend on voluntary support, and particularly when great employers of labour are suffering from grave industrial depression, the position naturally cannot be free from anxiety. The School has no funds whatever to finance research work except the ad hoc grants for particular investigations provided by such bodies as the Medical Research Council, the Empire Marketing Board, and the Department of Scientific and Industrial Research. Additional funds are needed at the earliest possible moment if the great programme which the School has set itself is not to be curtailed.

The overall structure of the LSHTM has therefore continued in much the same way until the present day, with an increasing emphasis on the *public health* component(s) in recent years; the small *clinical* 'appendage' continued to be given a low profile throughout. Present financial constraints are as much – if not more – in evidence as they were in 1931!

'The Ross Institute and Hospital for Tropical Diseases'

A letter signed by H H Asquith* and 32 others (including Sir James Cantlie) which appealed for public donations towards a new Institute in honour of Sir Ronald Ross, appeared in *The Times* for 1923[20]. The value of Ross' discovery, especially in relation to the recently constructed Panama canal, was given prominence. In the letter, Ross was placed on a pedestal with Pasteur, Lister, Jenner and Golgi; the suggested name for the proposed monument to the discoverer of the mosquito-man cycle of *Plasmodium* sp was the 'Ronald Ross Clinique for Tropical Diseases and Hygiene'. In a strongly supportive leading article, *The Times*[21] claimed:

> Such an institute, as we are assured, will in no way compete with the work now being accomplished at the Schools of Tropical Medicine in London and Liverpool. These bodies are engaged for the most part in the education of young graduates; the aim of the new foundation will be research alone.

---

* Herbert Henry Asquith, KG, LLD, DCL, KC, FRS (1852–1928) was Chancellor of the Exchequer 1905–8, Prime Minister and First Lord of the Treasury 1908–16. He was created 1st Earl of Oxford and Asquith in 1925.

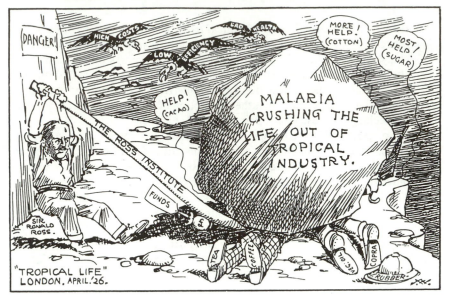

Fig 10.1: A cartoon aimed at attracting funds for the proposed Ross Institute and Hospital for Tropical Diseases in 1926. Below it the following text appears [*Tropical Life* 1926; 22: 54–55]:

WANTED – A BIGGER FULCRUM.
ONE TEN TIMES THE PRESENT SIZE PREFERRED.

Close observers will notice that there is more in the above picture than meets the eye. That, for instance, sugar, cacao, and cotton, as well as tea, rubber, and the other industries shown are in the picture, as proved by their calls for help. But so completely are they hidden under the stone that even the genius of the artist cannot make them visible. If those, therefore, interested in and dependent on these and other tropical industries, wish to be clear of trouble and remain so they must support the appeal of the Ross Institute and Hospital for Tropical Diseases and remember the letter to *The Times* signed by Mr. Asquith, now the Earl of Oxford, and thirty-two others of international fame. It is only by keeping the trouble of malaria at bay that they can hope to increase their output and lower their costs, and so, still speaking of sugar, cacao and cotton especially, be able to keep going even at the present low level of prices and to maintain the high standard now looked for in these industries, using these products as their raw material. If you think that malaria is of minor consequence, we would remind you and all our other readers of what Sir Ronald Ross himself told the planters in Ceylon as recently as January 30 last, when he said "all planters should have a malariologist, their work can only be done by experts; furthermore, all planters must unite and work for the common good. It may be that you have no malaria at the moment, but you may have an outbreak to-morrow, or next year, or at any moment. Remember the terrible outbreak of malaria in the Punjab in 1908. The death-rate in India was 1,300,000 per annum through malaria among a population of 300,000,000. This is an enormous figure, and if you wish to prevent its coming your way, even on a modified scale, you have got to spend money. There is no choice left for you, other than "Money or Malaria."

260

'The Ross Institute and Hospital for Tropical Diseases' was in due course established at Putney and was opened by the Prince of Wales in July 1926. The major drawback concerning the institute was that no endowment fund was set up; therefore recurrent appeals for funding had to be undertaken (fig 10.1). In addition, there were not of course enough *tropical* cases in London to justify a second Hospital for Tropical Diseases, despite minority views to the contrary.

The Ross Institute was never a viable enterprise. Its activities did in fact overlap with the LSHTM and the Hospital for Tropical Diseases, and not surprisingly it continually suffered financial problems. Ross himself who became Director-in-Chief of the institute died (in the hospital) in 1932. After his death approaches were made (initially through Sir Philip Manson-Bahr) to remove the Institute to the LSHTM[1]. Negotiations followed in 1933, and on 1 January 1934, the Institute became incorporated into the LSHTM[22]; the following is an account of these events seen

---

So much for the tropical side of the appeal, which also considerably affects all dwellers in the temperate zones to-day. We (in the temperate zones) cannot do without the foodstuffs and raw material which the hotter countries alone can supply. Were those supplies to cease, our population must shrink by 50 per cent at least, and perhaps more, and the world would be held up because production in, and consequently trade with, the tropics would be checked owing to the lack of labour. And to-day, what amounts to the same thing is that the low out-put and high costs of what we are now receiving owing to the indifferent health and heavy infant mortality, on account of chronic malaria, and other causes arising from this trouble, result in a great waste of lives and a reduced output from those who manage to survive.

Sir Malcolm Watson (well known for his long years of work as Dr. Malcolm Watson, and his books "Rural Sanitation in the Tropics," and especially "The Prevention of Malaria in the F.M.S.") told the Royal Society of Tropical Medicine, that in Singapore the health officers saved some 35,000 lives in twelve years who otherwise would have died from malarial trouble. Quinine and general sanitation failed. This success was achieved by a direct attack on the mosquito ... Yet Malaya has a rich anopheline fauna; a fauna which reaches up into Assam, where the great tea gardens are situated. In Assam, as in the Malay States, no amount of quinine and general sanitation is of any avail to stamp out malaria, nothing will suffice but a direct attack on the mosquito; this alone can give the desired results. And, as it has proved to be in these two typically tropical areas, so it is elsewhere. If the West Indies want to produce cacao to pay against the Gold Coast; if West Africa wants to compete in palm-oil production with Sumatra, or vice versa, or East Africa to turn out cotton, coffee and sisal, on an ever increasing scale, against long established and very experienced competitors, they must eliminate malaria, not only to increase their output and lower the cost per ton with the labour already existing, but also, and especially, to increase the labour supplies everywhere by raising the birth-rate and saving the babies when they do come. Help along these lines can only be looked for if the appeal for the Ross Institute and Hospital for Tropical Diseases, Putney Heath, London, S.W.15, receives the support that it thoroughly deserves, not to do themselves good but to confer benefits on everybody around.

261

through the eyes of a *British Medical Journal* reporter[23]:

> A printed memorandum on the proposed amalgamation of the Ross Institute and Hospital for Tropical Diseases with the London School of Hygiene and Tropical Medicine has been issued this week by Sir Charles McLeod, chairman of the Institute. On the death of Sir Ronald Ross he considered it his duty to make a special inquiry into the organization of the Institute, so as to ensure that it would be a worthy memorial to a great man, but before that could be completed there came a proposal for amalgamation with the London School of Hygiene and Tropical Medicine. The question was first raised by the Goldsmiths' Company, which, before giving a grant to the Institute, asked for an assurance from the honorary treasurer, Lord Queenborough, that there was no overlapping of the activities of the School and the Institute. At an informal meeting between Sir Austen Chamberlain, the late Sir Walter Fletcher, members of the Board of Management of the School, and Lord Queenborough and Sir Charles McLeod, representing the Institute, it became clear that overlapping occurred widely in the field from which support for both bodies was obtained, and that possibly there was overlapping in other activities. Since that date there have been a number of discussions. Early in their course a large measure of agreement was found, both on fundamentals and on details, and an assurance given that in the event of amalgamation the School would accord the work of the Institute its fullest support, both for its own sake and as a memorial to Sir Ronald Ross.
>
> 'As a result of these discussions, the Board of Management of the School and the Executive Committee of the Ross Institute have decided on the desirability of the amalgamation; and I am issuing this memorandum to explain to members of the Institute the reasons which have induced me to come to the conclusion that amalgamation should take place, how it will affect the objects for which the Ross Institute was founded, and something of the School and its associated hospital with which amalgamation is proposed.'
>
> Sir Charles McLeod recalls particularly that in the re-organization which led to the creation in London of a great School of Hygiene that would be of value not only to Britain and the British Empire, but to every part of the temperate and tropical zones, *the long association of the London School of Tropical Medicine and the Seamen's Hospital Society was preserved by a special agreement, which provided that research and clinical instruction should be carried on in their Hospital for Tropical Diseases in Endsleigh Gardens, a few minutes' walk from the School* [my italics]. Turning to the origin of the Ross Institute, he describes how, in addition to being a memorial to Sir Ronald Ross, the fundamental idea was again work for the benefit of mankind. Although the histories of the London School of Hygiene and Tropical Medicine and the Ross Institute have been different, and although each has been developed on somewhat different lines, their fundamental objects, he says, have been identical, and their spheres of work are found to be complementary. Sir Charles McLeod then explains

how carefully the memory of Ronald Ross is being preserved in the process of amalgamation:

On the front of the School the name of Ronald Ross has been carved among the immortals of hygiene and tropical medicine, as a reminder for all time in the capital of the Empire of the great work which he did for the Empire and for humanity. Secondly, there will be established within the School, as a permanent memorial to Sir Ronald Ross, a department to be known by the name of the 'Ross Institute of Tropical Hygiene.' Thirdly, on all official correspondence of the London School of Hygiene and Tropical Medicine there will appear the words 'Incorporating the Ross Institute.' Fourthly, to ensure the continuation of the policy of the Institute, two members of the Institute will be placed on the Court of Governors, and one on the Board of Management of the School. Fifthly, for the administration of the department called the Ross Institute of Tropical Hygiene, a special standing committee will be created, composed of members of the Board of Management, the Dean, and additional members having relevant experience. Sixthly, to signalize the amalgamation, the Board of the Seamen's Hospital Society has decided to call a ward, in its special tropical hospital in Endsleigh Gardens, 'The Ross Ward.'

For the work of Sir Aldo Castellani the Board of Management of the School will provide laboratory accommodation, and he will take with him his laboratory staff; he will be appointed to the staff of the School with a title of 'Director'. [Castellani was also to join the staff of the 'Tropical Hospital of the SHS' – where the patients of the institute were to be received[22]]. The appointment of Director of Tropical Hygiene at the School, which has been vacant since the death of Sir Andrew Balfour, will be filled by Sir Malcolm Watson.

We take this opportunity of recording that Sir Austen Chamberlain, chairman of the Court of Governors of the London School of Hygiene and Tropical Medicine, has lately received from Mr. W.J. Courtauld a large sum of money in aid of the tropical side of the work of the school, and that, in recognition of this gift, the senate of the University of London has conferred on Professor R.T. Leiper the title of 'William Julien Courtauld Professor of Helminthology.'

The Lancet's report added[22]:

> ... The pathological work now being carried on at the institute will be continued in the pathological department of the Hospital for Tropical Diseases. By the closing down of the hospital beds at Putney and by the ultimate sale of the property, economies will be effected, while the work will go on not only without interruption but with increased vigour derived from a wise fusion.

The amalgamation was marked by a reception which was held at the LSHTM on 29 June 1934[24]:

... Over 600 people were present. In the absence of Sir Austen Chamberlain, the guests were received by Sir Herbert Read, Sir Charles McLeod, and Dr. W.W. Jameson, the Dean of the school.

The ceremony of the evening was the unveiling by Lord Athlone, Chancellor of the University of London, of a tablet containing a medallion of Manson by Dr. Paul Richer, the gift of Lady Manson and family, and a bust of Sir Ronald Ross, presented by the sculptor, Lady Welby. Lord Athlone referred sympathetically to the collaboration between Manson and Ross, and quoted the letter dated March 21st, 1898, in which Ross wrote to Manson: 'My one wish is that you were here to share with me the pleasure which I have experienced yesterday and to-day in seeing your induction being verified step by step.' Manson Lord Athlone described as a great doctor, a humane being, and a thinker. He spoke of Ronald Ross's devotion to the cause of preventing disease, and pointed out that 'the problem of antimalaria work is not a biological problem alone; it is also largely a sanitary and engineering problem. It is one which must be dealt with not only by governments and municipalities, but by everybody, from the director of public health to the person responsible for labour in any industry and even to a chief of a village, all working in co-operation. The measures for stamping out this dreadful, wasteful disease must go forward everywhere with determination, with courage, and with high hope. That way lies the true path along which the workers in this school must go if they are to give Ross a real reward for his sacrifice and his labours, and do real honour to his memory.'

After the ceremony the guests had an opportunity of seeing a large number of exhibits and demonstrations, showing the work being done by the various departments of the school.

Amongst those exhibits (which are listed in the report) was one from the 'Division of *Clinical* Tropical Medicine; Dr G Carmichael Low demonstrated facilities for the teaching of tropical diseases, in which he included maps and charts'.

Shortly afterwards, an annual Mosquito Day luncheon was instituted at the LSHTM[25]. This had in fact been held previously on 20 August, the anniversary of Ross' discovery in 1897; but because this date proved an inconvenient one, it was transferred to 13 May – Ross' birthday:

On Monday last Mosquito Day was celebrated by a luncheon in honour of Patrick Manson and Ronald Ross, held at the London School of Hygiene and Tropical Medicine. Since the amalgamation of the Ross Institute with the School it has been considered fitting that the name of Manson should be linked with that of Ross in holding what has been for some years an annual celebration, and the day will in future be May 13th. Sir Austen Chamberlain, chairman of the governors of the School, who presided, spoke of the foundation of the Institute and of the School, and of the work which both were doing in the control of malaria. He recalled that his father, Joseph Chamberlain, had sought out Manson to be his medical adviser at the Colonial Office. Sir George Newman, speaking as the oldest personal friend of Sir Ronald Ross present at the gathering, said he could name no other discovery of life-saving value which had been so promptly appreciated by the persons interested. It had been shown that the work of science could be translated both into the saving of lives and the economic production of rubber and tea.

This convivial occasion remained viable until 1939; *The Lancet* reported the proceedings of the last of these luncheons to be held before the outbreak of the Second World War (1939–45)[26]:

... This year about 130 people were present, with Mr. Neville Chamberlain [then the British Prime Minister] in the chair. Mr. A. Chester Beatty paid tribute to Manson and Ross and to the London School of Hygiene and Tropical Medicine and the Ross Institute for the part they have played in the industrial and agricultural development of the British Empire. He regretted, however, that 'when some of the heads of the agricultural and mining companies are approached on the subject of the work of these institutions and are asked for contributions, they look upon the matter as if they were asked to contribute to a charity.' Later he quoted figures comparing the total production value of the various industries affected by research in tropical medicine and the contributions they made to medical research institutions. A most important factor for companies operating in unhealthy countries was, he said, the increased turnover in skilled labour due to illness, which had resulted in great loss of capital. Therefore he emphasised that these institutions should be looked upon as 'research laboratories for enterprises operating in unhealthy countries subject to malaria and other tropical diseases.' Whereas expenditure on metallurgical experiments had been large, that on research into the health problems of the places where the companies were operating, said Mr. Beatty, had constantly been inadequate. He mentioned how, after several companies in the copper belt of Northern Rhodesia had implemented the recommendations of Sir Malcolm Watson, the number of cases of malaria decreased from 90 per 1000 in 1929 to 15 per 1000 in 1938. The death-rate in the copper belt, 6.4 per 1000, was now less than half that in Kensington (where admittedly there were older people living). One rubber estate in Malaya had an acreage of 1632 in 1911, 2650 in 1923, and 6801 in 1932. In 1911 the death-rate was 232 per 1000, in 1923 it was 3, in 1932 it was 1.1, and in 1938 it was down to 0.08. In 1911 the European staff were unhealthy and were unable to have their families with them. In 1923 there was almost no sickness and the staff had their families. Mr. Beatty added that the school was doing not less important work for the temperate regions, being perhaps the greatest research and teaching school of hygiene in the world. – Sir Robert Annan said that the mining industry values the institute and realises that to do so is sound policy and good business. Mr. Neville Chamberlain said that there are extensive tropical areas still to be exploited for which the support of the school is necessary. He considered it a sound investment and urged mining and industrial enterprises to use it: *his presence was, he remarked, an indication of the importance that the Government attaches to the school* [my italics].

Conclusions

The LSHTM had therefore been set up in response to the Athlone Report; it was supported by a substantial American financial donation. The SHS backed out of the School's administration and the hospital was subsequently left 'high and dry'. But Britain still had a vast Empire and 'tropical' diseases remained important. The overall emphasis had shifted from a solely *clinical* one (targetted at the individual) or a preventive one (dominated by 'sanitation' and hygiene) in the nineteenth century, to a research orientation. Management of individual patients in the tropics was considered of lesser importance by the late 1920s. Public health was stressed as the major raison d'etre of the LSHTM from the outset. Assurances had been made from several quarters that the LSHTM required a close *clinical* link, and that a hospital in 'close proximity' was essential to its activities. Regrettably nothing came of this (chapter 12), and in retrospect, the day the Rockefeller Foundation's gift was accepted was the saddest one so far for *clinical* tropical medicine in Britain; it was the 'parting of the ways'. It was also a sad day however, for tropical medicine generally. Basic science in this discipline requires a strong *clinical* input; although supportive lip-service has subsequently been forthcoming from the LSHTM, that has in practice been the sum total of its support for this discipline. Furthermore, over the 60 years of separation, the controversial debate – *clinical* versus *primary health care (hygiene)* – has become disseminated throughout the 'Third world' (and indeed the whole world) and has continued in an unproductive way. A *balance* is obviously required, and if London had shown the way in the 1920s, this might very well have been achieved!

The Ross Institute was an expensive failure; the concept was flawed, especially from the clinical viewpoint – London certainly did *not* require a second hospital devoted to 'tropical' diseases. In the end, by being incorporated into the LSHTM, it gave increased strength to that institute but was a further 'nail in the coffin' for academic *clinical* tropical medicine.

11

The Second World War (1939–1945) – and after

So be it, Lord; thy throne shall never, like earth's proud empires, pass away . . .

John Ellerton (1826–93)

The Endsleigh Gardens building was closed by the Ministry of Health in 1939 – on the first day of the evacuation order and a fortnight before the onset of hostilities; it was not until 9 months later that the first German bomb was dropped on London. Manson-Bahr[1] recalls that a great deal of valuable material, apparatus, and case-notes were lost at this time; in fact, perhaps two-thirds of the latter completely disappeared. A year later, the building was occupied for several weeks by detachments of the Free French. On 17 May 1941 the building was badly bombed and in part destroyed; it was eventually taken over by the Ministry of Pensions.

During 1941, the Governing Board of the SHS reserved 10 beds at the Dreadnought Hospital, Greenwich (Plate 61) for 'tropical cases'. Clinical demonstrations were held there from time to time; but this building was bombed on 9 occasions and the difficulties involved in clinical teaching became virtually insuperable. Patients were also accommodated, however, in the newly rebuilt Albert Dock Hospital; the foundation stone had been laid on 13 July 1937 by the Right Hon Lord Ritchie of Dundee, Chairman of the Port of London Authority and it was opened in 1938 by Queen Mary. This hospital was, surprisingly, not damaged during the war. The numbers of patients who came to London with tropical diseases increased during these years. An out-patient department (two sessions weekly) was set up at the LSHTM by Dr W E Cooke[1,2]. Manson-Bahr recalled that numerous patients who were 'lying in hospitals in various tropical centres within the Empire' were evacuated to London, where it was assumed, incorrectly, that good diagnostic and treatment facilities still existed. *The Lancet* recorded, optimistically, in June 1941[3]:

> Lord Moyne, Secretary of State for the Colonies, has announced that a committee under the chairmanship of Mr. G.H. Hall, parliamentary secretary to the Colonial Office, is to be appointed to examine a plan

for the establishment in London of a tropical diseases hospital and centre where clinical research and training, including the training of women in tropical nursing, will be carried out.

In 1942 a decision was taken to discontinue regular courses of instruction at the LSHTM and to replace them with short intensive 14-day courses; British Medical Officers and some from the Allied Military Forces attended – in 1942–43 the total was 921. Towards the end of 1941, clinical instruction began in hospitals which were not run by the SHS – as far afield as Dartford. Dr A W Wingfield of the Dreadnought Hospital apparently played an important part in the organisation of these courses. Clinical demonstrations were held at the Albert Dock and Dreadnought Hospitals, and occasionally at St Mary's, the Ministry of Pensions Hospital (Roehampton), and the RAMC College, Millbank; a bus service which started at the LSHTM was used for members of these classes.

The position regarding formal training in tropical medicine in London, and also in Britain overall, was summarized in 1943:[4]

> A diploma in tropical medicine is required by those seeking medical appointments in the tropics. Three bodies normally grant such diplomas: Liverpool and Edinburgh Universities and the English Conjoint Board. Courses normally held at the London School of Hygiene and Tropical Medicine and the Liverpool School of Tropical Medicine have now been suspended until the end of the war and no regular courses have been held recently for the Edinburgh diploma; future courses at Edinburgh will depend on the demand and on the staff available. Examinations for the Conjoint diploma have been cancelled for the duration of the war.
>
> Intensive courses in tropical medicine and parasitology, each lasting a fortnight, have been provided at both the Liverpool and London Schools, however; these are designed mainly for medical officers of our own and allied Services, though civilians may also attend them by special arrangement. About forty candidates can be accepted at a time, and new courses begin every three weeks.

During the war, many members of staff served with HM Forces abroad. Lt-Col H E Shortt served in India. Lt-Col J A Sinton, VC, became consultant in malaria for the Middle-east. Dr F Murgatroyd – later to become Professor of Clinical Tropical Medicine at the LSHTM – became Lt-Col, RAMC and consultant to the Army in West Africa. Brigadier (later Sir) Neil Hamilton Fairley (Plate 62) – of the Hospital for Tropical Diseases – became consulting physician to the Australian Forces, and carried out a research programme at Cairns, Queensland which involved the use of mepacrine in malaria. Manson-Bahr[1] noted that mepacrine had been used at the Hospital for Tropical Diseases (amongst other hospitals) during the 1930s, but that a prejudice against its use had grown up in Britain; this was based on a suspicion that serious side-effects – eg acute hepatic necrosis – were significant limiting factors to its use[1]. In May 1942 when Java fell to the Japanese and supplies of quinine came to an end mepacrine simply had to be used because there was no alternative. Japanese soldiers taken prisoner at this time possessed liberal supplies of this chemotherapeutic agent!

The state of medical care in the colonies

But the problems facing tropical medicine were not confined to London. Concern was also increasing about the state of medical care in the Colonies which some felt was being neglected during the war years [5]:

> Our colonial empire, as distinct from the dependencies and mandated territories administered by the dominions, is inhabited by 60 million people, two-thirds of whom live in Tropical Africa, and the remainder mostly in the West Indies, Ceylon, Hong-Kong and Malaya. The colonies are administered by more than forty separate governments, and are responsible for an enormous volume of trade: in 1939 the value of exports amounted to more than £4 per head of population, the imports to £3 10s. About a quarter of the average expenditure is on social services; but since the revenues in many colonies are small in relation to their size, while the field of social service to be covered is very large, the sum is grossly inadequate.
>
> . . . last year, with the passing of the Colonial Welfare and Development Act, opportunities for raising the standard of living among the native populations have been greatly increased. This act authorises the expenditure of up to £5 million a year for ten years, with an additional yearly grant of half a million for research. Lord MOYNE [speaking in a House of Lords debate], said that but for the war the expenditure authorised might have been much higher. Last year the fall of France made it necessary to convert every available penny into aeroplanes and arms; but this year it is felt that war or no war we must not let the peoples of the colonies – many of whom already live at too low a standard – suffer from the disorganising effects of war. The obligation is the greater because the colonies have been so generous in offering us help, amounting already to more than £20 million. Some have offered their surplus revenues as a gift for the prosecution of the war. Lord Moyne, uneasy about accepting these generous offers from the poorer colonies, has proposed that they should be accepted as loans, to be repaid in time to come, for post-war development. The effects of the war on the various colonies have been uneven; a few produce materials which are in demand, and they are in a state of unwonted prosperity, especially Malaya and Northern Rhodesia; in others, such as the West Indies, there has been no serious interruption of their usual economy; but a few – especially Malta and Cyprus – are cut off from their ordinary trade; and some have lost their overseas markets through lack of shipping space – West Africa, for example, cannot dispose of cocoa and palm products,

East Africa of sisal, Palestine of oranges or Jamaica of bananas. The home government has helped in these difficulties by buying up crops or financing the growers in other ways.

... now the aim is to carry on all [social programmes] that were in progress [at the outbreak of war] and to plan ahead for others. Much of the personnel, of course, has been seconded for military service, but recruitment has been officially approved and young doctors are advised that service in the colonial empire is of as much national importance as service in the forces.

After a survey of the various research projects currently underway in various parts of the Colonial Empire this leader-writer concluded:

... the health and welfare services of the colonies have not been allowed to drift backwards since war broke out. At the moment developmental work which requires imported machinery or essential war materials cannot be undertaken, owing to difficulties of supply and shipping and because personnel is difficult to obtain; but everything is being done to increase local industries in the colonies, to get them to undertake production of their own necessities, and to extend their internal markets. They are to be encouraged to grow more foodstuffs of the right kind and to improve housing and sanitation; meanwhile the training of agricultural demonstrators, health workers and others to educate the community in matters affecting their social well-being is also proceeding. All this will help to raise the standard of living. Moreover Lord MOYNE is encouraging the colonial governments to put forward any schemes for development, especially in social welfare, which do not require imported material, and is able to assure them that the money to finance them will be forthcoming. He is specially anxious that schemes for development should be drawn up which can be put into action as soon as the war ends. ... This may well be the beginning of a new era in colonial government which will end for ever the charge of our enemies that our colonies are neglected estates.

The following report of some parliamentary proceedings in November 1941 is also revealing[6]:

In the ... debate on the Address which was devoted to colonial affairs, much stress was laid on nutrition for, as Mr. J.A.E. De ROTHSCHILD pointed out, vitamins and protein are equally necessary to black and white. Yet the malnutrition in parts of our Empire is still our greatest social folly. Mr. NOEL BAKER thought that we had made progress but in too many colonies there was still too much poverty, ignorance and preventable diseases. Exploitation of labour and of national resources were not only a social crime but also a social waste, and the Colonial Development and Welfare Act passed last year was our first effective stop to check the waste. He was glad that the Colonial Office was planning for the future but there were urgent tasks lying to hand. The tsetse fly in Africa [although still a popular subject, there were many far more important problems] was one, and he suggested that we should cooperate at once with our Free French and Belgian allies, put up a sum of money from our Colonial Development Fund, and call in the health section of the League of Nations to organise research and make a start on practical work. Dr. H.B. MORGAN, who was brought up in the West Indies, raised a medical storm with his speech on conditions there. As a doctor, he said, he had seen too many people playing with bandages rather than dealing with the general conditions which underlie the sores, and he was pessimistic about any benevolent policy unless the people on the spot were given a chance, with whatever reservations were necessary to have some say in the control of local affairs. He inveighed against a system which exported produce and imported heavily taxed food, while income-tax remained as low as 3d to 2s 6d in the £. When he visited Barbados in 1939 the people were living in a black cesspool of disease – yaws, hookworm, syphilis, malaria and tuberculosis. The Rockefeller Medical Commission had found instances of hookworm in two or three parishes in Trinidad amounting to 80–90% of the agricultural population. The doctors in the West Indies are blamed for a medical policy with which they have nothing to do; instead of a unified medical service a doctor may not move from one parish to another, while some of the hospitals he had seen were a disgrace. Mr. CREECH JONES . . . said that our knowledge of [the colonial] economic and social problems was hampered by a lack of vital statistics. He urged the need for an expansion of the social services department of the Colonial Office and said he would like to see a larger number of expert women with understanding and drive brought into it. He too stressed the need for the exhibition of greater vigour in the whole field of preventive medicine.

Mr. G.H. HALL, parliamentary secretary for the colonies, said that at the beginning of the war we were approaching a critical period in colonial history, and while the war had in one sense delayed the crisis, in another sense it had hastened it. The public conscience had been awakened to the need to take a more constructive interest in the social, economic and spiritual welfare of the colonial peoples who were now solidly behind us in our war effort. *Our duty was to improve their lot, to develop their resources so as to raise their standard of life, and to enable them to take an ever-increasing responsibility in ordering their own affairs* [my italics].

Health of the expatriate employee

Some idea of the state of 'travel medicine' in 1943 is provided by the following *Lancet* annotation[7]:

A report from the medical department of a commercial airline operating a service from Bathurst, West Africa, down the Coast to Lagos, thence inland through the Sudan to Egypt (a distance of almost 5000 miles) and finally to India, shows how knowledge can be used to prevent disease. The first 2000 miles took in the semi-jungle country of the West Coast of Africa where although the temperature rarely exceeded 90° F. the humidity was always high, the rainfall reaching in some parts 200 in. a year and the humidity in others not falling below 90% for several months on end. Crossing the African continent the temperature increased but humidity fell, until in the Sudan and Egypt real desert conditions were encountered with average maximum temperatures of 110–115° F. and wide diurnal variations of 60–80° F., while in the Persian Gulf temperatures reached as much as 127° F.

Candidates for service . . . were carefully selected and the age-limits were set at 18–45 years. A full clinical examination was supplemented by blood-counts, serological tests and X-ray examination of the lungs. Some 16% of applicants were rejected, the chief causes being cardiovascular diseases (20%), visual defects (12%), genito-urinary diseases (11%), and respiratory conditions (10%); those having a history of repeated attacks of venereal disease, chronic alcoholism or peptic ulcer were also regarded as unsuitable types. Accepted applicants were inoculated against smallpox, the enteric fevers, tetanus, yellow fever and cholera, and were provided with mosquito nets, anti-mosquito clothing, a sun helmet, and a supply of quinine and mosquito-repellant before sailing. Of the men sent to Africa less than 3% returned for medical reasons and none of these was seriously incapacitated. In Africa, hospital-bed accommodation was provided for 10% of the personnel, but in fact 1% sufficed. In large stations a medical and surgical officer was provided for each 600 men, but a doctor was posted to each station even when the numbers there were small. Well-trained laboratory staffs and adequately equipped hospitals with properly planned departments, including laundry services, played their part.

In West Africa, where malaria is rife, military statistics suggested that an attack-rate of 100% per annum, and in some parts even 200%, might be anticipated. However, apart from an outbreak in the first few weeks of hurried assembly – when 46 out of 284 men were attacked, and almost 2000 days of work were lost by 300 men in 11 weeks – the malaria-rate proved extremely low. In September, 1942, there was only one case among 1400 employees and in October only 3 among 1800. This was attributed to the aggressive antimalarial measures applied at all the stations of the line. Besides the personal protective measures taken by the staff, all quarters and accommodation were screened and maintenance men were employed whose sole duties were to keep the screening in order. Antimosquito locks of adequate proportions were provided for all entrances, which were kept to the minimum, and all doors were fitted with automatic spring-closing devices. Quarters were sprayed daily and the adjacent native quarters were similarly treated. Oiling, dusting and drainage of potential breeding areas were also carried out and continuous maintenance gangs looked after these works; some 45 miles of ditches were dug in one station alone. Flying personnel had blood-examinations before every flight and the value of this was proven by the fact that in nearly every instance where positive smears were obtained the subject developed a clinical attack within 24 to 48 hours. In the treatment of the acute attacks various combinations of drugs were tried without any striking differences in the therapeutic results, and finally a routine course of quinine, gr. 30 daily for 2 days, followed by mepacrine hydrochloride, 0.3 g. daily for 5 days, was adopted. Almost all the infections were malignant tertian and it was not considered that anything was lost by the omission of pamaquin from the treatment. Quinine and mepacrine were used in suppressive treatment and no evidence was forthcoming that mepacrine diminished tolerance to altitude.

Gastro-intestinal diseases were next in frequency to malaria, and were well controlled by the screening of messes, kitchens and latrines against flies. Before this was done some 20% of the personnel at one station contracted diarrhoea once or twice a month; and in another station the rate fell from 30% to 0 on the installation of flush toilets and the screening of quarters and kitchens. The importance of periodic examinations of all native food handlers was shown by the fact that 28% of the natives were found to be carriers of E[ntamoeba] histolytica.

Psychiatric problems, often stressed as a cause of trouble in the tropics, were found to be relatively unimportant; but all the personnel were volunteers and their living conditions and food were unusually good. Surgery presented no special difficulties and sepsis was not more common than in temperate regions. The medical staff was convinced that the climate as such had no deleterious effect on health and it was the unanimous opinion that good health can be maintained in the tropics provided preventive measures against disease are aggressively applied.

The future of clinical tropical medicine in London towards the end of the war

In 1944 consideration of the future of the discipline – clinical tropical medicine – in London again came to the fore. In a forward-looking review which stressed the importance of tropical medicine to the Empire, an anonymous contributor to *The Lancet* wrote as follows[8]:

a progressive and enlightened colonial policy in postwar years ought to make provision for still more extensive and intensive research in the treatment and prevention of tropical diseases.

In the metropolis the onus of this work will assuredly fall upon the London School of Hygiene and Tropical Medicine, and if the school is to add to its lustre in teaching and research, the more abstruse and theoretical technical subjects, such as protozoology, helminthology and medical entomology, must be linked to practical clinical medicine. *Such a school without an affiliated hospital may be likened to a ship without a rudder* [my italics]. That is the position today. The Hospital for Tropical Diseases, upon which this service has so far devolved, has been destroyed by enemy action and it will be necessary to reorganise it in a modernised form. Unless this is done within a reasonable time the study of tropical medicine in London may languish, which is unthinkable. It is obviously impossible to stock a hospital in London with representative cases of all known tropical diseases, but it has been amply demonstrated in the past that enough clinical tropical cases are always available to provide material for clinical teaching and clinical research, if full use is made of the opportunities London's central position affords.

. . . The aim should be to create an institution to which patients from the tropics may turn for specialised treatment, and where the diagnosis and treatment of tropical disease are understood and provided for. The hospital should be staffed by doctors who have been specially trained in tropical medicine, have had practical experience in the tropics, and have spent some years studying tropical problems. In the hospital there should usually be found cases of malaria, leishmaniasis, amoebiasis, sprue and the many intestinal affections which are prone to affect travellers in tropical lands. Experience has shown that patients invalided from the tropics cannot discriminate tropical from non-tropical affections, so that sufferers from all manner of diseases tend to seek treatment in such an institution, and its hospital service inevitably becomes a cross-section of what may be called the practice of medicine in the tropics. Herein lies the practical value of a tropical hospital of this kind. It provides an excellent means of instruction by the comparative method, the chief value of which lies in the sphere of differential diagnosis, with special emphasis on the parasitological and biochemical aspects of the case. The clinical features of malaria, for instance, can be contrasted with those of many other forms of pyrexia, splenomegaly and anaemia which are encountered in routine practice.

Clinical demonstration must be backed up by microscopic preparations of the parasites, slides illustrating changes in the blood-picture and pathological exhibits. The pictorial method of teaching, excellently displayed in the Wellcome Museum, lends itself particularly to the study of tropical disease. The equipment of the clinical teacher should therefore include not only a rich assortment of microscopic preparations but also pathological drawings, and whenever possible, cinematograph films. The main manifestations of amoebiasis, for example, embrace considerations of modern methods of investigation of intestinal disease and invite comparison with other forms of colitis and many other affections of the large intestine, such as malignant disease and diverticulitis. Many other examples will suggest themselves to those who have practised in the tropics; thus sprue and sprue-like diseases provide a never-ending topic for discussion. Then there are biochemical considerations. In no other department of medicine are these so significant as in the severe anaemias which are constant concomitants or sequelae of tropical fevers.

. . . Several circumstances in the present situation must be carefully considered in planning the teaching of the future. First and foremost is the opening up of the tropics and many parts of Africa and Asia,

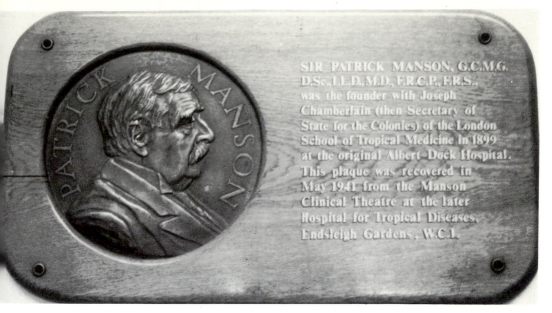

50. Plaque commemorating Sir Patrick Manson – now at the Albert Dock Hospital

51. The staff of the Hospital for Tropical Diseases in 1930

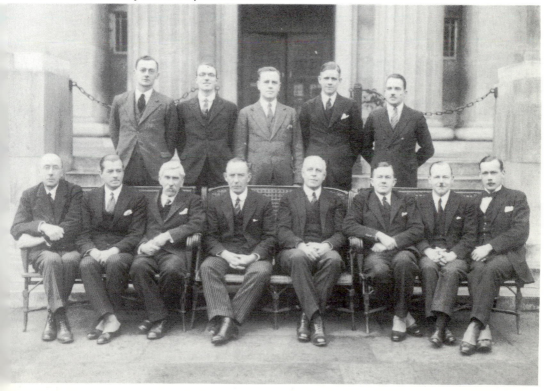

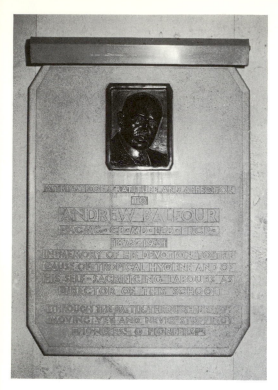

52. Plaque commemorating Sir Andrew Balfour
- at the LSHTM

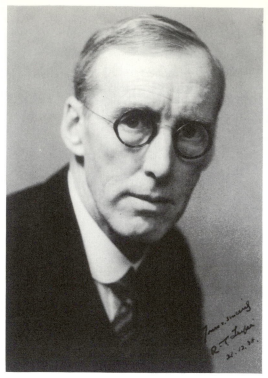

53. Professor Robert Leiper

54. The seal of the LSHTM

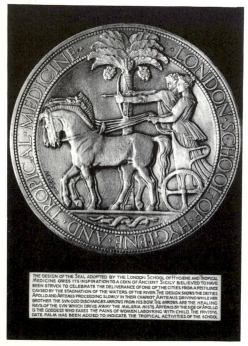

55. Foundation stone of the LSHTM

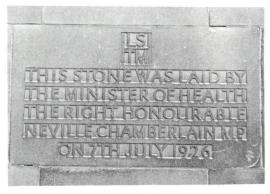

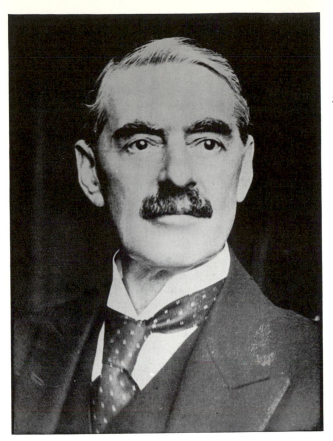

56. Mr Neville Chamberlain MP,
Minister of Health - in 1926

57. (*below*) The London School of
Hygiene and Tropical Medicine
building under construction
in 1927

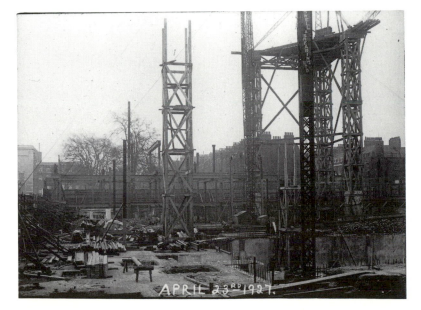

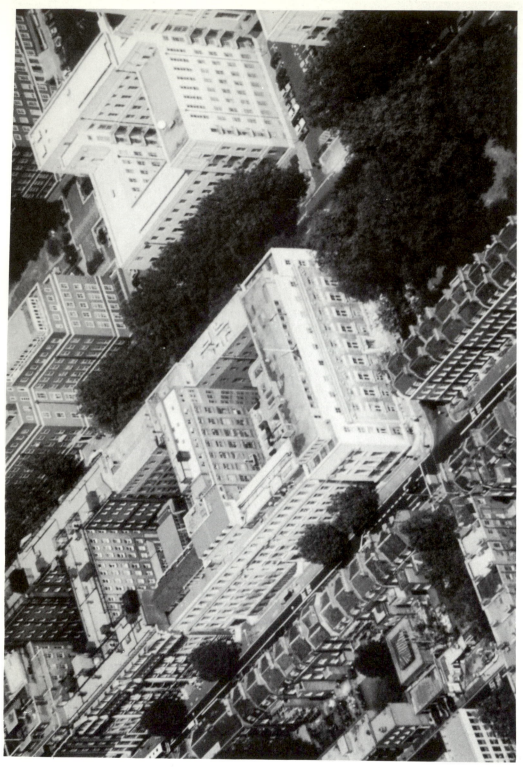

58. London School of Hygiene and Tropical Medicine (LSHTM) in 1990

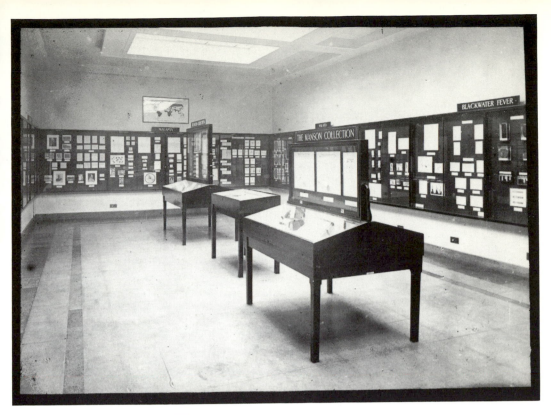

59. The museum of the new LSHTM in 1929

60. An exhibit in the new LSHTM in 1929.

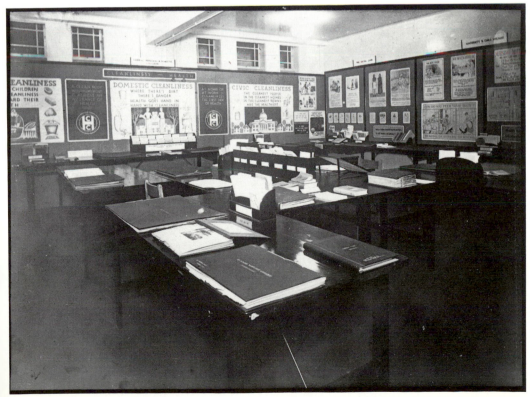

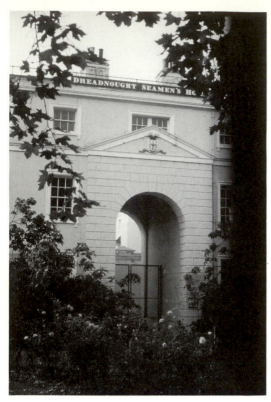

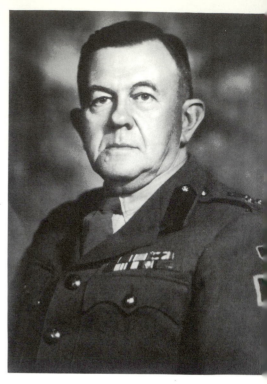

61. The Dreadnought Hospital, Greenwich
   - used for tropical medicine in 1939–45

62. Sir Neil Hamilton Fairley

63. Hospital for Tropical Diseases, 23, Devonshire Street W1 - building used in the late 1940s (left)

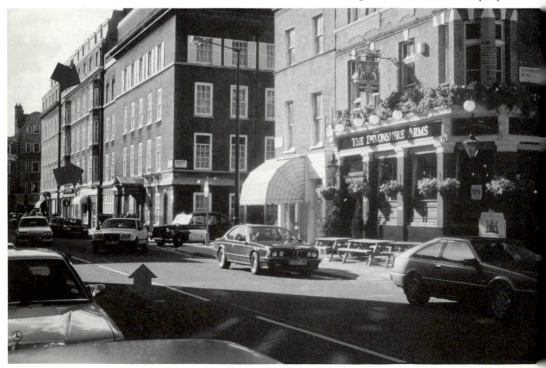

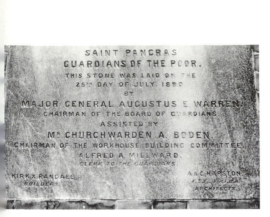

64. Foundation Stone of the rebuilt workhouse –
later to become St Pancras Hospital – in 1890

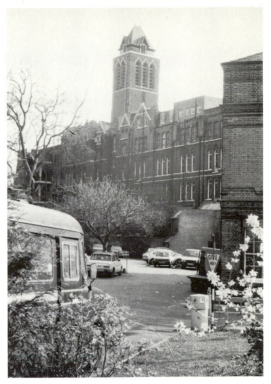

65. The Infirmary (now the South wing
of St Pancras Hospital)

66. The opening ceremony at the Hospital for Tropical Diseases - St Pancras, in 1951

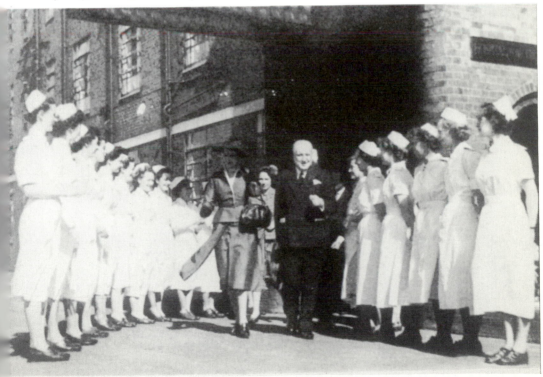

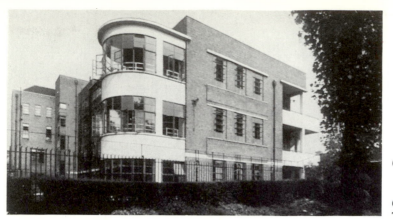

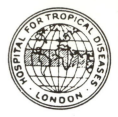

67a

67a & b. Hospital for
Tropical Diseases, St Pancras
- with letter-head

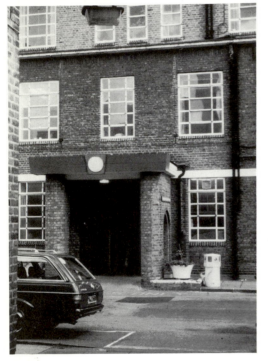

67b

68. St Pancras Old Church

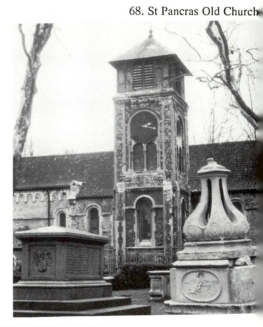

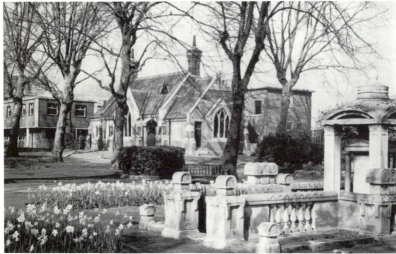

69. St Pancras
Coroner's Court

which have hitherto been almost inaccessible, by developments in air travel. These facilities will doubtlessly bring from the tropics many more patients who require immediate transfer to temperate climates and special methods of investigation and treatment for their recovery. Far from reducing the number of tropical cases available in London, air travel is likely to increase them. Moreover, air travel should enable members of the staff of the central London hospital to visit other medical centres in the Middle East, in West, Central and East Africa, and even in India and the Far East from time to time to study new methods of diagnosis and treatment. This will undoubtedly lead to much closer cooperation in teaching and research with schools of medicine and laboratory workers in other lands, to their mutual benefit.

These many-sided developments will necessitate reorganisation of the clinical teaching staffs. No longer will it be possible for tropical consultants, engaged in busy and exacting consulting practice with many divided loyalties and duties, to conduct the main teaching in clinical tropical medicine. It is therefore necessary to envisage setting up a unit system in this such as is already established in other branches of medicine. A prime consideration will be the appointment of a full-time clinical teacher. Many duties will devolve on him. The institution of a chair of tropical medicine in the London school might solve many of the inherent difficulties of the present situation. A director of studies may also be needed for overseas students, who urgently desire such assistance. This officer should be well versed in modern medicine and should be able to direct research in special cases. The aspirations of overseas students, especially Africans and Indians, require special consideration in this respect. In addition to the teaching of postgraduates in tropical medicine, due attention may have to be paid to special students from the tropics and elsewhere overseas who come to London to work for higher degrees. In this direction this hospital for tropical diseases may well act as the tropical associate of the British Postgraduate Medical School.

In choosing a site for a new Hospital for Tropical Diseases due consideration must be given to the amenities afforded by the Port of London, whither normally the greatest number of tropical cases tend to gravitate. The hospital should be planned on broad lines and should have enough beds to provide ample material for instruction in clinical tropical medicine, bearing in mind likely future developments in this rapidly expanding field of medicine.

Wise thoughts indeed, and how sad that more attention was not paid at the time to this perceptive writer! In 1944, a report by the Inter-Departmental Committee on Medical Schools, under the Chairmanship of W M (later Sir William) Goodenough, was published. Tropical Medicine (in London) did not come out of this awfully well as the following extract indicates[1]:

While a man may acquire a considerable amount of theoretical knowledge and become reasonable proficient in certain laboratory processes, it is abundantly clear that he cannot be given an adequate training in tropical medicine in this country. We therefore suggest that, having obtained his theoretical and laboratory instruction here, a student wishing to specialize in tropical medicine and hygiene should be required to hold approved hospital appointments in tropical countries as part of the prescribed postgraduate training and experience in this branch of medicine. It is likely that such a development would prove very popular in the Colonies and it would furnish British students with excellent experience, not only of tropical diseases, but of clinical work generally.

This seems on the face of it sound advice, but it does represent a somewhat rigid viewpoint!

With the dark days of war now relegated to the past, the *Royal Society of Tropical Medicine and Hygiene* devoted one of its ordinary meetings in 1945 to the teaching of tropical medicine in the years ahead[9,10]; the evening's proceedings were opened by Dr L Everard Napier:

. . . in the United States of America [he said] a serious attempt is being made both to improve the teaching of the subject to the undergraduate and also to develop its postgraduate teaching. In Great Britain, however, tropical medicine appears to have been relegated to the place of a specialty about which the general practitioner need know nothing and with which the ordinary student need not be burdened. These shortcomings require remedying urgently. To avoid overloading the undergraduate curriculum the student should be introduced in his premedical years to selected parasites of man, and the essential clinical diagnostic methods used in tropical medicine should be included in the teaching of clinical pathology. This would leave the pathology, symptomatology, and therapeutics of important tropical diseases to be taught in the systematic lectures on medicine and in the clinical departments as the occasion arose. At this stage it seems entirely wrong to segregate tropical medicine as it had been segregated in the past and to teach the student virtually nothing of the pathology, symptomatology, and therapeutics of tropical diseases. Tropical diseases furthermore could provide excellent examples for teaching the general principles of preventive medicine. Scarcity of clinical material must not be used as an excuse for avoiding clinical teaching; the student of general medicine fails to see examples of many diseases which he will be expected to diagnose and treat later in his practice. Much can be done by the use of lantern slides and cinema films. The future will also bring an increasing number of tropical diseases among those whom the war has taken to the tropics, while rapid air transport may allow cases of tropical disease to enter the country unsuspected during the incubation period. Interest in tropical medicine must be fostered by all means. Short-term exchanges of personnel, research-workers, and teachers between this country and the tropics should be encouraged. As an artificial way of maintaining interest in tropical diseases examining bodies should demand a sound knowledge of the commoner tropical diseases. Turning to postgraduate teaching Dr. Napier said there are few if any places in the world where one can see a better selection of tropical diseases than in London, but owing to the war there is at present no suitable hospital where the available clinical material can be collected; a crying need today is for a 'tropical medical centre'. Special provision should be made for those who are proposing to specialise in tropical hygiene. Dr. Napier ended by emphasising the necessity for making the undergraduate and his teachers conscious of the existence of tropical diseases, and for the early establishment of a hospital in London that would act as a centre for teaching and research in tropical medicine; meanwhile the society should prepare a memorandum on the teaching of tropical medicine and try to obtain representation on all committees considering the matter.

Following this useful overview, several other viewpoints were expressed from the audience:

Sir PHILIP MANSON-BAHR thought that the medical student's burdens should be not increased, but agreed that more emphasis should be laid in the premedical studies on the parasites associated with disease in man. He disagreed with the statement that tropical medicine is entirely neglected in the present undergraduate curriculum, pointing out that in practically every medical school in London lectures on tropical diseases are already given to the undergraduate, and that in the examinations of the last few years questions on the more important diseases have always been included. In the postgraduate courses it is also necessary to avoid overloading the curriculum. *The best days of teaching tropical medicine were those when the tropical school was a compact self-contained unit, with the laboratory and clinical work closely linked* [my italics]; a plethora of visiting lecturers, however specialised their knowledge, leads to overlapping and overloading of the curriculum. In teaching tropical medicine differential diagnosis is most important, and the practical value of microscopy cannot be overstressed. Any difficulty of obtaining clinical material would largely be overcome if the general hospitals were more willing to transfer tropical cases to a tropical hospital for teaching purposes.

And other opinions followed:

Prof. R.M. GORDON also agreed that the course in zoology should include the simpler parasitology of man, and that the teaching of tropical medicine should be extended, especially in the undergraduate's final year. The graduate student would then require an amplification of his general knowledge, and such teaching would be well covered by the present DTM&H course, which does not make a specialist but only a good practitioner for the tropics. He did not believe that the situation in which tropical medicine finds itself in London now that the war is over necessarily means that the subject is in danger throughout the country; the Liverpool School flourished during the war and is confident of its own future. The dearth of living material in this country for the teaching of parasitology and entomology necessitates the artificial maintenance of strains. This involves much labour, and loss of a strain is a disaster unless it is maintained in more than one place; some institution, such as the Wellcome Laboratories of Tropical Medicine, should interest itself in this matter. The Colonial Office and all firms operating in the tropics should insist on a diploma in tropical medicine for their medical officers.

Dr. G. [later Sir George] MACDONALD supported broadening the undergraduate curriculum to include more instruction in tropical medicine. He did not admit that the teaching of tropical medicine in London is in a parlous state, but he urged the restoration of facilities lost directly owing to the war and deplored that, outside the special group of those intimately concerned with tropical medicine, interest in the subject has been lost, even the writers of the Goodenough report failing to consider the matter seriously. There must be a centre of clinical research in London to replace that lost in the war, but on a better and more fully equipped scale, and it should co-operate with the existing School of Tropical Medicine as now constituted. Postgraduate teaching in tropical medicine should round off a general medical education and fit the student to practise medicine in the tropics, rather than create a specialist; the specialist requires, in addition to special knowledge of tropical diseases, a high qualification in general clinical medicine. Similarly those specialising in tropical hygiene should hold a DPH as a basis, supplemented by a DTM&H and experience overseas before taking up independent work in tropical hygiene. The society should form a policy committee to examine and foster the development, teaching, and standards required in tropical medicine and hygiene.

Lieut.-Colonel VERE HODGE, while agreeing that the establishment of an Imperial centre for tropical medicine should be the ultimate object, thought that immediate steps are required to deal with the large numbers of repatriates who may be returning with latent tropical infections; after a long absence from home these persons will not want to be sequestrated in special centres, and this will necessitate a number of tropical units throughout the country. The limitations of teaching tropical medicine in this country will make it necessary to have subsidiary centres abroad, but even short courses in this country would give practitioners going abroad an advantage. Three types of teaching in tropical medicine are required – first, undergraduate training; secondly, short courses for those going abroad for the first time; and thirdly, diploma courses for those who already have some experience in the tropics.

Lieut.-Colonel W.R.M. [later Lieut.General Sir Robert] DREW thought that undergraduate teaching in London has always been well balanced; ordinary students have a good grounding in tropical parasitology and the Conjoint Board examinations always include one question on tropical diseases. Early in the war the DGAMS [Director General of Army

Medical Services] approached the deans of the various medical schools, as a result of which special emphasis has been given to instruction in tropical medicine, and voluntary courses have also been given. In addition a hundred short courses for the Services have been held at Millbank. In any curriculum a proper balance of subjects is necessary. The centralisation of cases should offer no difficulty.

Dr. H.S. STANNUS suggested that, taking into account the rapidity of modern transport and the proposed development of the Colonies, regional centres should be established in the tropics to which students, after a preliminary education in this country, could go for further instruction before practising in the respective regions. There should also be interchanges of teachers between this country and the tropics.

Dr. H.C. TROWELL agreed with Dr. Stannus and remarked that general principles of medicine are more important than special practice, since the most important and lethal diseases even in the tropics are the cosmopolitan diseases.

Sir RICKARD CHRISTOPHERS, FRS strongly supported the suggestion for the re-establishment of a tropical centre in London.

A building in Devonshire Street

The talk about a 'tropical centre' for London was of course little more than 'hot-air', and in order to get going at all after the gloomy war years, the tropical physicians with the assistance of the SHS, took over a building which had been used as a 'Harley Street' nursing home (Plate 63), but which was to prove in practice extremely inadequate[1]. In early 1946, the matter was deemed sufficiently important to warrant discussion in the House of Commons[11]:

... Mr. CREECH JONES said one item in the Estimate [for Colonial and Middle Eastern Services] was concerned with the Seamen's Hospital Society in London. It represented the balance of a loan to enable the Society to re-establish in London a hospital for tropical diseases. At present hardly any accomodation was available for patients suffering from these diseases. It was desirable that patients should be treated near the School of Hygiene and Tropical Medicine in Central London. The tropical diseases hospital in Endsleigh Gardens, which was requisitioned by the Ministry of Health in 1939, was now declared by the Ministry to be unsuitable for use as a hospital. It was proposed to go ahead with a new tropical diseases hospital, but it was only at the planning stage. As an interim measure the Seamen's Hospital Society had acquired 23, Devonshire Street, which had accommodation to provide a maximum of 40 beds. The Society had not the funds to meet this cost and the Treasury had agreed that a short loan of £60,000 should be made. The Government now asked that a second loan should be available. He hoped this would be repaid comparatively soon.

Dr. MORGAN said there were already four institutions in London dealing with tropical diseases – the Seamen's Hospital in Greenwich, the Postgraduate Medical School, the hospital which used to exist in Endsleigh Gardens, and the School of Hygiene and Tropical Medicine. This temporary grant was a waste of money. It would be better at present to use beds in ordinary hospitals instead of lending money to reconstruct an old house in Devonshire Street. Mr. OLIVER STANLEY was surprised that it was worth while to make this loan seeing that it had to be repaid at the end of the year. While he was at the Colonial Office a small committee considered a long-term project concerning tropical diseases. They were in search of sites, but there was no question of a reconditioned house. The aim was "something much bigger and better."

Replying, Mr. CREECH JONES said a big tropical diseases hospital was being planned. In the interim it was proposed that 23, Devonshire Street should be acquired. That was a modern building and would give the Seamen's Hospital Society a nursing home which could be readily transformed into a hospital.

The House approved the Estimate.

The following notice appeared in *The Lancet* for 4 January 1947[12]:

Hospital for Tropical Diseases, London
This hospital, which was closed during the war, has now been reopened at 23, Devonshire Street, W.1 (Tel.: Welbeck 8371). The hospital is open to all patients suffering from tropical diseases. There is an outpatient department, for which appointments should be made by telephone or letter.

The move had to be taken because there was 'a flood of returning prisoners of war from the Far East for whose care some provision [had] to be made'[1]. A brief insight into the functioning of this 'hospital' is provided in the visitor's book (fig 11.1); the date indicates however, that there had been a significant degree of tardiness in the public announcement that the institution had reopened. Unfortunately there were only 47 beds, and the rooms and passages were so narrow that no systematic clinical teaching was possible; clinical demonstrations had to be given wherever room was available, and lectures were given at the Wellcome Institute. Also, there were no 'back-up' facilities, and the staff had to look to other hospitals for support. It was in fact a small 'private clinic'. At no time could this be considered anything more than temporary accommodation.

Manson-Bahr, in company with the other tropical physicians, continued to be unhappy with the *status quo* and he had some interesting comments to make in his Presidential Address to the *Royal Society of Tropical Medicine and Hygiene* in 1947[15]; he began with a historical overview of the discipline, and continued:

. . . But the late war struck two severe blows [to tropical medicine in

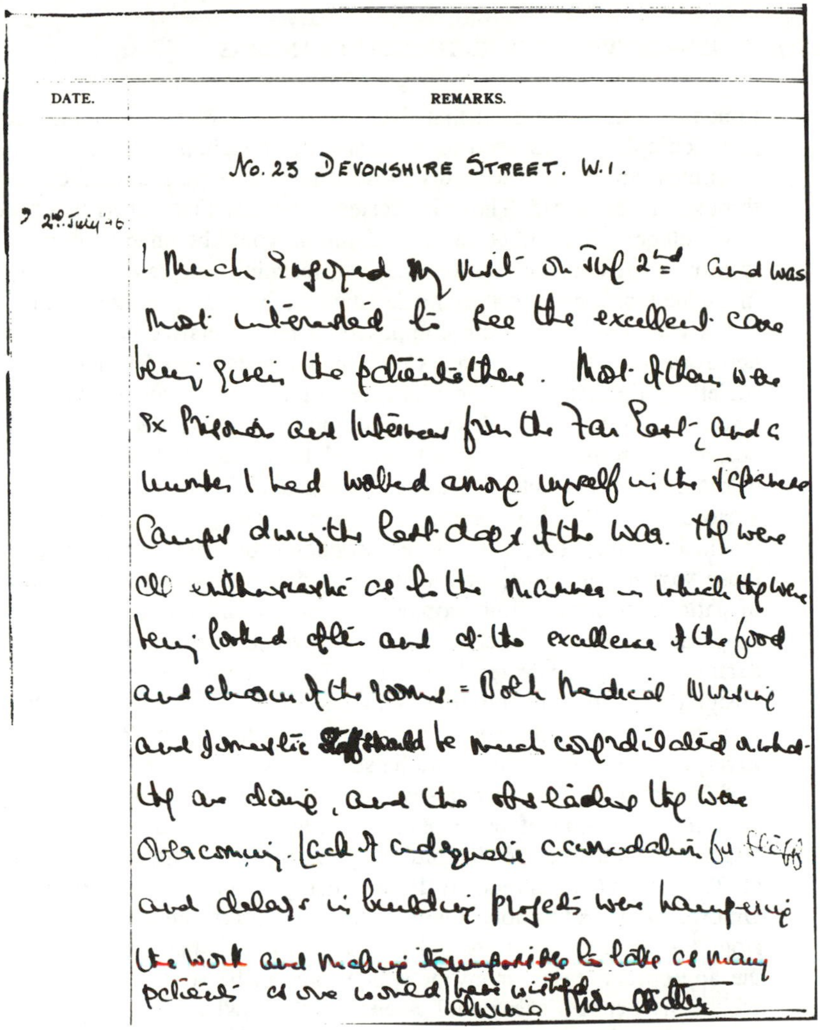

DATE.	REMARKS.

No. 23 Devonshire Street. W.1.

2nd July '46

[handwritten text reproduced in print below]

Fig 11.1: Entry in the visitors book by Countess (Edwina) Mountbatten of Burma (1901–1960)[13,14] – in which she expressed her satisfaction at the state of the hospital which had recently been re-established in this building:

SEAMEN'S HOSPITAL SOCIETY –
Hospital for Tropical Diseases – 1946
No 23, Devonshire Street, W1
2nd July 1946

I much enjoyed my visit on Jul 2nd and was most interested to see the excellent care being given the patients there. Most of them were ex prisoners and internees from the Far East, and a number I had worked among myself in the Japanese Camps during the last days of the war. They were all enthusiastic as to the manner in which they were being looked after and of the excellence of the food and cleanness of the rooms. Both medical nursing and domestic staff should be much congratulated on what they are doing, and the obstacles they were overcoming. Lack of adequate accommodation for staff and delays in building projects were hampering the work and making it impossible to take as many patients as one would have wished.

Edwina Mountbatten

London] at its very heart: first, because of the threat of bombing, it had to be completely removed to various other hospitals – which destroyed its clinical unity – and secondly most of its staff were scattered on service throughout the world. Those interested soon saw that unless this process of disintegration could be reversed London would be unable after the war to resume the contribution to treatment, teaching, and research in tropical medicine that it had worthily made since the beginning of the century.

Early in 1945 a meeting composed of representatives of Government departments, Dominion and Colonial interests, the Services, learned societies, and academic, hospital, and other bodies concerned met and made recommendations. It was agreed on the highest level that a suitable hospital of some 200–300 beds should be established, near and linked to the academic teaching school and research laboratories and forming a closely knit tropical centre. Thus the teaching of tropical medicine would be centralised, with close association between the clinicians and those working in the related academic sciences, while the concentration of patients suffering from tropical diseases would not only increase the scope and value of clinical teaching but would also provide material for detailed or large-scale research. In addition, such a centre would attract postgraduates from all countries and form one of the focal points of tropical medicine. Harmonious cooperation with the other great British centre at Liverpool was envisaged, while liaison with various research laboratories in different parts of the tropics would enable workers to be interchanged. Pending realisation of these plans, an attempt was made to fill the gap left by the closure of the old hospital by acquiring a nursing-home at 23, Devonshire Street, W.1, and using it as a temporary hospital. Unfortunately, admirable though this temporary hospital has proved from the standpoint of its individual patients, it has not room for all the appropriate cases, many of which have to be sent to other hospitals within the Seamen's Hospital Society and elsewhere. Moreover, it does not possess the space and facilities required for teaching large classes of students nor for research laboratories worthy of the clinical material on hand. Notwithstanding these difficulties, large classes of medical and nursing students are receiving instruction in tropical diseases; but the waste and trouble caused by the present dispersion of patients is considerable, and the need for the formation of a single centre is great.

Unhappily, hope for the major scheme now burns less bright. Controls, and the need for reducing capital expenditure, seem to make the possibility of building remote, while uncertainty about the exact pattern of our future health service and economic status possibly has a restraining influence on planning and development. Nevertheless there are cogent reasons for pressing on without further delays. Though tropical disease must be studied in the tropics, it must also be studied, against an academic background, in major scientific centres, of which London is outstandingly suited to the purpose. Today the greater movement of peoples and the rapidity of modern transport are bringing about a virtual contraction of the world that is bound to increase the interest taken in tropical diseases and necessitate further study and instruction in tropical medicine. Likewise the development of new agricultural and commercial undertakings in the Colonies whose importance for the welfare of Colonial people and for the very survival of our Commonwealth needs little emphasis, and the obligations that we owe to the Colonial peoples, make the restoration of every facility for treatment, research, and teaching in tropical medicine a matter of true urgency. Like Sir PHILIP MANSON-BAHR [wrote the leader writer], we trust therefore that some way will be found to enable the principal city of the Commonwealth to resume its proper part in advancing and disseminating knowledge of clinical tropical medicine.

In the first post-war 'five-year plan' of the LSHTM, Hamilton Fairley expressed himself strongly[16]:

The supreme consideration from the clinical side is the establishment of a modern Hospital for Diseases of the Tropics in the vicinity of the London School of Hygiene and Tropical Medicine.

Although the Devonshire Street hospital proved seriously inadequate, these were days of austerity, funding was difficult to obtain, and future prospects for clinical tropical medicine gloomy. But when the National Health Service came into being in 1948, new hope arose that a hospital to cover the speciality would be provided under the aegis of that body[17]:

... Mr IVOR THOMAS asked the Minister of Health what plans he had for the creation of a tropical diseases hospital in London worthy of the imperial responsibilities of the United Kingdom.
— Mr. [Aneurin] BEVAN replied: It is proposed to develop a tropical diseases centre as a unit of the University College Hospital group. The Colonial Secretary and I are most anxious to ensure that development shall be worthy of the object in view, and shall take place as rapidly as building and other difficulties permit.

The LSHTM's second post-war 'five-year plan' however, makes this comment[16]:

By arrangement with University College Hospital accommodation has been made available for a professorial teaching unit in clinical tropical medicine at St. Pancras Hospital. It is anticipated that the transfer from the Hospital for Tropical Diseases in Devonshire Street to the new unit will take place in 1951. This will increase the number of beds available for teaching purposes ... It is hoped that ultimately a hospital devoted solely to the treatment of tropical diseases will be built, and so administered that all cases of tropical disease in London and the Home Counties will be admitted there rather than scattered over a number of London teaching hospitals, as is now the case.

Unfortunately the envisaged 'tropical diseases centre' (the Imperial Hospital for Tropical Diseases) had not materialised. *Clinical* medicine was therefore to go its own way and become increasingly detached from the LSHTM (chapter 12). Perhaps the only significant strategy to forge a 'loose-link' between the two was the creation of a chair of *Clinical* Tropical Medicine at the LSHTM; the first occupant was Professor (later Sir) Neil Hamilton Fairley FRS. Others have followed, some more *clinically* oriented than others!

Following preliminary discussions (see above) a definite decision was ultimately taken by University College Hospital to offer the vacant building on the St Pancras Hospital site (chapter 12). This was subsequently accepted by the tropical physicians. Despite all of these uncertainties, the teaching of tropical medicine – with a distinctly *clinical* orientation – did continue to receive serious attention as is made clear in the following leading article in the *British Medical Journal* for 1949[18]:

> At the present time there are three centres in this country at which post-graduate courses of instruction in tropical medicine are given: these are in London, Liverpool, and Edinburgh. The length of the courses is about five months, and the students then sit an examination for a diploma in tropical medicine and hygiene. That in London is conducted by the Conjoint Board, and those in the other centres by the universities concerned. Their original purpose was to fit medical men for clinical practice in the Tropics, essentially to familiarize them with a variety of diseases of which they learn little or nothing in the ordinary qualifying medical curriculum in this country. Among the diseases which are of more peculiarly tropical distribution those due to protozoa, to spirochaetes, and to helminths are of very great importance. The study of these cannot be confined to the more rigidly clinical aspects of their diagnosis and treatment; it entails an introduction to subjects largely foreign to the graduate in medicine in this country. It is impossible to understand the parasitic diseases of man without a sound knowledge of the parasites causing them and of the vectors which convey these parasites. The student's course of study must therefore include clinical parasitology and medical entomology and zoology in order to give him sufficient knowledge to undertake ordinary tropical practice. The basic requirements of the curriculum are thus wide, and not least of the difficulties for the student is the acquirement of an extensive new vocabulary.

The writer then emphasised the importance of:

> . . . skill in the technical examinations which are necessary for diagnosis and for the control of treatment. The help of a laboratory, so easy to obtain in this country, is but rarely available in the Tropics, and the medical

practitioner there must be his own clinical laboratory technician. To give him confidence in his ability to do this work a large proportion of his time in training must be spent in the laboratory if he is to acquire the necessary technical proficiency. The need for this is great, for teachers have found that many postgraduate students coming for training cannot even use a microscope competently. In addition to essential instruction in tropical diseases the three courses now include a wide range of subjects such as ethnology, nutrition, sanitary engineering, field surveying, public health practice, epidemiology, and vital statistics. That adequate knowledge of each of these can be acquired by the student in so limited a period is doubtful, and in the attempt to absorb it there is a very real danger that the facts necessary for the ordinary practice of his profession may be obscured.

. . . the primary object is to equip the medical graduate for his immediate duty as a general practitioner in the Tropics, and a preliminary course of study might well be limited to this. After experience in the Tropics the practitioner would have first-hand knowledge of the medical problems of his own district, and he would know which were capable of solution by his own efforts. Armed with this knowledge, he would be in a far better position to seek and to assimilate a wider range of information to this end. Those who advocate a preliminary course of instruction in tropical medicine of rigidly limited scope and of severely practical aspect have a strong case. At a later date medical officers with practical experience in the field could take a more advanced course of study. The preliminary course might be followed by an examination, which would in effect afford a certificate of competence to practise medicine in the Tropics. The advanced course would be much less stereotyped and could be varied to meet the needs of individuals; an examination after this course might be dispensed with.

Tropical diseases in London following World War II

As had been anticipated (see above) large numbers of ex-servicemen who had experienced tropical exposure during the 1939–45 war returned with diseases with which the average medical practitioner was unfamiliar. Clearly, not all of them could be managed at one of the 'tropical diseases centres'. Descriptions of many of the illnesses experienced by prisoners-of-war in South-East Asia, especially those who had worked on the Burma-Siam Railway, have been described in war-time diaries[19,20]. An excellent example of one chronic illness from which they suffered can be found in an account published in 1949 from The Ministry of Pensions Tropical Diseases Unit, Queen Mary's Hospital, Roehampton[21].

It was subsequently noted without exception in a series of *several hundred cases* [my italics] that this type of creeping eruption . . . occurred only in ex-prisoners-of-war from the Far East, and that they had been held in captivity

285

in grossly insanitary conditions in Burma and Siam, with one case from Java.

This report clearly refers to persisting *Strongyloides stercoralis* infection, for which at that time there was no effective chemotherapy.

Care of leprosy patients

The HTD became involved at this time with the management of leprosy patients at an isolation hospital in Surrey[22]. (The only existing hospital in Britain at this time was the 'Homes of St Giles' in Essex – which had been opened in 1913[23]). In the immediate post-war era, there was a large influx of people indigenous to the tropics, to Britain. Fears that the disease was 'infectious' were wide-spread and cases could not be managed at the HTD. In 1951 the Minister of Health made leprosy a notifiable disease, after deciding in 1950 that a special hospital was required for these patients. This was constructed in the grounds of the Redhill-Reigate Hospital, Surrey and was named the 'Jordan Hospital'[22]; opened in 1950, it had 18 beds (later increased to 24) and was staffed by the HTD and administered by University College Hospital (chapter 12). Outpatients with leprosy were and still are seen at the HTD, as are in-patients. The Jordan Hospital was closed in 1967.

12

Removal to Old St Pancras; the itinerant saga continues

St Pancras Hospital, NW1 (and its environs) possesses an interesting and colourful history[1-3]. In the same era that London dockland provided the milieu for the formation of the SHS, in 1821 (chapter 3), so north London (with its massive problem of sick poor) became a site for the foundation of a 'public' hospital. The social conscience of the nineteenth century had been aroused!

The 'Directors of the Poor' were appointed in 1804[2]; their task was to remove from the Vestry [St Pancras became a Borough only in 1900, when one of the first councillors (formerly a member of the Vestry Committee) was George Bernard Shaw[3,4]] the administration of poor relief. However, administration of the Poor Laws subsequently went from bad to worse[5]. The *workhouse* (erected in 1809 under an Act passed by George III) became terribly overcrowded. Pauperism escalated, and by 1832, following an agricultural decline, accompanied by famine, disease, and various epidemics the Government of the day at last became concerned. The social scene of the time has been portrayed by Charles Dickens (who lived temporarily in Johnson Street, Somers Town) in *Oliver Twist* and others of his novels[2]. In 1834 an Act was passed appointing Poor Law Commissioners; they remained in power until 1847, and were succeeded by the Poor Law Board which was in turn displaced by the Local Government Board in 1871, and in 1919 by the Ministry of Health[2]. From the 1860s onwards, there were various inquiries and Royal Commissions and the first of the Acts (Metropolitan Poor Law Act 1867) gave the Poor Law Board the authority to provide hospitals for the poor[5]. The 1867 Act was however slow to make an impact; there were asylums for the mentally ill, and fever hospitals for patients with infectious diseases which were provided by the Metropolitan Asylums Board (chapter 3) but it was almost 20 years later that the St Pancras Infirmary was opened (on the workhouse site). The workhouse and infirmary were quite separate, however, the former being run by a master and the latter by a medical superintendent – who was junior in rank to the master. The 1867 Act was in fact the first to acknowledge the

State's duty in providing such hospitals; it was an important foundation-stone in the much later development of the National Health Service[5,6]. In the 1870s and 1880s 'pauper' hospitals became 'public' hospitals, and in London every citizen was then entitled to free medical treatment. The present workhouse buildings were established under the aegis of the Guardians of the Poor; Plate 64 shows the foundation stone – which was laid in 1890. Thereafter the old workhouse became St Pancras Hospital with its attached Infirmary – built in 1884 – (now the South Wing) (Plate 65). Between 1929 and 1948 the London County Council transformed the St Pancras Workhouse into a modern hospital; the North Wing was opened as a Mental Observation Unit in 1937.

It was not inappropriate then that *clinical* tropical medicine was to move to a site which had been so closely associated with the great social awakening of the mid-nineteenth century – led by Wilberforce, Chadwick and others (chapter 1). With the introduction of the National Health Service on 5 July 1948, responsibility for St Pancras Hospital was transferred from the London County Council (LCC) to University College Hospital; 19 years previously it had passed from the Poor Law Board of Guardians to the LCC.

Fig 12.1 shows a plan of the St Pancras Hospital site in 1935. As part of a project to replace the old workhouse buildings one by one, a proposed obstetric hospital was erected and completed immediately before World War II. This building was never actually used; many potential patients were evacuated to the country in 1939 and it lay empty throughout the dark days between 1939 and 1945. After the war, the obstetricians (who had been designated as the first occupants of the building) decided that their discipline should be sited at University College Hospital. One of their main objections to the St Pancras site was that it was insanitary; the St Pancras railway stables were situated on the opposite side of the Grand Union Canal, and flies were present in abundance. The building was therefore placed at the disposal of the tropical physicians then located at Devonshire Street. Despite a great deal of bomb damage to the site, this building, shortly to become the Hospital for Tropical Diseases (HTD), survived the war intact. Now identified as the future home of *clinical* tropical medicine in London the following notices appeared in 1951[7]:

> ... In 1939, when war broke out once more, the [Endsleigh Gardens] hospital closed and distributed its patients among the other Seamen's hospitals. As a result its clinical unity was lost, and most of its staff were soon scattered in the Services throughout the world. It was clear that unless this process of disintegration was reversed London could not resume its contribution to tropical medicine after the war, and in 1945 a representative committee recommended that a hospital should be established near to and linked with the academic teaching school and research laboratories to form

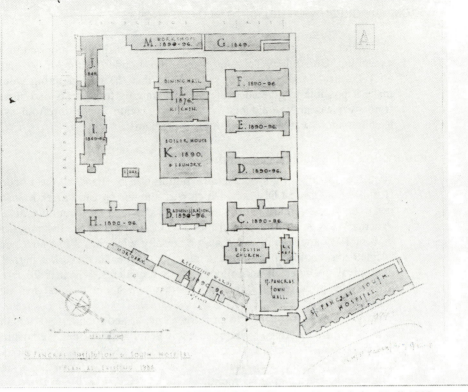

Fig 12.1: Architect's plan (dated 1935) of the St Pancras Hospital site. Until 1929 this had been the St Pancras Workhouse; St Pancras South Hospital was previously the Infirmary. Blocks J, M and G were subsequently demolished by the LCC. Block F was replaced by the building which was to become the *Hospital for Tropical Diseases* in 1951. A great deal of bomb damage occurred on the site; the St Pancras Town Hall was completely demolished.

a closely knit tropical diseases centre. Building a new hospital would obviously take time, so a temporary hospital was opened in Devonshire Street, to replace the Endsleigh Gardens premises which had been damaged by a landmine. Unfortunately the building was too small to hold all the appropriate cases; it had neither the space nor the equipment for teaching large classes; and it lacked research laboratories worthy of the potential clinical material.

The hospital has now made a third move, and the Duchess of Kent opened its new building, in the grounds of St. Pancras Hospital, on May 24 [Plate 66]. This was built in 1939 as a maternity home [Plates 67a & b], though it was never used for that purpose; it will have beds for 68 patients and ample space for teaching and research. Under the N.H.S. it is included in the University College Hospital Group, and the Seamen's Society thus relinquishes its control after more than 50 years.

At the opening, the Minister of Health [The Rt Hon Aneurin Bevan] said there was an erroneous impression that no new hospitals are being built and no new beds provided. There may have to be some postponement

289

of schemes, but this occasion proved that the hospital's programme is expanding. Dr. Andrew Topping, dean of the London School of [Hygiene and] Tropical Medicine, expressed a hope that the new building would make it possible to give adequate clinical training to students and nurses from overseas and would put London once again in the forefront as a teaching and research centre in tropical medicine.

and the following enthusiastic report[8]:

With the opening of a spacious new building in St. Pancras, the London Hospital for Tropical Diseases, which was founded by Sir Patrick Manson just over half a century ago, enters upon a new era. The building, in St. Pancras Way, adjacent to the former L.C.C. hospital of St. Pancras, was built in 1939 and was intended as a maternity wing, but it has now been adapted and equipped in the most modern manner to serve the purpose of tropical medicine. It accommodates 68 in-patients, which is 20 more than at the premises in Devonshire Street which the hospital has just vacated. . . .

At St. Pancras it is hoped to carry on in better and roomier quarters the clinical researches which have for so many years distinguished the hospital and the school. The move will enable the London School of Hygiene and Tropical Medicine to introduce a longer course of eight months, which will include four continuous months at the hospital. It will make it easier for hospitality to be offered to medical men from home or overseas who wish to devote their attention to this specialty, and it is hoped to bring about a wider interchange of doctors, students, and nurses with hospitals and schools abroad. The hospital will be the yellow-fever inoculation centre for south-east England, and a mobile vaccination team will visit the London docks to inoculate ships' crews making only a few hours' stay. The new hospital, which is only a mile or so from the London School of Hygiene and Tropical Medicine, was opened by the Duchess of Kent on Empire Day. It is one of the University College group of hospitals.

At the time of the opening the 68 beds (9 of them private) were situated on the second and third floors. The first floor was named the *Manson Ward* and the second the *Chamberlain Ward*. There was a pathology laboratory (on the ground floor), a small operating theatre, laboratories, and a postgraduate lecture theatre (on the third floor). Table 12.1 gives the names of the medical staff of the HTD at that time. Although considerably happier than they had been at Devonshire Street, they were not all content with their position under the University College Hospital 'umbrella'; this in fact led to a great deal of dissatisfaction in the early days and they still strove for autonomy. Statistics indicate that the HTD was well used in the early days on the St Pancras site. In 1958, for example, the average bed occupancy was 58, and 1868 discharges/deaths were recorded; by

Table 12.1 – Medical staff of the Hospital for Tropical Diseases in 1951

Consulting Physicians
>G Carmichael Low, MD, FRCP, 7 Kent House, Kensington Court, W8.
>Sir Philip Manson Bahr, CMG, DSO, MD, FRCP, DTM&H, 149 Harley Street, W1
>F M R Walshe, OBE, MD, DSc, FRCP, FRS, 11/12 Wimpole Street, W1

Consulting Surgeons
>T Pomfret Kilner, CBE, MB, FRCS, Churchill Hospital, Oxford
>Sir Archibald H McIndoe, CBE, MS, FRCS, 149 Harley Street, W1

Consulting Radiologist
>G R Mather Cordiner, CVO, MB, ChB, DMRE, 7 Upper Wimpole Street, W1

Consultant Staff

Physicians
>Sir Neil Hamilton Fairley, KBE, DSc, FRCP, DTM&H, FRS, 73 Harley Street, W1
>Professor F Murgatroyd, MD, FRCP, DTM, 73 Harley Street, W1
>Sir George McRobert, CIE, MD, FRCP, 55 Harley Street, W1

Surgeons
>C Naunton Morgan, FRCS, 149 Harley Street, W1
>H R I Wolfe, MS, FRCS, 16 Thornton Way, NW11

Ophthalmic Surgeon
>Colonel E W O'G Kirwan, CIE, MD, FRCSI, 33 Wimpole Street, W1

Anaesthetists
>C Langton Hewer, MRCP, DA, 33 Stormont Road, N6
>J Truscott Hunter, MRCS, LRCP, DA, FFARCS, 11 Mansfield Street, W1
>G S Organe, MB, ChB, DA, 17 Burghley Road, SW19
>Consultant Staff of University College Hospital are available when required.

First Assistant in Tropical Medicine
>A W Woodruff, MD, MRCP, DTM&H

Medical Registrars
>W H Jopling, MRCP, DTM&H
>D Lawrence, MD, DTM&H

Medical Registrar for Pathology
>Miss Minnie Gosden, OBE, MB, BS, DTM

1961 the respective figures were 54 and 1540. In 1960 there were 2530 'new' outpatient appointments with a total of 5304; in 1961 the respective figures were 2496 and 4887.

The long association of the SHS with 'tropical' medicine had thus ended. Not only the HTD, but the Dreadnought Hospital (Greenwich), the Albert Dock Hospital (rebuilt in 1937–38), and the Angas Home had entered the National Health Service on 5 July 1948. The SHS did however continue with the administration of the three other institutions for some years. The facilities which were now available at the newly sited hospital were referred to in a parliamentary debate the following year[9]:

> . . . Colonel J.H. HARRISON drew attention to the facilities offered by the Hospital for Tropical Diseases in St. Pancras Way, London, N.W.1. He had tried, but not with much success, to interest the British Medical Association in the improvement of the health of those who had been prisoners of war in the Far East. He asked whether it was not possible for a specialist in tropical diseases periodically to visit provincial centres with publicity beforehand to all local doctors so that they could send him as out-patients men who thought they still had traces of tropical diseases. He asked whether the Government could ensure that the 900 men who were now prisoners in Korea would, on their return, be properly tested to see whether they were suffering from tropical diseases.
>
> Miss P. HORNSBY-SMITH assured Colonel Harrison that the Ministry was ready to do anything possible to bring the facilities of the Hospital for Tropical Diseases to the attention of such persons. The Minister of Pensions was also ready to see that the facilities open to war pensioners were brought to their attention. She said the Ministry had no evidence of unusual prevalence of tropical diseases in this country. It had taken special measures in connexion with malaria, and the Chief Medical Officer of the Ministry of Health shortly after the war had circulated all doctors on the possibility of unrecognized relapses in patients who might have had malaria. A practitioner could refer a patient to the local general hospital, and if it were in the South of England it in turn could send him to the Hospital for Tropical Diseases. It had always been intended that this hospital should be a consultative centre for specialized treatment in tropical diseases, and senior administrative medical officers of the regional boards were well aware of its facilities. It was not easy to send out specialists on tour, but Miss Hornsby-Smith would see whether the regional hospital board in the district for which Colonel Harrison spoke had any evidence of a particular need.

Continuing importance of tropical medicine in Britain

The war which was currently raging in South-east Asia, clearly raised the 'index of awareness' of tropical disease in Britain and the *British Medical Journal* devoted a leading article to the subject in 1953[10]:

> The presence of our forces in the Far East, particularly those fighting in Korea and Malaya, must renew the interest of the practitioner in this country in diseases of the Tropics. In particular he should be aware of those which may persist in Europeans after their return to Britain. Attacks

of malaria, especially of benign tertian (*P[lasmodium] vivax*) malaria, may occur in men home from these areas. The measures now taken by the Army authorities include the daily administration of proguanil ('paludrine') for the prevention of illness due to malaria, replacing the mepacrine so well known during the 1939–45 war. This prophylaxis has proved extremely efficient in suppressing the manifestations of malaria while the drug is being taken regularly. However, unhappily no drug has so far been found which can safely be given to prevent a B.T. [*P.vivax*] malaria infection. It follows that when the suppressive drug is stopped on leaving the Far East a suppressed infection may come into the open as an actual attack of B.T. malaria in a period of anything from a few days to nine or ten months after a man's return home. These are the cases that the doctor in this country may meet, and the difficulties in diagnosis are not lessened by the fact that the patient has not suffered from malaria while overseas, and that he has remained well for a considerable period after his return home and re-entry into civil life.

The writer proceeded to underline the importance of suspecting malaria:

> . . . A first and elementary step in its investigation should always be an examination of blood films for malaria parasites. Any treatment in advance of this blood examination is most undesirable, as it may vitiate the diagnosis. The inferential, or 'therapeutic', diagnosis of malaria is unwarrantable when a simple blood examination will put the matter beyond doubt. If the prompt examination of blood films is impossible, at least the films themselves can usually be made before treatment is begun, and subsequently studied to make the diagnosis. Perfectly satisfactory thick blood films have been made in exceptional circumstances on pieces of window glass. Once diagnosed an attack of benign tertian malaria becomes a matter of minor significance. The infection can rapidly be controlled, and furthermore it can be completely eradicated within a week or two in a high proportion of cases; in any event it spontaneously disappears within, at most, two years of its acquisition. Under such conditions the disability resulting from it is transitory and trivial.

And intestinal parasitic infections also received attention:

> . . . These occur wherever sanitation is defective. Worm infections of the bowel in otherwise healthy Europeans are of little significance. While aesthetically unpleasant, they rarely cause ill-health. True hookworm disease occurs only in debilitated populations suffering from heavy infestations superimposed on malnutrition and the avitaminoses; it is not seen in the well-nourished. The eradication of roundworms and of hookworms, if these are present, is quite a simple matter.
>
> Of the protozoal infections of the bowel amoebic dysentery is by far the most important. Persistently recurring diarrhoea, sometimes with the passage of blood and mucus (dysentery), should raise suspicion of

Entamoeba histolytica. Its detection rests on examination of the stools by an experienced pathologist. As in malaria, and indeed any other parasitic infection, the diagnosis is established only on recovery of the parasite, and 'therapeutic' diagnosis is to be deprecated. Emetine, though very remarkable in treatment, should find no place in diagnosis.

A well-known and not very uncommon complication of old-standing amoebic dysentery is amoebic liver abscess. It may appear some years after repatriation to the temperate climates, and it must be considered as a possibility whenever an increasing lesion of the liver with acute ill-health makes its appearance after sojourn abroad. Occasionally an amoebic liver abscess develops in a person who gives no clear history of previous diarrhoea or dysentery; early diagnosis then is one of the most difficult in the field of tropical medicine.

If efficiently diagnosed and treated the after-effects of amoebic dysentery or of a complicating amoebic liver abscess are as a rule negligible. It is therefore a prime duty of the physician in this country to be alert for these readily controllable and eradicable malarial and dysenteric infections in ex-Service men.

The extent of interest in this article was reflected in subsequent correspondence to the journal[11–13].

Old St Pancras

The immediate surroundings of the present HTD building are interesting on several counts. A mere 'stone's throw' away is St Pancras Old Church (Plate 68). This ancient site of Christianity was first recorded in two deeds dated 1160–1180[3]; the altar stone has been dated 6th century and was possibly used by St Augustine. It is likely that the Church had its origins in the 4th century – possibly 313 or 314 AD. It is possible that this was the last church in England from which the bell tolled for Latin Mass after the Reformation; as a result it is said many Roman Catholics subsequently chose to be interred in the St Pancras Churchyard[2]. It fell into disrepair after the new St Pancras Church in Euston Road was opened in 1822. The church was extensively renovated in 1848, and further restorations were carried out in 1888 and 1925[3]. It was badly damaged during World War II (1939–45). Within the building are many items of interest including several seventeenth and eighteenth century tombs.

A large part of the local burial ground, but not the oldest portions, was appropriated by the Midland Railway Company in the mid-1860s[2]. Considerable public concern arose at this time because many graves were disturbed during the construction of the railway. The ecclesiastical architect in charge was A W Blomfield[14], and he found himself at the centre of this controversy; one of his young assistants Thomas Hardy

(1840–1928) (later to abandon architecture, and subsequently to become a major novelist and poet) – seems to have successfully resolved the matter on his behalf, and made sure that everything was reverently done thereafter. Hardy in fact wrote two poems recalling these events[15] – 'In the Cemetery', and 'The Levelled Churchyard':

O Passenger, pray list and catch
  Our sighs and piteous groans,
Half stifled in this jumbled patch
  Of wrenched memorial stones!

We late-lamented, resting here,
  Are mixed to human jam,
And each to each exclaims in fear,
  'I know not which I am!'

The wicked people have annexed
  The verses on the good;
A roaring drunkard sports the text
  Teetotal Tommy should!

Where we are huddled none can trace,
  And if our names remain,
They pave some path or porch or place
  Where we have never lain!

Here's not a modest maiden elf
  But dreads the final Trumpet,
Lest half of her should rise herself,
  And half some sturdy strumpet!

From restorations of Thy fane,
  From smoothings of Thy sward,
From zealous Churchmen's pick and plane
  Deliver us O Lord! Amen!

500 headstones were subsequently relocated and a re-interment service was conducted on 3 July 1866 by the Bishop of London[2].

This graveyard contains the remains of many individuals of interest and importance – including princes, ambassadors, marshals, statesmen, musicians (including Johann Christian Bach (the 'London' Bach) – 1735–82), ecclesiastical dignitaries, painters, sculptors, architects (including Sir John Soane, FRS (1803–87) – architect of the Bank of England), wits and sages, and numerous members of noble English and Irish families[2].

Table 12.2 – Location of clinical tropical medicine in London
between 1821 and the present day

1	1821–1831	HMS 'Grampus', Greenwich
2	1831–1857	HMS 'Dreadnought', Greenwich
3	1857–1870	HMS 'Caledonia' (Renamed 'Dreadnought'), Greenwich
4	1870–1890	Greenwich Hospital-Infirmary/Somerset Ward, Greenwich
5	1890–1899	Greenwich Hospital and Branch Hospital, Royal Victoria & Albert Docks
6	1899–1920*	Albert Dock Hospital
7	1920–1939*	23 Gordon Street, WC1 (Endsleigh Gardens)
8	1939–1944	Dreadnought Hospital, Greenwich
9	1944–1951	23 Devonshire Street, W1
10	1951–present	St Pancras Hospital (University College Hospital), NW1

* Hospital and school in close proximity; LSHTM established in 1924 and opened in 1929

Buried here also is the longest of the few survivors from the Black Hole of Calcutta – which took place on the night of 20 June 1756 – (who died aged 90 years), and Mary Wollstonecraft [Godwin] (1759–97)[16,17] mother of Mary Shelley (the wife of Percy Bysshe Shelley the poet), and a pioneer of women's rights. An Act was passed in 1875 enabling the Vestry to acquire and lay out the grounds as a public garden; this was opened by Baroness Burdett-Coutts – who laid the foundation stone of the sundial memorial – on 28 June 1877[2].

The train-shed of St Pancras Station was completed in 1867 and the station opened on 1 October 1868; the accompanying hotel (with 400 rooms) was opened to the public for the first time on 5 May 1873. In 1889 the Midland Railway Company acquired more of Somers Town. After constructing the railway and St Pancras Station, an extensive goods station and yard was established. Another building which lies in close proximity to the HTD is the St Pancras Coroner's Court (Plate 69), the foundation stone of which was laid on 15 December 1886 – 'to commemorate the erection of these buildings in accordance with the joint recommendation of the Sanitary Committee and the Parliamentary General Services Committee'. Another landmark which lies a very short way from the HTD is the Grand Union (Junction) Canal, which was constructed between 1793 and 1805.

An itinerant specialty

Table 12.2 summarizes the various locations of *clinical* tropical medicine in London between 1821 and the present day. This has indeed been an itinerant discipline! Manson-Bahr wrote in 1956[18]:

> In recounting the chequered history of this institution [the HTD, and clinical tropical medicine] a venture one would have thought essential to the greatest of all tropical Empires, there runs the thread of insecurity . . . The hospital became the whipping boy of medical politics . . . The Board of the SHS was always a representative body of admirals whose interest lay in the sailor, but *not* in tropical medicine . . .

This seems a little unfair to the SHS, for other bodies were more responsible for the relative neglect of the *clinical* discipline. The next siting of the HTD is unknown; negotiations are presently underway to remove it to University College Hospital (see below) – but this will doubtless be some way off.

Geographical separation from the LSHTM: the greatest disaster

Looked at with hindsight, the greatest disaster which befell tropical medicine in London was the geographical separation brought about by the opening of the new LSHTM building at Keppel Street in 1929. This separated the *clinical* discipline from the basic sciences (and hygiene). When viewed retrospectively this clearly reflected the growing dominance of public health (hygiene/sanitation) in Britain over the previous 50 years. What the Athlone Committee (chapter 10) had in mind is not entirely clear – tropical medicine was not discussed – but the formation of the 'non-clinical' LSHTM (via the generosity of the Rockefeller Trust) left the *clinical* discipline largely where it was before the foundation of the LSTM in 1899. Significant efforts were made over the years to counteract this but to no avail[18]:

> i) In 1921 Manson urged the SHS to purchase a plot of land on Euston Road to build a Tropical Hospital there; this was not carried out however and the Society of Friends building now occupies the site,
>
> ii) In 1930 Sir Andrew Balfour and Sir Cooper Perry planned to establish an Imperial Hospital in Keppel Street – opposite the LSHTM,

and iii) In 1943 (Sir) Neil Hamilton-Fairley suggested the creation of a 'tropical centre' at Greenwich – which was to become the national 'Mecca' for the study and management of tropical disease.

But the 'Imperial Hospital for Tropical Diseases' never emerged; it was not to be![19]

Postscript: why did tropical medicine emerge around 1900 as a separate specialty?

It is now clear that both positive and negative factors accounted for the timing of the foundation of 'Tropical Medicine'. On the positive side the following were influential:

i) The relatively sudden onset of Colonial expansion; this was without doubt the dominant reason. The discipline had been required for the success of Empire and Raj[20],

ii) The recent establishment of the 'germ theory' of disease,

iii) The discovery of vector-borne parasitoses (by Manson, Ross and others),

and iv) The establishment in 1898 of a Tropical Section of the British Medical Association (at the Edinburgh meeting); a far wider interest in the discipline developed, both throughout the medical profession, and also beyond.

On the negative side the following factors were clearly important:

i) Most 'tropical' diseases had formerly existed in temperate countries – including northern Europe and northern America – also, where they constituted a major problem. Examples of these were cholera, typhoid, malaria and smallpox (chapter 1),

ii) High mortality rates resulting from communicable disease in the tropics were considered unavoidable; the white man would never be able to live safely and/or work satisfactorily in a tropical country,

iii) The 'miasmatic' theory of disease had so far prevailed; there was therefore widespread pessimism that the environment could ever be adequately improved (eg in West Africa) to counteract disease,

and iv) British medical officers serving in tropical countries had, as their sole duty, the care of the health of the expatriate community; *research* into this group of diseases assumed a very low priority.

It is now fashionable to be hyper-critical of the Chamberlain/Manson discipline and to denounce it as 'constructive imperialism' which was centred on state promotion of railways and research – to 'open up' the colonies to private capital and individual initiative'; there are however, two sides to the story! It has also been suggested that colonial doctors were medical 'operatives' or 'agents of imperialism'[21]. Some would rather agree with Ross, that the Empire had done more for tropical medicine than tropical medicine had done for the Empire[22]! As a specialty, tropical medicine lacked a clinical identity; it was in some ways closer to being a biological discipline, due to its dependence on morphology and natural history, and was structured around parasite life-cycles[22]. [The LSTM in fact became linked in 1905 with University College, London via a shared chair in protozoology.]

Management of disease in the tropics had however, come a very long way at the time of the removal to the present site in 1951, but as a specific discipline it was already in decline; it is salutary to recall that when the Manson-Chamberlain collaboration led to the first tropical teaching hospital in London in 1899, the only effective chemotherapeutic agents which were available were quinine (for malaria), ipecacuanha (amoebiasis), and mercury (syphilis and yaws). Some recollections of the major advances achieved during the first half of the twentieth century were recorded by Manson-Bahr in his Manson Oration to the Royal Society of Tropical Medicine and Hygiene in 1958[23].

But the future not only of the hospital but the subspecialty itself remains clouded by uncertainty[24]. During 1991, two clear options for a definitive location for the Hospital for Tropical Diseases (HTD) emerged: (i) the old Dental Hospital at University College Hospital (UCH) (together with a few beds in the Hospital proper), and (ii) block 8 (a Victorian 'pavilion' built in 1871 overlooking the River Thames at Westminster) of St Thomas' Hospital. To many, the latter alternative seemed the ideal (and obvious) venue and one which the pioneers of the specialty too, would have favoured. However, at a meeting of the HTD Medical Committee held on 21 January 1992[25], the UCH option received the higher number of votes! In the judgement of this writer, if this goes ahead the identity of HTD (the 'flagship' of the specialty, 'tropical medicine') is likely to be lost forever, and Manson's achievement (like that of the British Empire) will become a mere memory from a bygone era.

Appendix 1

Admissions (with outcome), and finances during the days of the SHS hospital-ships

Table A.1 summarizes the numbers of in-patient and out-patient admissions during the 49 years of the Greenwich hospital-ships. During this period well over 100,000 sailors were admitted to one of the 3 vessels. During the 40 year period ending 1861, the breakdown of admissions was as follows: 3428 from Her Majesty's navy, 1798 from the Honourable East India Company's service, and 79,683 from the merchant vessels of different nations[1]. The respective totals up to 31 January 1871 were: 3586, 1798, and 99,491[2]. Their provenance was as follows[3]:

> The patients of different nations received were in the following proportion:
> – Englishmen, 39,734; Scotchmen, 8199; Irishmen, 6035; Frenchmen, 249; Germans, 913; Russians, 871; Prussians, 1346; Dutchmen, 233; Danes, 907; Swedes and Norwegians, 2299; Italians, 639; Portuguese, 520; Spaniards, 313; East Indians, 1142; West Indians, 1167; British Americans, 918; United States, 1322; South Americans, 149; Africans, 391; Turks, 16; Greeks, 64; New Zealanders, 35; New South Wales, 36; South Sea Islanders, 226; Chinese, 42; born at sea, 137; total, 67,903.

A later breakdown (up to 31 January 1871) which does not change the proportions significantly, is given by McBride[2]; the overall total to that date was 104,875. Table A.2 summarizes the outcome of these admissions during four periods during which figures are extant.

Reports in *The Lancet* summarize some of the donations to the SHS; table A.3 gives details of overall receipts and expenditure. Amongst the early gifts and legacies were the following: His Excellency Keying, the High Commissioner to the Emperor of China – £187.10.0[4]; His Majesty the King of Sweden – one hundred guineas[5]; the gentlemen forming the Royal Victoria Yacht Club, on their dissolution – £95.0.0[6]; legacies from Mr Benjamin Hill – £300, Mr Boucher – £100 and Lady Colville – £10; the Emperor of Russia, and other potentiates, the Emperor of France – 400 francs annually, the King of Denmark – £50.0.0, a legacy from

Table A.1 – In-patient and out-patient admissions*
for the 3 hospital-ships – March 1821 to 1871

Date (year)	Time span (mths)	In-patients (total)	Out-patients (total)	Date of *The Lancet* report
1831	–	[14,328]	–	–
1832	12	2017[16,345]	954[3029]	–
1847	12	2509	1629	13 February
1848	3	957[56,175]	555	22 January
"	3	756		5 August
"	12	2712	1941	26 August
1849	12	>2500		7 April
1850	12	2239		2 March
1852	3	768[65,373]	372	17 January
"	3	700	338	17 April
"	3	828[67,053]	412	16 October
1853	3	738	129	22 January
"	12	2366[67,903]	–	22 October
"	12	2316	1554	19 February
1854	12	2563	1458	4 February
"	3	862[70,928]	347	22 April
1856	–	2050[75,603]	1658	–
1857	12	1851	1658	7 March
"	–	[77,454]	–	–
1858	3	654[80,198]	400	17 July
1861	12	1779[84,909]	1202[48,788]	2 March
1870	–	[102,863]	–	–
1871	12	2179	1358	11 February
"	–	[104,875]	–	–

* Cumulative numbers from March 1821 are given in parentheses. When a reference to a report in *The Lancet* is not cited, the figure is derived from McBride[1].

Miss Hardwicke of £605.0.0[7]; legacies from Captain Johnson – £50.0.0, Colonel Purchase – £138.0.0, Miss Palmer – £200.0.0, a donation from an able seaman of the *Imaum* – £1.8.0, and one from the Emperors of France and Russia[8]; His Highness the Viceroy of Egypt £100.0.0[9]; Mr De Berg, the Russian Consul-General in London – £131.8.8 'being the amount of contributions from the Governments of several provinces of the Grand Duchy of Finland, and collections from Finnish merchants and captains, in aid of the fund for the reconstruction of the hospital, so long established afloat off Greenwich', and an annual subscription from the Grand Duchy of Finland, by consent of the Emperor of Russia, of £20.0.0[10].

Table A.2 – Outcome of in-patients at the 3 hospital-ships

	1821*	1831 –32*	1855 –57*	1860 –61+	1870 –71*
Discharged at own request, cured	168	828	1229	942	990
Discharged:					
fit for duty/relieved	–	6	168	162	267
convalescent	–	354	208	415	462
not cured	–	27	11	68	53
Absent, from Surgeon's leave	20	56	60	25	22
Discharged to ships:					
cured	79	311	–	–	–
fit for duty	–	7	–	–	–
convalescent	–	208	–	–	–
not cured	–	14	–	–	–
to ships found by the SHS	30	32	0	–	–
Conveyed to their Homes	14	5	9	4	9
Without Certificates of good conduct	–	2	64	33	94
Expelled	10	14	23	24	2
Died	3	141	111	82	110
Under cure, and convalescent	89	193	167	171	170
TOTAL	**413**	**2198**	**2050**	**1926**	**2179**

* Derived from McBride[1].   + *The Lancet* (2 March 1861).

Table A.3 – Receipts and expenditure for the 3 hospital-ships

Date (year)	Time span (mths)	Total receipts	Total expenditure	Date of *The Lancet* report
1848	3	£2031.17.1	–	5 August
"	12	£9025.13.9	£5387.5.4	26 August
1850	12	£8264.0.0	–	2 March
1852	3	£1252.12.1	£1622.2.2	17 January
"	3	£1182.18.1	£1380.13.8	16 October
1853	3	£1639.0.0	£2058.0.0	22 January
"	12	£8135.14.11	£17,716.11.4	19 February
1854	12	£10,638.17.6	–	4 February
"	3	£2697.17.3	£3235.17.3	22 April
1857	12	£21,125.0.0	£<20,000.0.0	14 February
1858	3	£11,522.1.10	–	17 July
1861	12	£8187.8.11	£7514.12.5	2 March

The cost of removal in 1870 from the second *Dreadnought* to the Infirmary of the Greenwich Hospital was £1990[11]; overall expenditure for that year was ' . . . somewhat reduced by certain payments received from the Admiralty for the care and maintenance of a few Greenwich Hospital pensioners, who were too ill or too helpless to be removed when the building was handed over to the Society[11]'. The report for this year also forecast a likely increase in numbers of outpatients in the forthcoming years:

> . . . as the hospital is situated in a thickly populated district, and no general hospital exists nearer than London-bridge – a distance of about four miles.

Appendix 2

Case-reports of medical and surgical illnesses on board the hospital-ships

An account of some of the diseases which were common on the hospital ships can be found in chapter 3. Scurvy was a major problem; from 1839 until 1867, the SHS campaigned for the inclusion of citrus fruit in the sailors' diet[1]. In 1844 the Merchant Seamen's Act recommended that a Scale of Medicines should be drawn up and this would include lime juice; however this did not apparently apply to those sailing to European and the Mediterranean posts. On 20 August 1867, a bill which was introduced by the Duke of Richmond, President of the Board of Trade, was given Royal assent. Seamen were to be be given lime juice daily; this should, it was stipulated, be purchased from a bonded warehouse and certified (by an Inspector of lime juice) to contain 15% proof spirit.

The seamen came from all over the world, many of them from Asia. Therefore, many were admitted to the *Dreadnought* with tropical ailments; indeed these diseases were sufficiently common for the SHS to consider the desirability of providing special accommodation[1].

Typhus occurred on the *Dreadnought* between 1842–47[1]. Smallpox was never a major problem however, despite the fact that it proved to be so on shore.

Venereal disease was rife amongst the sailors; there were 'over a thousand known prostitutes in the Chatham and Woolwich area and some eighteen thousand in the streets of London'; it was estimated that at least one third of them were diseased'[1].

Accidents were commonplace, both on board ship, in the ship-building yards, and in other industries on both sides of the Thames[1]. Cases were admitted to the *Dreadnought* because there was no other hospital in the area; Guy's and St Thomas' Hospitals had previously been used but they were too distant and many of the injured men would not survive the journey. Accident cases in the Greenwich and Woolwich areas were also sometimes admitted as emergencies, because there was a general lack of hospital accommodation in south-east London.

304

Many case-reports giving detailed *clinical* descriptions of patients admitted to the hospital-ships have survived, some of them in the columns of *The Lancet*. Many are of surgical or orthopaedic conditions. Several give accounts of serious trauma involving the limbs[2-5], central nervous system[6], and in one case the diaphragm[6]. Post-traumatic infections frequently produced difficult problems. Amputation of a leg for scrofula is the subject of a case-report[7]. Excision of the femoral head in 'hip-joint disease' is the subject of another[8]. A patient under the care of Mr George Busk had a 'strumous ulceration' of the tongue and throat which required tracheostomy[9]. Strangulated hernia figures prominently[10,11]. A fungal infection of the testicle, associated with deposits of 'encephaloid cancer' in the liver is described[12]. A case of urethral stricture is recorded[5].

Medical entities are also covered. Two reports are devoted to cholera[13,14]. Typhus[15], diphtheria[16] and tetanus[17] are recorded. Scurvy is the subject of two case-reports (see above)[18,19]. A case of purpuric fever seems to have presented a diagnostic challenge[20]; suppressed variola was one suggestion! A joint study with the Metropolitan Free (later the Royal Free) Hospital documented the value of zinc phosphate in epilepsy[21]. And an anaesthetic death, caused by chloroform, was documented[22].

References

Preface

1. Singer C. Notes on some early references to tropical diseases. *Ann Trop Med Parasit* 1912; 6: 87-101, 379-403.
2. Nova et Vetera: early references to tropical medicine. *Br Med J* 1913; i: 1331-1332.
3. Ryle JA. 'Tropical' diseases. *Lancet* 1946; ii: 61.
4. Cockburn A, Cockburn E (eds). *Mummies, disease and ancient cultures.* Cambridge: Cambridge University Press 1980: 243.
5. *The Times.* Teaching the world to stay healthy. *The Times, London* 1985; 29 October: 26.
6. Balfour A. Some British and American pioneers in tropical medicine and hygiene. *Trans R Soc Trop Med Hyg* 1925; 19: 189-231.
7. Patten C. Britain's role and responsibility for health in the tropics. *Trans R Soc Trop Med Hyg* 1988; 82: 660-664.
8. Cook GC. Early history of clinical tropical medicine in London. *J Roy Soc Med* 1990; 83: 38-41.

Chapter 1

1. Balfour A. Some British and American pioneers in tropical medicine and hygiene. *Trans R Soc Trop Med Hyg* 1925; 19: 189–231.
2. Singer C, Underwood EA. *A short history of medicine* 2nd ed. Oxford: Oxford University Press 1962: 854.
3. Cook GC. The great malaria problem: where is the light at the end of the tunnel? *J Infect* 1989; 18: 1–10.
4. Bruce-Chwatt LJ, Zulueta J de. *The rise and fall of malaria in Europe: a historico-epidemiological study.* Oxford: Oxford University Press 1980: 240.
5. Bruce-Chwatt LJ. Three hundred and fifty years of the Peruvian fever tree bark. *Br Med J* 1988; 296: 1486–1487.
6. Dewhurst K. *Dr. Thomas Sydenham (1624–1689): his life and original writings.* London: Wellcome Historical Medical Library 1966: 101–125 and 131–139.
7. Howell M, Ford P. The head that wore a crown. In: *The ghost disease and twelve other stories of detective work in the medical field.* Harmondsworth, Middlesex: Penguin 1986; 281–305.
8. Browne SG. Leprosy in the Bible. In: Palmer B (ed). *Medicine and the Bible.* Exeter: Paternoster Press 1986: 101–125.
9. Richards P. Leprosy: myth, melodrama and mediaevalism. *J R Coll Physns Lond*

1990; 24: 55–62.

10. Møller-Christensen V. *Bone changes in leprosy*. Copenhagen: Munksgaad 1961: 51.

11. Morris RJ. *Cholera 1832: the social response to an epidemic*. London: Croom Helm 1976: 228.

12. Pelling M. *Cholera, fever and English medicine 1825–1865*. Oxford: Oxford University Press 1978: 342.

13. Snow J. *On the mode of communication of cholera*. London: John Churchill 1849: 31.

14. Richardson BW. John Snow, MD: a representative of medical science and art of the Victorian era. *The Asclepiad* 1887; 4: 274–300.

15. Chave SPW. Henry Whitehead and cholera in Broad Street. *Med Hist* 1958 2: 92–108.

16. Howell M, Ford P. Death in the parish. In: *The ghost disease and twelve other stories of detective work in the medical field*. Harmondsworth, Middlesex: Penguin 1986: 138–164.

17. Howell M, Ford P. The visitor from a far country. In: *The ghost disease and twelve other stories of detective work in the medical field*. Harmondsworth, Middlesex: Penguin 1986: 191–209.

18. Shrewsbury JFD. *A history of bubonic plague in the British Isles*. Cambridge: Cambridge University Press 1970: 661.

19. Wilson FP. *The plague in Shakespeare's London*. Oxford: Oxford University Press 1927: 228.

20. Bell WG. *The Great Plague in London in 1665*. London: John Lane The Bodley head Ltd. 1924: 374.

21. Defoe D. *A journal of the Plague Year*. London: Penguin 1986: 256.

22. Zwanenberg DV. The last epidemic of plague in England? Suffolk 1906–1918. *Med Hist* 1970; 14: 63–74.

23. Zinsser H. *Rats, lice and history: the biography of a bacillus*. London: Macmillan 1985: 301.

24. Luckin B. Evaluating the sanitary revolution: typhus and typhoid in London, 1851–1900. In: Woods R, Woodward J (eds). *Urban disease and mortality in nineteenth-century England*. London: Batsford Academic and Educational Ltd 1984: 102–119.

25. Booth C. The conquest of smallpox. *Quart J Med* 1985; 57: 811–823.

26. Fenner F, Henderson DA, Arita I, Ježek Z, Ladnyi ID (eds). *Smallpox and its eradication*. Geneva: WHO 1988: 1460.

27. Hopkins DR. *Princes and peasants: smallpox in history*. Chicago, London: University of Chicago Press 1983: 380.

28. Baxby D. *Jenner's smallpox vaccine: the riddle of vaccinia virus and its origin*. London: Heinemann 1981: 214.

29. Dubos R, Dubos J. *The white plague: tuberculosis, man, and society*. New Brunswick, London: Rutgers University Press. 1987: 277.

30. Smith FB. *The retreat of tuberculosis 1850–1950*. London: Croom Helm 1988: 271.
31. Scott HH. *Some notable epidemics*. London: Edward Arnold 1934: 272.
32. McTavish JR. Antipyretic treatment and typhoid fever: 1860–1900. *J Hist Med* 1987; 42: 486–506.
33. Federspiel JF. *The Ballad of Typhoid Mary*. London: Andre Deutsch 1984: 172.
34. Soper GA. The curious career of Typhoid Mary. *Bull NY Acad Med* 1939; 15: 698–712.
35. Finer SE. *The life and times of Sir Edwin Chadwick*. London, New York: Methuen 1952: 555.
36. Lewis RA. *Edwin Chadwick and the public health movement 1832–1854*. London: Longmans, Green and Co 1952: 411.
37. Wohl AS. *Endangered lives: public health in Victorian Britain*. London: Methuen 1983: 440.
38. Webster C. *The Victorian public health legacy: a challenge to the future*. Birmingham: The Public Health Alliance 1990: 18.

Chapter 2

1. Balfour A. Some British and American pioneers in tropical medicine and hygiene. *Trans R Soc Trop Med Hyg* 1925; 19: 189–231.
2. Scott HH. *A history of tropical medicine*. London: Edward Arnold 1939; 2 vols: 1219.
3. *Dictionary of National Biography: from the beginnings to 1921*. London: Oxford University Press 1903: 1456.
4. Kunitz SJ. Making a long story short: a note on men's height and mortality in England from the first through the nineteenth centuries. *Med Hist* 1987; 31: 269–280.
5. Dunn RS. *Sugar and slaves: the rise of the plantar class in the English West Indies, 1624–1713*. Chapel Hill: The University of North Carolina Press 1972: 359.
6. Booth CC. William Hillary: a pupil of Boerhaave. *Med Hist* 1963; 7: 297–316.
7. Cook GC. The small-intestine and its role in chronic diarrhoeal disease in the tropics. In: Gracey M (ed). *Diarrhea*. Boca Raton: CRC Press 1991: 127–161
8. McGrigor J. *The Autobiography and Services of Sir James McGrigor, Bart*. London: Longman, Green, Longman & Roberts. 1861: 201.
9. Cantlie N. *A history of the Army Medical Department*. Edinburgh: Churchill Livingstone 1974; 1: 519.
10. Neal JB. The history of the Royal Army Medical College. *J Roy Army Med Corps* 1957; 103: 1–10.

11. McLaughlin R. *The Royal Army Medical Corps*. London: Leo Cooper, Ltd 1972: 121.

12. Milne GP (ed). *Aberdeen Medico-Chirurgical Society: a bicentennial history 1789–1989*. Aberdeen: Aberdeen University Press 1989: 313.

13. Burgess NRH. Millbank from medieval times to the present. *J Roy Army Med Corps* 1978; 124: 96–104.

14. Arnold D. Introduction: disease, medicine and empire. In: Arnold D (ed). *Imperial medicine and indigenous societies*. Manchester: Manchester University Press 1988: 1–26.

15. Arnold D. Smallpox and colonial medicine in nineteenth-century India. In: Arnold D (ed). *Imperial medicine and indigenous societies*. Manchester: Manchester University Press 1988: 45–65.

16. Catanach IJ. Plague and the tensions of empire: India 1896–1918. In: Arnold D (ed). *Imperial medicine and indigenous societies*. Manchester: Manchester University Press 1988: 149–171.

17. Crawford DG. *A history of the Indian Medical Service 1600–1913*. London: W Thacker & Co 1914; 2: 535.

18. Keevil JJ. *Medicine and the Navy 1200–1900*. Edinburgh, London: E & S Livingstone 1963; 4: 300.

19. Fayrer J. *Recollections of my life*. Edinburgh, London: William Blackwood and Sons 1890: 508.

20. Ernst W. The European insane in British India, 1800–1858: a case-study in psychiatry and colonial rule. In: Arnold D (ed). *Imperial medicine and indigenous societies*. Manchester: Manchester University Press 1988: 27–44.

21. Winterbottom T. *An account of the Native Africans in the neighbourhood of Sierra Leone; to which is added an account of the present state of medicine among them*. London: John Hatchard 1803 (second edition 1969); 2 vols: 362 + 283.

22. Thorp E. *Ladder of bones*. London: Jonathan Cape; 1956: 320.

23. *The Lancet*. One hundred years ago. *Lancet* 1913; i: 455–456.

24. Porterfield JS. Yellow fever in west Africa: a retrospective glance. *Br Med J* 1989; 299: 1555–1557.

25. Gelfand M. *Livingstone the doctor: his life and travels*. Oxford: Basil Blackwell 1957: 333.

26. Jeal T. *Livingstone*. London: Heinemann 1973: 427.

27. Manton J. *Elizabeth Garrett Anderson*. London: Methuen 1965: 382.

28. Howard C. *Mary Kingsley*. London: Hutchinson 1957: 231.

29. Frank K. *A voyager out: the life of Mary Kingsley*. London: Corgi books 1988: 364.

30. Joyce RB. *Sir William MacGregor*. London: Oxford University Press 1971: 484.

31. Keevil JJ. *Medicine and the Navy 1200–1900*. Edinburgh, London: E & S Livingstone 1961; 3: 402.

32. Roddis LH. *James Lind: founder of nautical medicine*. New York: Henry Schuman 1950: 177.

33. Cook E. *The Life of Florence Nightingale*. London: MacMillan & Co. 1913; 2 vols: 507 + 510.

34. Woodham-Smith C. *Florence Nightingale, 1820–1910*. London: Constable 1950: 615.

35. Mackay D. *In the wake of Cook: exploration, science and empire, 1780–1801*. London: Croom Helm 1985: 216.

Chapter 3

1. McBride AG. *The history of the Dreadnought Seamens Hospital at Greenwich*. Chartham: Seamens Hospital Management Committee, Greenwich 1970: 36.

2. Rodger NAM. *The wooden world: an anatomy of the Georgian navy*. Yeovil: Fontana Press 1988: 445.

3. Pollock J. *Wilberforce*. London: Constable 1977: 368.

4. Manson-Bahr P. *History of the School of Tropical Medicine in London (1899–1949)*. London: HK Lewis 1956: 15–21.

5. *Minutes, Seamen's Hospital Society*: book 1 pp 1–2, 8–12 (meetings 8 March and 11 April 1821).

6. To correspondents. *Lancet* 1828; 11 October :64.

7. Seaman's Hospital Society. *Lancet* 1828; 25 October : 113.

8. Budd G. *On Diseases of the liver*. London: John Churchill 1845: 399.

9. Muller R. *Worms and disease: a manual of medical helminthology*. London: Heinemann 1975: 161.

10. Power d'Arcy. George Busk. In: *Plarr's lives of the fellows of the Royal College of Surgeons of England*. Bristol: John Wright 1930: 174–176.

11. Wood BA. The 'Neanderthals' of the College of Surgeons. *Ann R Coll Surg Engl*. 1979; 61: 385–389.

12. Reader J. *Missing links: the hunt for earliest man*. London: Penguin 1988: 8, 11–12.

13. Seamen's Hospital Ship. *Lancet* 1849; ii: 55.

14. The Seamen's Hospital. *Lancet* 1853; i: 216.

15. Seamen's Hospital Society. – cholera on the river. *Lancet* 1853; ii: 406.

16. *The Lancet* 1857; i: 152.

17. Seamen's Hospital Society. *Lancet* 1857; i: 208.

18. The Old "Dreadnought". *Lancet* 1857; i: 281.

19. Seamen's Hospital, "Dreadnought". *Lancet* 1857; ii: 305.

20. Tudor J. The hygienic condition of the "Dreadnought" hospital ship in the year 1857–58 as exemplified by the result of surgical operations. *Lancet* 1859; i: 361–362.

21. Ward S. Analysis of 1000 consecutive cases admitted into the Seamen's Hospital, "Dreadnought". *Lancet* 1860; ii: 78–79.

22. The Seamen's Hospital Society. *Lancet* 1865; i: 245.
23. The Seamen's Hospital Society. *Lancet* 1868; ii: 266.
24. The "Dreadnought". *Lancet* 1870; i: 425.
25. *The Lancet* 1867; ii: 110.
26. Seamen's Hospital, Cardiff. *Lancet* 1870; i: 426.
27. Seamen's Hospital, Cardiff. *Lancet* 1870; i: 508.
28. The "Dreadnought" small-pox hospital. *Lancet* 1871; i: 545.
29. Powell A. *The Metropolitan Asylums Board and its work, 1867–1930*. London: Metropolitan Asylums Board 1930: 106.
30. Burne J. *Dartford's capital river: paddle steamers, personalities and smallpox boats*. Buckingham: Barracuda Books Ltd 1989: 120.
31. The "Dreadnought" convalescent hospital. *Lancet* 1871; i: 623.
32. The "Dreadnought" small-pox hospital. *Lancet* 1871; i: 725.
33. The "Dreadnought" small-pox convalescent hospital. *Lancet* 1871; ii: 408.
34. The cholera: the Port of London. *Lancet* 1871; ii: 413.
35. Disused small-pox hospitals. *Lancet* 1871; ii: 588.
36. Seamen's Hospital Society. *Lancet* 1870; i: 560–561.
37. The Seamen's Hospital, Greenwich. *Lancet* 1872; ii: 56.
38. The Seamen's Hospital. *Lancet* 1872; ii: 235.
39. *The Lancet* 1873; ii: 459–460.
40. The Seamen's Hospital. *Lancet* 1873; ii: 644.
41. Seamen's Hospital Society. *Lancet* 1874; i: 100.
42. The Seamen's Hospital. *Lancet* 1874; ii: 639.
43. *The Lancet* 1874; i: 527.
44. The Seamen's Hospital Society. *Lancet* 1875; i: 249.
45. The Seamen's Hospital. *Lancet* 1875; i: 555.
46. *The Lancet* 1876; i: 684.
47. The Seamen's Hospital. *Lancet* 1878; i: 248.
48. The Seamen's Hospital Society. *Lancet* 1880; ii: 705.
49. The Seamen's Hospital. *Lancet* 1880; i: 813–814.
50. Seamen's Hospital, Greenwich. *Lancet* 1877; i: 289.
51. The Seamen's Hospital. *Lancet* 1877; i: 921.
52. The Seamen's Hospital. *Lancet* 1878; ii: 164.
53. The Seamen's Hospital Society. *Lancet* 1879; i: 824–825.
54. Naval and Military Hygiene. *Lancet* 1891; ii: 452.
55. The Seamen's Hospital Society. *Illustrated London News* 1889; 27 July: 115.
56. The Seamen's Hospital Society. *Lancet* 1890; i: 1337.
57. The Seamen's Hospital Society. *Lancet* 1891; i: 466.
58. Seamen's Hospital Society. *Lancet* 1891; ii: 905.
59. Seamen's Hospital Society. *Lancet* 1892; ii: 554.
60. The medical staff of the Seamen's Hospital Society. *Lancet* 1897; ii: 1556.
61. Matthews J. *Welcome aboard: the story of the Seamen's Hospital Society and the Dreadnought*. Buckingham : Baron 1992: 148.

Chapter 4

1.   Alcock A. Patrick Manson, 1844–1922. *Trans R Soc trop Med Hyg* 1922; 16: 1–15.
2.   Manson-Bahr PH, Alcock A. *The life and work of Sir Patrick Manson.* London, Toronto: Cassell and Co Ltd. 1927: 273.
3.   Manson-Bahr P. The Manson saga, 3rd October 1844 – 9th April 1922. *Trans R Soc trop Med Hyg* 1945; 38: 401 – 417.
4.   Manson-Bahr P. *Patrick Manson: the father of tropical medicine.* London, Edinburgh: Thomas Nelson and Sons Ltd. 1962: 192.
5.   Guppy HB. A reminiscence of Sir Patrick Manson at Amoy. *Trans R Soc trop Med Hyg* 1925; 18: 385–386.
6.   Manson P. Remarks on an operation for abscess of the liver. *Br Med J* 1892; i: 163–167.
7.   Manson P. Notes on sprue. *Med Rep Imperial Maritime Customs, China* 1880; special series no. 2 (19th issue): 33–37.
8.   Cook GC. Tropical sprue: implications of Manson's concept. *J R Coll Physcs Lond* 1978; 12: 329–349.
9.   Chernin E. Patrick Manson (1844–1922) and the transmission of filariasis. *Am J trop Med Hyg* 1977; 26: 1065–1070.
10. Cobbold TS. Discovery of the adult representative of microscopic filariae. *Lancet* 1877; ii: 70–71.
11. Cobbold TS. On Filaria Bancrofti. *Lancet* 1877; ii: 495–496.
12. Manson P. Remarks on lymph-scrotum, elephantiasis and chyluria. *Med Rep Imperial Maritime Customs, China* 1875; no. 27 (part 6): 1–14.
13. Manson-Bahr P. A commentary on the diary kept by Patrick Manson in China and now conserved at Manson House. *Trans R Soc trop Med Hyg* 1935; 29: 79–90.
14. Manson P. Further observations on filaria sanguinis hominis. *Med Rep Imperial Maritime Customs, China* 1877; special series no. 2 (14th issue): 1–26.
15. Manson P. On the development of the *Filaria sanguinis hominis*, and on the Mosquito considered as a Nurse. *J Linn Soc, Zoology* 1879; 14: 304–311.
16. Manson P. The metamorphosis of *Filaria sanguinis hominis* in the mosquito. *Trans Linn Soc, Zoology* 1884; 2: 367–388.
17. Low GC. A recent observation on filaria nocturna in Culex: probable mode of infection of man. *Br Med J* 1900; i: 1456–1457.
18. Manson P. On the periodicity of filarial migrations to and from the circulation. *Med Rep Imperial Maritime Customs, China* 1881; special series no 2 (22nd issue): 63–68.
19. Manson P. Notes on filaria disease. *Med Rep Imperial Maritime Customs, China* 1882; special series no 2 (23rd issue): 1–16.
20. Manson P. On filarial periodicity. *Br Med J* 1899; ii: 644–646.

21. Manson P. Distoma ringeri and parasitical haemoptysis. *Med Rep Imperial Maritime Customs, China* 1881; special series no 2 (22nd issue): 55–62.

22. Scott HH. Patrick Manson (1844–1922). In: *A history of tropical medicine.* London: Arnold 1939: 1068–1076.

23. Manson P. On the operative treatment of hepatitis and hepatic abscess. *Med Rep Imperial Maritime Customs, China* 1883; special series no 2 (26th issue): 50–63.

24. Cantlie N, Seaver G. *Sir James Cantlie: a romance in medicine.* London: John Murray 1939: 279.

25. Stewart JC. *The quality of mercy: the lives of Sir James and Lady Cantlie.* London: George Allen and Unwin 1983: 277.

26. Manson P. On the nature and significance of the crescentic and flagellated bodies in malarial blood. *Br Med J* 1894; ii: 1306–1308.

27. Lankester ER. Discoveries in tropical medicine. *Nature, Lond* 1922; 109: 549 & 812–813.

28. Ross R. Malaria and mosquitoes. *Nature, Lond* 1900; 61: 522–527.

29. Ross R. *Memoirs: with a full account of the great malaria problem and its solution.* London: John Murray 1923: 547.

30. Manson P, Daniels CW. Remarks on a case of trypanosomiasis. *Br Med J* 1903; i: 1249–1252.

31. Lyons M. Sleeping sickness, colonial medicine and imperialism: some connections in the Belgian Congo. In: Macleod R, Lewis M (eds). *Disease, medicine, and Empire: perspectives on western medicine and the experience of European expansion.* London, New York: Routledge 1988: 242–256.

32. Manson P. The necessity for special education in tropical medicine. *Lancet* 1897; ii: 842–845.

33. Manson P. The need for special training in tropical disease. *J trop Med* 1899; 2: 57–62.

34. *The Lancet* 1897; i: 1226.

35. Reviews and notices of books. *Lancet* 1898; i: 1694–1695.

36. Reviews. *Br Med J* 1898; ii: 157–158.

37. Cushing H. *The life of Sir William Osler.* Oxford: The Clarendon Press 1926: vol 1: 642–643.

38. The late Sir Patrick Manson: memorial service in St Paul's. *Br Med J* 1922; i: 664.

39. *The Times, London* 1922; 10 April: 15 & 16.

40. Obituary. Sir Patrick Manson. *Lancet* 1922; i: 767–769.

41. Obituary. Sir Patrick Manson. *Br Med J* 1922; i: 623–626 & 702–703.

Chapter 5

1. Manson-Bahr P. *History of the School of Tropical Medicine in London (1899–1949).* London: HK Lewis 1956: 328.

2. Manson-Bahr PH, Alcock A. *The life and work of Sir Patrick Manson.* London, Toronto: Cassell and Co Ltd. 1927: 273.

3. Instruction in tropical diseases. *Br Med J* 1898; ii: 224.
4. A school for tropical diseases. *Br Med J* 1898; ii; 200–201.
5. *Minutes, Seamen's Hospital Society*: book 13. pp 97–103 (meeting 14 October 1898).
6. *Minutes, Seamen's Hospital Society*: book 13. pp 142–146 (meeting 10 March 1899).
7. Instruction in tropical diseases. *Br Med J* 1898; ii: 1565.
8. Tropical diseases. *Lancet* 1898; ii: 1448.
9. The school of tropical medicine. *Br Med J* 1898; ii: 1637.
10. The school of tropical medicine. *Br Med J* 1898; ii: 1832.
11. *Colonies: Miscellaneous: Papers relating to the investigation of malaria and other tropical diseases and the establishment of Schools of Tropical Medicine.* Presented to both Houses of Parliament by Command of His Majesty. June 1903. pp 1–13.
12. Mr Chamberlain at Birmingham. *The Times, London* 1892; 21 March: 8.
13. The study of tropical medicine. *Lancet* 1899; i: 1319.
14. Mr Chamberlain and the colonies. *The Times, London* 1899; 11 May: 8.
15. Rotberg RI. *The founder: Cecil Rhodes and the pursuit of power.* New York, Oxford: Oxford University Press 1988: 800.

Chapter 6

1. Manson-Bahr PH, Alcock A. *The life and work of Sir Patrick Manson.* London, Toronto: Cassell & Co Ltd. 1927: 273.
2. Curnow J. 'Beri-beri and erroneous diagnoses.' *Lancet* 1897; ii: 1143.
3. Instruction in tropical diseases. *Lancet* 1897; ii: 1266.
4. Burdett HC. A school for tropical diseases in London. *The Times, London* 1898; 11 July: 12.
5. Leading article. *The Times, London* 1898; 11 July: 11.
6. The teaching of tropical diseases in London. *Lancet* 1898; ii: 158.
7. Curnow J, Anderson J, Turner GR. A proposed school for tropical diseases. *Lancet* 1898; ii: 227.
8. Royal College of Physicians of London. *Lancet* 1898; ii: 1224–1225.
9. Instruction in tropical medicine. *Lancet* 1898; ii: 1346.
10. Instruction in tropical medicine. *Lancet* 1898; ii: 1416–1417.
11. The new school of tropical medicine. *Lancet* 1898; ii: 1496.
12. A tropical school of medicine. *Lancet* 1898; ii: 1499–1500.
13. The suggested school of tropical medicine. *Lancet* 1898; ii: 1560.
14. Crookshank EM. Instruction in tropical medicine. *Lancet* 1898; ii: 1579.
15. 'A school of tropical medicine.' *Lancet* 1898; ii: 1574–1575.
16. Roberts W, Duckworth D, Fayrer J, *et al.* The proposed school for tropical medicine. *Lancet* 1898; ii: 1654–1655.
17. Leading article. *The Times, London* 1898; 16 December: 9.
18. Curnow J. The proposed school of tropical medicine. *Lancet* 1898; ii: 1660–1661.

19.	Michelli P. The proposed school of tropical medicine. *Lancet* 1898; ii: 1661.

20.	Hutchinson J. The proposed school of tropical medicine. *The Times, London* 1898; 15 December: 7.

21.	Netley as a school for tropical medicine. *Lancet* 1898; ii: 1805–1806.

22.	Corlette CE. The proposed school of tropical medicine. *Br Med J* 1898; ii: 1844–1846.

23.	Baker O. The School for Tropical Diseases. *The Times, London* 1898; 21 December: 7.

24.	Curnow J, Anderson J, Turner GR. School for Tropical Diseases. *The Times, London* 1898; 23 December: 8.

25.	Howard R. The proposed school for tropical diseases. *The Times, London* 1898; 24 December: 4.

26.	Corlette CE. The proposed school of medicine for tropical diseases. *The Times, London* 1898; 28 December: 6.

27.	Curnow J, Anderson J, Turner GR. The Seamen's Hospital Society and its visiting staff. *Lancet* 1898; ii: 1736–1737.

28.	Manson P. 'The Seamen's Hospital Society and its visiting staff.' *Lancet* 1898; ii: 1815.

29.	'The Seamen's Hospital Society and its visiting staff.' *Lancet* 1899; i: 57–58.

30.	Anderson J. Netley and tropical disease. *The Times, London* 1899; 6 January: 6.

31.	Netley as a school for tropical medicine. *Lancet* 1899; i: 106–107.

32.	Cox HB. A school of tropical medicine. *Lancet* 1899; i: 187.

33.	Schools of tropical medicine in Liverpool and elsewhere. *Lancet* 1899; i: 181–182.

34.	Yarr MT. The proposed school of tropical medicine. *Lancet* 1899; i: 336.

35.	Eder MD. Instruction in tropical diseases. *Lancet* 1899; i: 988.

36.	Tylecote, JHL. 'Instruction in tropical diseases.' *Lancet* 1899; ii: 51.

37.	Parliamentary intelligence: The study of tropical diseases: statement by Mr Chamberlain. *Lancet* 1899; i: 806.

38.	*The Lancet. Lancet* 1899; i: 787.

39.	Seamen's Hospital Society. *Lancet* 1899; i: 1507.

40.	*Editorial. Lancet* 1899; i: 909.

41.	Broadbent WH. [see: *Lancet* 1898; ii: 1574].

Chapter 7

1.	*The Lancet* 1899; ii: 696.

2.	Manson-Bahr P. *History of the school of tropical medicine in London (1899–1949).* London: HK Lewis 1956: 328.

3.	*Minutes, Seamen's Hospital Society*: book 13 (meeting 9 June 1899): 174–179.

4.	*Minutes, Seamen's Hospital Society*: book 13 (meeting 8 September 1899): 199–202.

5.	MacGregor W. Some problems of tropical medicine. *Lancet* 1900; ii: 1055–1061.

6. Editorial. The opening of the London School of Tropical Medicine. *J trop Med* 1899; 2: 75–76.

7. *Minutes, Seamen's Hospital Society*: book 13 (meeting 13 October 1899): 203–210.

8. *Minutes, Seamen's Hospital Society*: book 13 (meeting 8 June 1900): 264–267.

9. Manson P. London School of Tropical Medicine: the need for special training in tropical disease. *J trop Med Hyg* 1899; 2: 57–62.

10. *Minutes, Seamen's Hospital Society*: book 13 (meeting 8 June 1900): 265–266.

11. *Minutes, Seamen's Hospital Society*: book 13 (meeting 26 April 1901): 343–347.

12. *Liverpool School of Tropical Medicine: historical record 1898–1920*. Liverpool: University Press 1920: 103.

13. Low GC. A retrospect of tropical medicine from 1894 to 1914. *Trans R Soc trop Med Hyg* 1929; 23: 213–232.

14. The study of tropical diseases in Liverpool. *Lancet* 1898; ii: 1495.

15. The Liverpool School of Tropical Medicine. *Lancet* 1899; i: 1174–1176.

16. Worboys M. Manson, Ross and colonial medical policy: tropical medicine in London and Liverpool, 1899–1914. In: Macleod R, Lewis M (eds). *Disease, medicine, and Empire: perspectives on western medicine and the experience of European expansion*. London, New York: Routledge 1988: 21–37.

17. Ross R. Tropical medicine – a crisis. *Br Med J* 1914; i: 319–321.

Chapter 8

1. Manson-Bahr P. *History of the School of Tropical Medicine in London (1899–1949)*. London: H K Lewis 1956: 328.

2. Medical news. *Lancet* 1901; i: 978.

3. MacGregor W. Some problems of tropical medicine. *Lancet* 1900; ii: 1055–1061.

4. London School of Tropical Medicine. *Lancet* 1901; ii: 1144–1145.

5. The London School of Tropical Medicine; its achievements and requirements. *Lancet* 1903; ii: 1676–1677.

6. The developments of tropical medicine. *Lancet* 1905; ii: 736–737.

7. The work of the London School of Tropical Medicine. *Lancet* 1905; ii: 1199.

8. Nuttall G H F. Scientific research in medicine. *Lancet* 1905; ii: 1155–1158.

9. Manson P. Recent advances in science and their bearing on medicine and surgery. *Lancet* 1908; ii: 991–997.

10. Osler W. The nation and the tropics. *Lancet* 1909; ii: 1401–1406.

11. Civil and military sanitation in the tropics. *Lancet* 1914; ii: 1384.

12. Health and life in the tropics. *Lancet* 1919; i: 644.

13. *The Lancet* 1902; i: 480.

14. The London School of tropical medicine. *Lancet* 1905; i: 1285–1286.

15. The dinner of the London School of Tropical Medicine. *Lancet* 1905; i: 1292–1293.

16. Leading article. *The Times, London* 1905; 11 May: 9.

17. Falkland Islands. Governor to Colonial Office 22 February 1904. *Public Records Office* CO885/9/no 170, no 54: 31.

18. The study of tropical diseases. *Lancet* 1912; i: 662–663.

19. The tropical diseases research fund. *Lancet* 1910; i: 738.

20. Parliamentary intelligence: Tropical Diseases Research Fund. *Lancet* 1911; i: 1741.

21. Parliamentary intelligence: Tropical Diseases Investigation. *Lancet* 1911; ii: 199.

22. Parliamentary intelligence: Tropical Diseases Research Fund. *Lancet* 1912; i: 550.

23. *Report of Seamen's Hospital Society meeting*. Mansion House, London: 28 February 1912 [*Ross archives: London School of Hygiene and Tropical Medicine*].

24. The study of tropical diseases: extent of government grants. *The Times, London* 1912; 29 February: 4.

25. Tropical medicine: the special fund for the London School: Mr A Chamberlain on the allocation. *The Times, London* 1913; 25 October: 5.

26. Parliamentary intelligence: Tropical Diseases Research fund. *Lancet* 1914; i: 1087.

27. Report of the tropical diseases research fund. *Lancet* 1914; i: 1272–1273.

28. *Minutes, Seamen's Hospital Society*: book 13 (meeting 10 May 1901): 348–350.

29. *Minutes, Seamen's Hospital Society*: book 13 (meeting 12 December 1902): 481–486.

30. Colonial office to Seamen's Hospital Society. 4 November 1904. *Public Records Office* CO885/9/no 173, no 6: 11.

31. Manson P. Foreward. *Journal of the London School of Tropical Medicine* 1911; 1: 1–2.

32. Manson P. Experimental proof of the mosquito-malaria theory. *Br Med J* 1990; ii: 949–951.

33. Lyons M. Sleeping sickness, colonial medicine and imperialism: some connections in the Belgian Congo. In: Macleod R, Lewis M. (eds) *Disease, medicine, and Empire: – perspectives on western medicine and the experience of European expansion*. London, New York: Routledge 1988: 242–256.

34. Leishman W B. On the possibility of the occurrence of trypanosomiasis in India. *Br Med J* 1903; i: 1252–1254 and ii: 1376–1377.

35. Manson P, Low G C. The Leishman-Donovan body and tropical splenomegaly. *Br Med J* 1904; i: 183–186.

36. Ross R. *Memoirs, with a full account of the great malaria problem and its solution*. London: John Murray 1923: 547.

37. Ross R. In: Scott H H. *A history of tropical medicine*. London: Arnold: 1086–1090.

38. Ross R. Observations on a condition necessary to the transformation of the malaria crescent. *Br Med J* 1897; i: 251–255.

39. Ross R. On some peculiar pigmented cells found in two mosquitos fed on malarial blood. *Br Med J* 1897; ii: 1786–1788.

40. Ross R. Pigmented cells in mosquitos. *Br Med J* 1898; i: 550–551.

41. Manson P. Surgeon-Major Ronald Ross's recent investigations on the mosquito-malaria theory. *Br Med J* 1898; i: 1575–1577.

42. Worboys M. Manson, Ross and colonial medical policy: tropical medicine in London and Liverpool, 1899–1914. In: MacLeod R, Lewis M (eds). *Disease, medicine, and Empire: – perspectives on western medicine and the experience of European expansion*. London, New York: Routledge 1988; 21–37.

43. Chernin E. Sir Ronald Ross vs. Sir Patrick Manson: a matter of libel. *J Hist Med* 1988; 43: 262–274.

44. Chernin E. Sir Ronald Ross, malaria, and the rewards of research. *Med Hist* 1988; 32: 119–141.

45. Leading article: A Ross Institute. *The Times, London* 1923; 22 June: 15.

46. Manson-Bahr P. The story of malaria: the drama and the actors. *Int Rev Trop Med* 1963; 2: 329–390.

47. Ross R. The work of Sir Patrick Manson. *Br Med J* 1922; i: 698–699.

48. Asquith HH. *et al*. Tropical diseases: the debt to Sir Ronald Ross: proposed institute as monument. *The Times, London* 1923; 22 June: 15.

49. The Ross Institute and the London School of Hygiene and Tropical Medicine. *Br Med J* 1933; ii: 245–246.

50. A valuable amalgamation. *Lancet* 1933; ii: 300.

51. *Minutes, Seamen's Hospital Society*, book 15 (meeting 10 October 1912): 126–129.

52. *Liverpool School of Tropical Medicine: historical record 1898–1920*. Liverpool: University Press 1920: 103.

53. Liverpool School of Tropical Medicine. *Br Med J* 1914; i: 324.

54. A school of tropical medicine in Australia. *Lancet* 1908; i: 904.

55. Tropical diseases. *Lancet* 1910; i: 897.

56. A school of tropical medicine for India. *Lancet* 1910; i: 1174.

57. Balfour A. A marine floating laboratory for the study of tropical medicine. *Lancet* 1910; ii: 55–56.

58. A floating school of tropical medicine. *Lancet* 1919; ii: 164.

59. School of tropical medicine. *Lancet* 1915; i: 510.

60. The Calcutta School of tropical medicine. *Lancet* 1928; ii: 842.

61. Cantlie N, Seaver G. *Sir James Cantlie: a romance in medicine*. London: John Murray 1939: 279.

62. Stewart JC. *The quality of mercy: the lives of Sir James and Lady Cantlie*. London: George Allen and Unwin 1983: 277.

63. *The Lancet* 1907; i: 605.

64. Low G C. The history of the foundation of the Society of Tropical Medicine and Hygiene. *Trans R Soc trop Med Hyg* 1928; 22: 197–202.

65. Low G C. A retrospect of tropical medicine from 1894 to 1914. *Trans R Soc trop Med Hyg* 1929; 23: 213–232.

Chapter 9

1. *Minutes, Seamen's Hospital Society*: book 15 (meeting 12 July 1917): 435–438.
2. *Minutes, Seamen's Hospital Society*: book 16 (meeting 9 January 1919): 31–36.
3. *Minutes, Seamen's Hospital Society*: book 16 (meeting 13 February 1919): 45–50.
4. *Minutes, Seamen's Hospital Society*: book 16 (meeting 22 May 1919): 75–80.
5. *Minutes, Seamen's Hospital Society*: book 16 (meeting 26 June 1919): 89–92.
6. A new hospital for tropical diseases. *Lancet* 1919; i: 946.
7. The teaching of tropical medicine. *Lancet* 1919; ii: 744.
8. The new hospital for tropical diseases in London. *Lancet* 1920; i: 210.
9. Manson-Bahr P. *History of the School of tropical medicine in London (1899–1949)*. London: HK Lewis 1956: 328.
10. *Minutes, Seamen's Hospital Society*: book 16 (meeting 12 February 1920): 161–165.
11. *Minutes, Seamen's Hospital Society*: book 16 (meeting 22 November 1920): 238–239.
12. The tropical disease prevention committee. *Lancet* 1920; i: 1370–1371.
13. Prevention of tropical diseases and the responsibility of London: presidential address. *Lancet* 1921; i: 538–539.
14. Tropical sanitation. *Lancet* 1921; ii: 144.
15. The tropical diseases library, London. *Lancet* 1923; i: 396.
16. Research in tropical disease: I. London School of Tropical Medicine. *Lancet* 1923; i: 1335.
17. Research in tropical disease: IV. The Wellcome Bureau of Scientific Research. *Lancet* 1923; ii: 137–138.
18. Research in tropical medicine. *Lancet* 1936; i: 558.
19. Training for research in tropical medicine. *Lancet* 1936; ii: 30.
20. Fellowships for research in tropical medicine. *Lancet* 1936; ii: 48.
21. Medical Research Council : tropical medicine. *Lancet* 1937; i: 711–712.
22. Diplomas in tropical medicine. *Lancet* 1923; ii: 427–428.
23. Balfour A. Education of Medical Officers for service in the tropics. (parts 1 & 2) *Lancet* 1928; i: 63–67 and 117–122.
24. Balfour A. The tropical field: its possibilities for medical women. *Lancet* 1928; ii: 721–723.
25. Leiper RT. Medical careers in the tropics. *Lancet* 1937; ii: 920–923.
26. The curse of the tropics (leading article). *Lancet* 1924; i: 855–856.
27. British Empire Exhibition, Wembley: health in the tropics. I *Lancet* 1924; i: 916–917.
28. British Empire Exhibition, Wembley: health in the tropics. II *Lancet* 1924; i: 1022–1023.
29. Anonymous. White men and work in the tropics. *Lancet* 1924; i: 51.

30. The effects of hot climate. *Lancet* 1935; i: 1226.

31. Acclimatisation in the tropics. *Lancet* 1924; ii: 32.

32. Royal Society of Medicine. Section of tropical diseases and parasitology: tropical neurasthenia. *Lancet* 1933; i: 302–303.

33. Deterioration in the tropics. *Lancet* 1933; i: 320.

34. Food and disease in the tropics. *Lancet* 1924; i: 142.

35. A diet scheme for the tropics. *Lancet* 1924; i: 610.

36. The dangers of life in the tropics. *Lancet* 1929; i: 1390.

37. Notes, comments, and abstracts: An Empire problem. *Lancet* 1933; i: 231.

38. Blacklock DB. House diseases in the tropics. *Lancet* 1935; i: 526–529.

39. The London School of Hygiene and Tropical Medicine. *Lancet* 1925; ii: 931.

40. London School of Hygiene and Tropical Medicine: presentation to Dr. Andrew Balfour. *Lancet* 1926; ii: 248.

41. Clark CM, Mackintosh JM. *The School and the site: a historical memoir to celebrate the twenty-fifth anniversary of the School.* London: HK Lewis 1954: 105.

Chapter 10.

1. Manson-Bahr P. *History of the School of Tropical Medicine in London (1899–1949).* London: HK Lewis 1956: 328.

2. Acheson R, Poole P. The London School of Hygiene and Tropical Medicine: a child of many parents. *Med Hist* 1991; 35: 385–408.

3. Postgraduate Medical Committee's Report. London: HMSO 1921: 23–24.

4. Leiper RT to Sheppard RL 15 November 1950. [*London School of Hygiene and Tropical Medicine Library*].

5. *Minutes, Seamen's Hospital Society*: book 16 (meeting 13 June 1921): 285.

6. The new institute of hygiene. *Br Med J* 1922; i: 361.

7. Clark CM, Mackintosh JM. *The School and the site: a historical memoir to celebrate the twenty-fifth anniversary of the School.* London: HK Lewis 1954: 105.

8. The London School of Hygiene and Tropical Medicine. *Lancet* 1925; ii: 931.

9. London School of Hygiene and Tropical Medicine. *Lancet* 1925; i: 1354.

10. London School of Hygiene and Tropical Medicine: laying of the foundation-stone. *Lancet* 1926; ii: 86–88.

11. Preventive medicine in London: the new school of hygiene and tropical medicine. *Lancet* 1929; ii: 148–150.

12. London School of Hygiene and Tropical Medicine: the opening of the new building. *Lancet* 1929; ii: 175–176.

13. Leading article: thinking aloud. *The Times, London* 1926; 21 October: 15.

14. Mond, Alfred. Future of voluntary hospitals: the London School of Tropical Medicine. *The Times, London* 1926; 22 October: 14.

15. Tropical Medicine and the London School. *Lancet* 1926; ii: 1280–1281.

16. The London School of Hygiene and Tropical Medicine. *Lancet* 1929; ii: 1155.
17. London School of Hygiene and Tropical Medicine. *Lancet* 1930; ii: 1246.
18. A short course in tropical medicine. *Lancet* 1931; ii: 85–86.
19. London School of Hygiene and Tropical Medicine. *Lancet* 1931; ii: 1308.
20. Asquith HH, *etal*. Tropical diseases: the debt to Sir Ronald Ross: proposed institute as monument. *The Times, London* 1923; 22 June: 15.
21. Leading article: A Ross Institute. *The Times, London* 1923; 22 June: 15.
22. A valuable amalgamation. *Lancet* 1933; ii: 300.
23. The Ross Institute and the London School of Hygiene and Tropical Medicine. *Br Med J* 1933; ii: 245–246.
24. London School of Hygiene and Tropical Medicine: Memorials to Manson and Ross. *Lancet* 1934; ii: 56.
25. Mosquito Day. *Lancet* 1935; i: 1194.
26. Medicine and industry in the tropics. *Lancet* 1939; i: 1189.

Chapter 11

1. Manson-Bahr P. *History of the School of tropical medicine in London (1899–1949)*. London: HK Lewis 1956: 328.
2. London School of Hygiene and Tropical Medicine. *Lancet* 1942; i: 432.
3. *The Lancet* 1941; i: 730.
4. Postgraduate study. *Lancet* 1943; ii: 269–270.
5. Colonial welfare begins its climb. *Lancet* 1941; ii: 399–400.
6. Parliament: From the press gallery: our colonial responsibilities. *Lancet* 1941; ii: 680–681.
7. Tropics not so unhealthy if –. *Lancet* 1943; ii: 451–452.
8. Reconstruction: tropical medicine and the future. *Lancet* 1944; i: 160.
9. Napier LE. Teaching of tropical medicine. *Trans R Soc trop Med Hyg* 1946; 39: 273–300.
10. Royal Society of tropical medicine and hygiene: teaching of tropical medicine. *Lancet* 1946; i: 16–17.
11. Tropical Diseases: temporary hospital premises. *Br Med J* 1946; i: 454.
12. Hospital for Tropical Diseases, London. *Lancet* 1947; i: 48.
13. Hough R. *Edwina: Countess Mountbatten of Burma*. London, Sydney: Sphere Books Ltd. 1985: 242.
14. Morgan J. *Edwina Mountbatten: a life of her own*. London: Harper Collins 1991: 509.
15. Clinical tropical medicine in London. *Lancet* 1947; ii: 658–659.
16. Clark CM, Mackintosh JM. *The School and the site: a historical memoir to celebrate the twenty-fifth anniversary of the School*. London: HK Lewis 1954: 105.
17. Tropical diseases centre for London. *Lancet* 1949; i: 329.
18. Teaching of tropical medicine. *Br Med J* 1949; ii: 525.

19.   Hardie R. *The Burma-Siam railway: The secret diary of Dr Robert Hardie 1942–45*. London: Imperial War Museum 1983: 181.

20.   Dunlop EE. *The war diaries of Weary Dunlop: Java and the Burma–Thailand Railway 1942–1945*. London: Viking Books 1989: 401.

21.   Caplan JP. Creeping eruption and intestinal strongyloidiasis. *Lancet* 1949; i: 396.

22.   Jopling WH. Leprosy in Great Britain and its nursing care. *Nursing Mirror* 1961; 16 January: i–iv.

23.   MacLeod JMH. Leprosy in Great Britain: the St. Giles Homes for British lepers. *Int J Lepr* 1935; 3: 67–70.

Chapter 12

1.   Palmer S. *St. Pancras; being antiquarian, topographical, and biographical memoranda relating to the extensive metropolitan parish of St. Pancras, Middlesex: with some account of the parish from its foundation*. London: Samuel Palmer and Field & Tuer 1870: 322.

2.   Denyer CH (ed). *St. Pancras through the centuries*. London: Le Play House Press 1935: 123.

3.   *London County Council: Survey of London. XIX Old St. Pancras and Kentish Town*. London: London County Council 1938: 173.

4.   Holroyd M. *Bernard Shaw. I. 1856–1898 The search for love*. London: Penguin Books 1990: 486.

5.   Mayer A. Christmas in the workhouse . . . *Health Social Service J* 1978: 1446–1453.

6.   Honigsbaum F. The evolution of the NHS. *Br Med J* 1990; 301: 694–699.

7.   London Hospital for Tropical Diseases. *Lancet* 1951; i: 1236.

8.   New hospital for tropical diseases. *Br Med J* 1951; i: 1251–1252.

9.   Facilities for treating tropical diseases in Britain. *Br Med J* 1952; i: 1360 .

10.   Tropical diseases in Britain. *Br Med J* 1953; i: 1096.

11.   Arnott WM. Tropical diseases in Britain. *Br Med J* 1953; i: 1219.

12.   Manson-Bahr P. Tropical diseases in Britain. *Br Med J* 1953; i: 1448.

13.   Nicol B. Tropical diseases in Britain. *Br Med J* 1953; ii: 288.

14.   James E. *Thomas Hardy 1840–1928*. London: The British Library 1990: 37.

15.   Radford B. *Midland line memories: a pictorial history of the Midland Railway main line between London (St Pancras) and Derby*. London: Bloomsbury Books 1988: 144.

16.   Richardson R. *Death, dissection and the destitute*. London: Penguin Books 1989: 426.

17.   St Clair W. *The Godwins and the Shelleys: the biography of a family*. London, Boston: Faber & Faber 1990: 572.

18.   Manson-Bahr P. *History of the school of tropical medicine in London (1899–1949)*. London: HK Lewis 1956: 328.

19.   Clark CM, Mackintosh JM. *The School and the site: a historical memoir*

to celebrate the twenty-fifth anniversary of the School. London: HK Lewis 1954: 105.

20. Bayly CA (ed.) *The Raj: India and the British 1600–1947*. London: National Portrait Gallery 1990: 432.

21. Lyons M. Sleeping sickness, colonial medicine and imperialism: some connections in the Belgian Congo. In: Macleod R, Lewis M (eds). *Disease, medicine, and Empire: perspectives on western medicine and the experience of European expansion*. London, New York: Routledge 1988: 242–256.

22. Worboys M. Manson, Ross and colonial medical policy. Tropical medicine in London and Liverpool 1899–1914. In: Macleod R, Lewis M (eds). *Disease, medicine, and Empire: perspectives on western medicine and the experience of European expansion*. London, New York: Routledge 1988: 21–37.

23. Manson-Bahr P. The march of tropical medicine during the last fifty years. *Trans R Soc trop Med Hyg* 1958; 52: 483–499.

24. Cook GC. Future structure of clinical tropical medicine in the United Kingdom. *Br Med J* 1982; 284: 1460–1461.

25. *Minutes, Hospital for Tropical Diseases*: meeting 21 January 1992.

Appendix 1

1. The Seamen's Hospital. *Lancet* 1861; i: 231.
2. McBride AG. *The history of the Dreadnought Seamens Hospital at Greenwich*. Chartham: Seamens Hospital Management Committee, Greenwich 1970: 36.
3. Seamen's Hospital. *Lancet* 1853; i: 191.
4. Seamen's Hospital Society. *Lancet* 1847; i: 190.
5. Seamen's Hospital Ship. *Lancet* 1848; ii: 252.
6. Seamen's Hospital Ship. *Lancet* 1848; ii: 167.
7. Seamen's Hospital Society. *Lancet* 1854; i: 147.
8. Seamen's Hospital Society. *Lancet* 1854; i: 459.
9. The Seamen's Hospital. *Lancet* 1862; ii: 193.
10. The Seamen's Hospital. *Lancet* 1865; ii: 418.
11. Seamen's Hospital Society. *Lancet* 1871; i: 205.

Appendix 2

1. McBride AG. *The history of the Dreadnought Seamens Hospital at Greenwich*. Chartham: Seamens Hospital Management Committee, Greenwich 1970: 36.
2. Dreadnought hospital ship, River Thames: cases requiring amputation, disease of the ankle, amputation. *Lancet* 1843; 14 October: 69–71.
3. Dreadnought hospital ship: case of curious injury to the knee. *Lancet* 1844; 8 June: 356.
4. Dreadnought hospital ship, River Thames: cases requiring amputation of the lower extremity. *Lancet* 1844; 6 July: 482–484.

5.	Seamen's Hospital Ship, 'Dreadnought': urethral stricture; amputation; necrosed bone; removal of tumours. *Lancet* 1856; i: 457.

6.	Dreadnought hospital-ship, River Thames: paralysis from lesion of the cerebral portion of the nervous system; paraplegia; rupture of the diaphragm. *Lancet* 1843; 12 August: 700–702.

7.	Dreadnought hospital ship, River Thames: scrofula, amputation of the leg. *Lancet* 1843; 28 October: 124.

8.	'Dreadnought' hospital ship: excision of head of femur with great trochanter for hip-joint disease; subsequent perforation of the floor of the acetabulum from extensive caries; death. *Lancet* 1869; ii: 507–508.

9.	Dreadnought hospital ship, River Thames: case of strumous ulceration of the tongue and throat, attended with a partial closure of the glottis. – tracheostomy. – recovery. *Lancet* 1844; 21 December: 384.

10.	Dreadnought hospital-ship, River Thames: cases of strangulated hernia. Operations. *Lancet* 1843; 26 August: 771–773.

11.	Dreadnought hospital ship: strangulated hernia. – operation. *Lancet* 1846; i: 282–284.

12.	'Dreadnought' Hospital: fungous disease of the testicle, associated with deposits of encephaloid cancer in the liver; sudden death. *Lancet* 1870; ii: 154–155.

13.	'Dreadnought' hospital ship: cholera and choleroid diarrhoea. *Lancet* 1859; ii: 137–138.

14.	Dreadnought hospital ship: two cases of cholera; recovery. *Lancet* 1868; ii: 77.

15.	Dreadnought Seamen's Hospital: case of acute petechial typhus. *Lancet* 1871; i: 408–409.

16.	Dreadnought Hospital: two cases of diphtheria, followed by recovery. *Lancet* 1859; i: 629.

17.	The Dreadnought Seamen's Hospital: a case of idiopathic tetanus. *Lancet* 1870; ii: 435.

18.	Dreadnought hospital ship: fatal case of scurvy; post-mortem examination. *Lancet* 1865; i: 594.

19.	Dreadnought Seamen's Hospital: five cases of scurvy. *Lancet* 1870; ii: 46–47.

20.	Dreadnought Seamen's Hospital: case of purpuric fever. *Lancet* 1871; i: 647.

21.	The 'Dreadnought' and Metropolitan Free Hospitals: phosphate of zinc in epilepsy. *Lancet* 1858; i: 119.

22.	'Dreadnought' hospital ship: death during the inhalation of chloroform. *Lancet* 1859; ii: 412.

Index

Important page references are given in **bold** type.
Plate numbers are cited in *parentheses*.

actinomycosis, eradication of, 119

Admiralty: granting of pendant by, 37; lease of Greenwich Hospital Infirmary by, 48–9; and tropical medicine, 297

Albert Dock years (of the LSTM): 1899–1920, **163–217**

Albert Dock Hospital, [*34*]; admission books of, [*40*]; diagnoses of cases at, 165; establishment of, 63–4; geographical location of, 106; history of, 67; laying of foundation stone, [*22*]; Manson, Patrick and, 75, 79; opening by Prince and Princess of Wales, 64; used for tropical cases during Second World War, 267; tropical medicine and, 88, 91, 94–5, 105, 110, 116, 126, 131, 141, 148, 151; wall-plaques at, [*36, 43*]

amoebiasis, 274; *see also*: liver abscess, amoebic

Amoy, China, 69–74

Amsterdam, School of Tropical Medicine at, 212

anaemia, tropical, 159

ancylostomiasis: diagnosis of, 133; disease caused by, 230, 238; eradication of, 222, 231, 242; *see also*: hookworm disease

Anderson, Elizabeth Garrett (1836–1917), 28

Anderson, John (1840–1910): 'acrimonious correspondence' regarding formation of LSTM, and, 107, 108, 110–2, 113–4, 115, 116, 121, 126, 134, 135–6, 138, 139; resignation from Dreadnought Hospital, 144–6; and SHS, 65

Angas Convalescent Home, of SHS, 66

Annals of Tropical Medicine and Parasitology: origin of, 212

Annesley, James (1780–1847), 20–1; illustrations in book, by, [*7*]

Antwerp, School of Tropical Medicine at, 212

Army Medical School, at Fort Pitt, Chatham, 17, 20, 102

Asquith, Herbert (1852–1928): appeal for public donations for 'Ross Institute and Hospital for Tropical Diseases', 259

Athlone Committee, role in British tropical medicine 242–3, 249, 297; report of, 242

Athlone, Earl of (1874–1957), 242

Australian Institute of Tropical Medicine 182, 191

Baccelli, Guido (1832–1916), 149

Bach, Johann Christian (1735–82): grave at Old St Pancras, 295

Bagshawe, Arthur, and Tropical Diseases Bureau, 243

Balfour, Andrew (1873–1931): appointed Director of LSHTM, 245; and clinical acumen of the pioneers xiv; death of, 258; and floating laboratory, 214–6; and historical perspective, xiv; presentation ceremony for, 239–40; plaque, commemorating, [52]; and removal of LSTM to central London, 219; tropical research and, 176–7, 233

Ballingall, George (1780–1855), 20, 21–2

Bedford College, University of London, 218

Belle Isle, hospital-ship, 39, 48, 52

beri-beri: at Amoy, China, 69; and British Empire, 222; history of, 22; at Liverpool, 159; in London, 107, 142, 163, 165; in Malay States, 168; at Royal Victoria Hospital, Netley, 139

Bidie, George (1830–1913), 20, 24–5

bilharzia, *see* schistosomiasis

Black Death, in Europe, 4–5

blackhole of Calcutta, last survivor of, 296

blackwater fever, 85, 165, 186, 222, 224, 238; *see also*: malaria

Board of Education: and official recognition of LSTM courses, 208–12

Boyce, Rubert (1863–1911), and foundation of Liverpool School of Tropical Medicine, 155, 156, 158, 160

Boyle, James (18?–18?), 27, 28

Branch Hospital, *see* Albert Dock Hospital

Brassey, Thomas (1836–1918): and fund-raising, 166–7; lecture at LSTM, 166–67

British Colonies: nutrition amongst indigenous inhabitants in, 270–1; state of medicine in, 269–71

British Empire Exhibition, Wembley, 229–31

British Medical Association, Edinburgh meeting of, 86, 87, 298

British Museum and library, 70, 245

British pioneers, and disease in the tropics, **13–32**; commemorated at LSHTM, 250; contributions to medicine in Africa, 25–9; in English 'Sugar Islands', 13–7; in India, 17–25; Scottish, origins of, 13

British Red Cross, 218

Broadbent, William (1835–1907), 120–1, 130–1, 132, 145

Bruce, David (1855–1931): and brucellosis research, 161; research on African trypanosomiasis, 161; and sleeping-sickness research, 187

Burdett, Henry (1847–1920): 'acrimonious correspondence', and, 105–6, 110, 111–6, 121–3, 126–8, 145; appeal for funds for LSTM, 103–5; donation to LSTM, 98; and formation of LSTM, 88, 103–5; report by, as Secretary of SHS, 58, 62

Busk, George (1807–86), 40; and discovery of *Fasciolopsis buski*, 40

Caledonia hospital-ship, 42, 43, 49, [18]; *see also: Dreadnought* hospital-ship

Cantlie, James (1851–1926), [38]; and annual dinner of LSTM, 192, 194; appointed to staff of LSTM, 149; and founding of Society of Tropical Medicine and Hygiene, 216; in Hong Kong, 74; lecture by, 175; and planning of LSTM, 93; and Ross Institute appeal, 259

Cardiff, hospital-ship at, 49–50

Carter, Henry (1831–97), 20, 23–4

Castellani, Aldo (1877–1971): and first Royal Society sleeping-sickness expedition, 201; laboratory accommodation at LSHTM, 263; student at LSTM, 199

Chadwick, Edwin (1800–90), 6, 11, 12, 250, 288, [5]; eponymous lectures, 174, 238

Chamberlain, Austen (1863–1937), 100, [44]; appeal cartoon, 195–6; cartoon of, 99; plaque, commemorating, [31]; and receipt of donation for LSHTM, 263; and reward to Ronald Ross, 203; speech at annual LSTM dinner, 192–4

Chamberlain, Joseph (1836–1914), [28]; collaboration with Manson, Patrick, **80–100**; Birmingham speech by, 96–7; cartoons of, 81, 82, 83, 99; decision in favour of Albert

Dock site, 140–4, 150; definition of democracy, 218; health of Europeans in tropical climates, 96; letter to Colonial Governors, 94–5; letter to medical schools, 91–3; letter to SHS Committee, 88; and Liverpool School of Tropical Medicine, 154–5, 157–8, 160; and Manson, Patrick, 78, 80, 85, 100, 101, 153; message to LSTM Annual Dinner, 1913, 192; and origin of LSTM, 105, 107–8, 152, 167, 219; plaque, commemorating, [31]; Secretary of State for the Colonies, 80, 81, 86; speech at charity dinner, 1899, 97–100; speech at fund-raising banquet, 1905, 178–9

Chamberlain, Neville (1869–1940), [56]; and future of voluntary hospitals, 254–5; laying of foundation stone, LSHTM, 247–9; and opening of LSHTM, 251; speech at Mosquito Day luncheon, 1939, 265–6

Charing Cross Hospital, 218

Charles, Havelock (1858–1934): appointed Dean LSTM, 200; and removal of LSTM to central London, 177, 218

Chevers, Norman (1818–86), 20, 22

Chinese Imperial Maritime Customs, 69

Chisholm, Colin (17?–1825), 15, 16

cholera: at Amoy, China, 69; and British expatriates abroad, 186, 231, 237, 272; discovery of cause of, 3–4; epidemics in England, 1, 3–4, 298; in India, 17, 25, 30; in indigenous inhabitants of tropics, 238; management of, 30; on River Thames, 39, 41, 48, 53, 305; -ships, 39, 41, 54; Snow, John, and cause of, 3–4, 25, 30; and tropical medicine teaching, 110, 119

cinchona: London pharmacopoeia 1677, 2; in treatment of malaria, 21, 31, 299

clinical medicine: in balance with preventive medicine xiv

clinical tropical medicine: division of,

established at LSHTM, 258; identity of, 154

Cobbold, Spencer (1828–86), 40, 70, 71, 72, 73

Colonial development: Royal Naval Medical Officers and, 81

Colonial Governors: letters from Chamberlain, Joseph to, 94–5, 154

Colonial Medical Officers: training of, in tropical medicine, 80–4, 87

Colonial Medical Service: career prospects and, 228; and training in tropical medicine, 91, 94–5, 124, 129, 140, 148, 219, 225

Colonial Office: financial contribution to LSTM, 104; and LSTM, 150, 151, 157, 158; representation on SHS Board of Management, 90

communicable (infectious) disease departments in UK: effect of HIV/AIDS on future of, xiv

Conjoint Board: qualifications in tropical medicine, 227

'constructive imperialism', and tropical medicine, 85, 298

'contagion' theory, of disease transmission, 5

Cook, Albert (1870–1951), and sleeping-sickness at Kampala, 201

Cook, James (1728–79), scientific explorer, 32

Cornish, William (1827–97), 20, 23

Crookshank, Edgar (1858–1928), 118–20, 132–4, 141, 148; importance of bacteriology in training programme, 118–20

Culex fatigans, and filaria transmission, 71, 72

Cunningham, David (1843–1914), 20, 24

Curnow, John (1846–1902): 'acrimonious correspondence' regarding foundation of LSTM, and, 101–2, 107–8, 111, 113–6, 123, 126–30, 134, 135–9; and diagnosis of cases admitted to Seamen's Hospital, 62; resignation from Dreadnought Hospital, 144–6; on SHS staff, 65 cyclops, and transmission of dracontiasis, 75

Daniels, Charles (1862–1927), [42]; editor, *The Journal of the London School of Tropical Medicine*, 199; physician at LSTM, 219; and research at Calcutta, 201; research on blackwater fever, in Africa 202; second medical tutor LSTM, 198; signature of, 199; and trypanosomiasis, 76
Davidson, Andrew (1833–1918), 30, 31–2
dengue, 1, 237
Devonport Nurses Home, 66
Devonport Pathological Laboratory, 66
Devonshire, hospital-ship, 39, 41
diet: importance of, in tropics, 234–7; recommendation in 'chronic dysentery' and colitis, 236–7
dispensaries (SHS): at East-India Dock Road, 65; at Gravesend, 65
Distoma ringeri, see Paragonimus westermani
distomiasis, 133
Dracunculus medinensis: (and guinea-worm infection), 75; *see also*: dracontiasis
dracontiasis (guinea-worm infection), 14, 152, 163, 165, 238
Dreadnought Hospital, Greenwich, [*19, 32, 61*]; administrative problems, 56–8, 167; correspondence from physicians at, 101–2, 107, 110, 111–6, 135–9; diagnoses of cases in, 61–3; facilities at, 55, 60–1; finances at, 57–8, 59–61, 167; fire at, 58; honorary medical staff of, 104–8, 110–8, 121–3, 144–5; medical staff of, 65–6, 75; and training of Colonial Office officers, 87, 109, 124–6, 143; and tropical medicine during Second World War; (1939–45), 267–8
Dreadnought Hospital-ships, Greenwich, [*16, 17, 18, 21*]; and cholera on River Thames, 41; use as cholera ship, 53–4; end of service at Greenwich, 48–9; facilities onboard,

39–40, 42–3; hygienic standards on, 43–7; medical admissions to, 46; medical diagnoses of cases admitted to, 46–7; medical staff, 43; use as smallpox hospital, 51–3, 54; surgical operations on, 43–7
dysentery: in Caribbean, 14; and death in the Colonies, 85, 230, 231, 238; differentiation of, 21; in England, 1, 31, 107, 128, 132, 133, 159, 165; in Great War, 176; in India, 17, 22, 23

East Indies, 173
ectoparasites, 238
Ehrlich, Paul (1854–1915), 188
elephantiasis, and lymphatic filariasis, 14, 70
Empire, British: Chamberlain, Joseph, and, 98, 218; disease in the, 186, 224, 237; nutrition amongst indigenous inhabitants of, 270–1; state of medical care in, 161, 269–71; tropical medicine and, 163, 184, 185, 188, 222, 298
Endsleigh Gardens, WC1, and LSTM/HTD: closed by Ministry of Health, 267, 296; description of facilities at, 220–1; first course at, 220; formal opening of LSTM at, by Duke of York, 220; loss of archival material, 267; removal of LSTM to, 218–21, 224, 296; staffing of, 219–21
Endsleigh Palace Hotel: purchased by SHS, 218
English 'Sugar Islands' (the Caribbean): pioneers in medicine in, 13–17; and slave trade, 14
Entamoeba coli, 24
Entamoeba histolytica, 273
enteric fevers, 1, 272
expatriate employees in the tropics: gastrointestinal infections in, 273; health of, 271–3; malaria in, 272–3; psychiatric problems in, 273

Fairley, Neil Hamilton, *see* Hamilton Fairley
Fayrer, Joseph (1824–1907), 20, 23, 123, 125, [*8*]

Filaria bancrofti (*nocturna*), 71, 72, 160
Filaria immitis, 71, 73
Filaria medinensis, 160
Filaria perstans: possible cause of sleeping-sickness, 76
Filaria sanguinis hominis, 24, 70, 71, 75; see also: *Filaria bancrofti*
filariasis, 24, 70–3, 133, 152, 160, 165, 222, 224
floating laboratory for studying tropical diseases: advocated by Balfour, Andrew, 214–5; opposed by Bruce and Low, 215–6
Foreign Office, 94, 150
Formosa (now Taiwan), 69
French schools of tropical medicine, 212
Fülleborn, Friedrich (1866–1933): student at LSTM, 199

General Medical Council; and tropical medicine training, 88, 95, 154
'germ-borne' disease: cholera, 4; dysentery, in Britain, 4; tropical medicine and, 298
Gilbert and Ellis Islands (now Republic of Kiribati): tropical disease and, 85
Glossina morsitans: described by Livingstone, David, 27
Godwin, Mary Wollstonecraft (1759–97), 296
Gold Coast (now Ghana): tropical disease and, 85, 89
Goodenough, William (1899–1951) and Inter-departmental Committee on Medical Schools, 275–6, 278
Grainger, James (1721–66), 15–6
Grampus, first SHS hospital-ship, 34, 35–40, 49, 58, 296, [*15*]
Grand Union (Junction) Canal, 296
Great Plague, of London, 5
Greenwich Hospital, [*20, 21*]; infirmary of, 48, 49, 51, 55, 56, 63; possible use by SHS, 48; removal to, from *Dreadnought* hospital-ship, 303; Somerset Ward of, 49, 55; see also: *Dreadnought* Hospital,

Greenwich; see also: Seamen's Hospital, Greenwich
Greenwich Hospital-ships, 35–49, 51–4; accident cases and, 305; anaesthetic death onboard, 305; cholera and, 305; diphtheria and, 305; epilepsy and, 305; expenditure of, 302–3; in-patient and out-patient admissions to, 300–1; medical diagnoses of in-patients, 304–5; orthopaedic problems and, 305; outcome of admissions, 302; provenance of patients onboard, 300; purpuric fever and, 305; scurvy and, 304, 305; smallpox and, 304; surgical diagnoses of in-patients, 304–5; tetanus and, 305; typhus and, 304, 305; venereal disease and, 304
Guardians of the Poor, the, 288
guinea-worm disease, see dracontiasis
Guy's Hospital, 126

Hamadryad, hospital-ship, 50
Hamburg, tropical school at, 160, 212, 256
Hamilton Fairley, Neil (1891–1966) [*51, 62*]; appointed to Chair of Clinical Tropical Medicine 284; consultant physician at HTD, 291; Member of Committee of Medical Research Council, 225; physician to Australian Forces, 268–9
Hardy, Thomas (1840–1928): involvement in railway construction at St Pancras, 294–5
Haslar, see Royal Naval Hospital, Haslar
health hazards of the tropics, 229–39
health in the tropics: exercise and, 232–3; hazards for the white man, 229–37; importance of diet on, 234–7; importance of vitamins, 235; indigenous population and, 237–8; influence of houses on, 238–9; neurasthenia and, 233–4; physiological adaptation and, 231–3; psychiatric problems and, 233–4
helminths: life-cycles of, 70–3, 152–3
'hepatitis', 17, 73, 165

Hillary, William (17?–1763), 15; description of tropical malabsorption, 15

Hong Kong, 69, 73, 74

Hong Kong Medical School; founded by Manson, Patrick, 74

hookworm disease, 14, 222, 271; see also: ancylostomiasis

Hospital for Tropical Diseases, London, [67]; accommodation at St Pancras Hospital site, 283–4; amalgamation with University College Hospital 283–4; bed occupancy at St Pancras site, 291; clinical material supplied by SHS 257; description of St Pancras building, 290; and Devonshire Street building, 279–83, [63]; at Endsleigh Gardens, 219–225, [49]; history of St Pancras building, 288–9; leprosy patients and, 286; medical staff in 1951, 291; mention of in Parliamentary debate, 292; opening of St Pancras building, by Duchess of Kent, 289, [66]; plans for future location of, 299; plans for new building after Second World War 267–8; plans for purpose-built premises near LSHTM, 297; removal to St Pancras, 288–91; separation from LSHTM, 297; staff of, during Second World War, 268–9; staff of, in 1930, [51]; temporary building at Devonshire Street, 279–83; urgent need for at end of Second World War, 273–5; visit by Mountbatten, Countess (Edwina), 281; see also: 'Ross Institute and Hospital for Tropical Diseases'

House of Commons: speech by Chamberlain, Joseph, 96–7

'humoral' theory of medicine, 14

Hutchinson, Jonathan (1828–1913): polyclinic and, 126, 131

Hygiene: increased emphasis on, xiv, 174–6, 223; teaching of, at LSHTM, 248; see also: London School of Hygiene and Tropical Medicine

'Imperial Hospital for Tropical Diseases': plans for, 297

India: Bengal Medical Service, forerunner of IMS, 20; conditions in, in 19th century, 17–9; Medical College, Bombay, 20; Medical College, Calcutta, and Rogers, Leonard, 20, 213–6; Medical College, Madras, 20; Sanitary Act, Bombay, 18; sanitary Commission in, 19; training of lady doctors for, 126, 227; Women's Medical Service for, 227

Indian Medical service (IMS), 17–25, 87, 95, 228, 256

Indian mutiny, 23

Industrial revolution, 33

infectious disease departments in UK: effect of HIV/AIDS on future of, xiv

Institute of State Medicine and University of London, 242

Inter-departmental Committee on Medical Schools, 275–6, 278

intestinal parasitic infections: importance of, in Britain, 293–4

Iphigenia, hospital-ship, 39, 40, 41

Jenner, Edward (1749–1823): awarded by Parliament, 7, 203, [3]; vaccination and, 6–7, 8, 30, 250

Johnson, James (1777–1845), 20, 21

Jones, Alfred (1845–1909): business interests of, 155; and foundation of the Liverpool School of Tropical Medicine, 154–5, 156, 158, 160, 223

Journal of the London School of Tropical Medicine, The, 199, 225

Kala azar, 202, 238

King George's Sanatorium for Sailors, 66

Kingsley, Mary (1862–1900), 27, 28–9

King's College Hospital, 143; Ross, appointed physician to, 203

King's College, London: and public health teaching, 247; tropical medicine instruction at, 107, 118–20, 132–3, 140–1, 147–8

Koch, Robert (1843–1910), 84–5, 105, 188, 201, 250

Lamb, George (1869–1911), 20, 24

Laveran, Alphonse (1845–1922): and discovery of *Plasmodium* sp, 24, 75, 85, 149, 188, 203, 230, 250

lectures on tropical medicine: by Manson, Patrick at St George's Hospital, 76–7, 87, 101, 102

Leiper, Robert (1881–1969), [*53*]; appointment to Chair of Helminthology at LSHTM, 263; and foundation of LSHTM, 243; and investigation of schistosomiasis in Egypt, 176; and *Journal of Helminthology*, 225; lecture on medical careers in the tropics, 227–9; and life-cycle of *Loa loa*, 75–6; researches in Africa, 202; on staff of LSTM, 198, 247

Leishmania sp, discovery of, 24

leishmaniasis, 231, 274; *see also*: Kala azar

Leishman, William (1865–1926), 192, 202, 250

leprosy: crusaders and, 2; in England, 2–3, 110, 119, 165; in Europe, 2–3; hospitals for, in Britain, 286; and stigma of disease, 286; in tropical countries, 14, 24, 32, 69, 186, 222, 230; world-wide distribution, 1

Lewis, Timothy (1841–86), 20, 24, 70, 250

Lind, James (1716–94): prevention of scurvy, 30, 31, 250, [*13*]

Lister, Joseph (1827–1912), 250; collaboration with Manson, 85; opening of Liverpool School of Tropical Medicine 154, 158

liver abscess, amoebic: in England, 109, 110, 132, 140, 165; in India, 17; Manson, Patrick and, 69, 73; *see also*: amoebiasis

Liverpool School of Tropical Medicine: foundation of, **154–62**; and *Annals of Tropical Medicine and Parasitology*, 212; and courses in tropical medicine, 143, 146; early years of, 212; expeditions to tropics, 159; financial support and, 159, 161, 190, 196; Government support and, 184–5; inauguration of, 154, 158-9, 197; and preventive medicine, 161, 174; work carried out at, 183

Livingstone, David (1813–73), 25–8, 183, [*9*]

Loa loa, 75–6

London School of Hygiene and Tropical Medicine (LSHTM), **242–59**, [*58*]; Board of Management of, 240–1; building of, [*57*]; commemoration of pioneers, on frieze, 250; completion and opening by Prince of Wales, 249–54; creation of Chair of Clinical Tropical Medicine at, 284; Hospital sub-committee set up, 240–1; establishment of clinical tropical medicine division, 258; field station in Southern Rhodesia, 246; first Annual Report of, 255–6; foundation departments at, 245; foundation of in 1924, xiii, 239–41; foundation stone, laying of by Chamberlain, Joseph, 247–9, [*55*]; hygiene, teaching of, xiii, 248; LSTM merged into, 239–40, 245–6; major public health centre for United Kingdom, xiii; Mosquito Day luncheons, 264–6; museum of, [*59, 60*]; opening of Ross Institute of Tropical Hygiene, 263–4; origins of, 245–6; post-Second World War plans, 283; research studentships at, 246; Rockefeller Foundation, and, 240, 242–6; seal of, 247, [*54*]; second Annual Report of, 256–7; teaching museum at, 246; third Annual Report of, 257–8; withdrawal of application for hospital site in Bloomsbury, 241

London School of Tropical Medicine (LSTM) [*33, 34, 35, 41, 49*]; and Albert Dock years, **163–212**; foundation of, **147–54**; origins of, **80–100**; removal to central London, **218–39**; admitted as School of the University of London, 177; and bacteriology, 105; clinical research conducted by, 200–2; correct venue for, 117–35, 140–4; courses at, 148–9; damage by

TNT explosion, 177; disadvantages of Albert Dock site, 108–9; established in London in 1899, xiii; facilities provided at, 148; finances for the first 12 years, 180; financial support and, 177–97; fund-raising dinner for, 1913, 192–4; fund-raising meetings for, 97–100, 186–92; fund-raising speech by Manson, Patrick, 188–90; Government support for, 90, 184, 185, 196; the Great War (1914–18), and, 176–7; inaccessibility of, 131, 163; laboratory at, [37]; merged into LSHTM, 239–40, 245–6; opening of, 147, 150; opening of extension by King George V, 163; provenance of students at, 150, 163–4; railway journey to, 163; research interests at, 224–5; Royal Society grant for, 90; student numbers at, 150, 163–4; teaching and courses at, 197–200; tropical expeditions from, 224–5; visit by King George V, 177; visit by Prince of Wales and Princess Royal, 177; visit by Queen Mary, 177

Lovell, Francis (1844–1916): appointed first Dean of LSTM, 197, 200; and fund-raising for LSTM, 167, 192; and LSTM, 167, 168; overseas visits by, 177; signature of, 199

Low, George (1872–1952), [46, 51]; appointed third tutor of LSTM, 198; consulting physician at HTD, 291; demonstration of *Leishmania* amastigotes, 202; elucidation of mosquito-man transmission of *Filaria (Wuchereria) bancrofti*, 201; and first Royal Society sleeping-sickness expedition, 201; and founding of Society of Tropical Medicine and Hygiene, 216; granted rank of Major IMS, 177; physician to LSTM, 219; and Roman Campagna expedition, 200–1; and teaching of tropical diseases, 264

Lugard, Frederick (1858–1945), 29

Lukis, Charles (1857–1917), 20, 25, 192

Macaulay, Zachary (1768–1835), 33

McGregor, William (1846–1919), 27, 29, [11]; address to LSTM, 149, 163–6; administrative appointments, 29; contributions to preventive medicine, 29; Ross, Ronald and, 207; training of indigenous students, 29

McGrigor, James (1771–1858), 15, 16–17, [6]; Army Medical Department and, 17

madura foot, 110, 119

malaria: in Africa, 32; and Amoy, China, 69; association with certain houses, 238; bleeding, in management of, 31; British Empire, and, 85, 186, 231, 237, 271, 272; in the Caribbean, 14; and Chaucer, 2; eminent individuals, as sufferers from, 1; in England, up to twentieth century, 1–2, 298; Jesuit missionaries and introduction of cinchona, 2; importance of in returned travellers, 139–40; in London in nineteenth century, 2; Manson, Patrick and, 73, 75, 77, 184, 230; mepacrine in management of, 268–9; problems in prophylaxis and management, 272–3; research and teaching on, in London 110, 133; research by LSTM staff, 200–1, [45, 46]; research in Africa, 92; Ross, Ronald and, 75, 92, 152, 159, 184, 202–3, 230; and Shakespeare, 2; at SHS hospitals, 107, 128–9, 163, 165

Malcolmson, John (17?–1844), 22

Manson, Patrick (1844–1922), **68–79**, [24, 25]; collaboration with Chamberlain, Joseph, **80–100**; and the London medical scene, 75–8; Aberdeen/Edinburgh Universities, and, 68; Amoy and, 69; appointed lecturer at London School of Tropical Medicine, 149; appointment as Medical Adviser to the Colonial Office, 85; birthplace of, [23]; candidature for Regius Chair of Medicine, Oxford, 78; China years, 68–74; Chinese Imperial Maritime Customs, and, 69; cottage at Chalfont St

Giles, Buckinghamshire, 86; demonstration of *Leishmania* amastigotes 202; demonstration of Ross' work on *Plasmodium* sp, 86; diary kept by, 71; early years in Scotland, 68; and Endsleigh Gardens building, 219; establishment of LSTM, 93, 98, 100, 101, 160, 161, 165, 167, 192; filaria research, 70–3; Formosa and, 69; foundation of Hong Kong Medical School, 74; and frieze at LSHTM, 250; fund-raising speeches for LSTM, 167–8, 188–90; graduation, 68; Hong Kong and, 74; honours, 78, 79; Huxley lecture at Charing Cross Hospital, 171; introductory address to LSTM, 150–4; involvement in 'acrimonious correspondence' 135–9; lecture at Charing Cross Hospital Medical School, 76; lecture at Livingstone College, 76; lecture to LSTM, 167–8; lecturer in tropical diseases, London School of Medicine for Women (Royal Free Hospital), 86; lectures at St George's Hospital Medical School, 76–7, 80, 87, 101–2; marriage to Henrietta Thurburn, 71; memorial service for, 79; mentor to Ross, Ronald, 204, 207; pioneer of tropical medicine, 32; plaques, commemorating, [*26, 27, 39, 50*]; presentation of portraits to, 194; Presidential Address to the Society of Tropical Medicine and Hygiene, 84–5; public addresses, 86; Queen Anne Street and, 75; removal to London, 75–8; representative on SHS Committee of Management, 90; retirement from LSTM, 194–5; on SHS medical staff, 65, 75; signature of, 199; support for Prout, William, 204–7; textbook on tropical diseases, 78; theory on malaria transmission, 73, 75, 77, 183, 230; trypanosomiasis and, 76, 201; views on formation of LSHTM, 243–4; views on Netley as venue for LSTM, 87

Manson-Bahr, Philip (1881–1966) [formerly P H Bahr] [*51*]; assis-

tant physician to LSTM, 219; consulting physician at HTD, 291; Presidential Address to the Royal Society of Tropical Medicine and Hygiene, 280–3; research on sprue in Ceylon, 195; SHS and tropical medicine, 33; views on Hospital for Tropical Diseases 220, 297

Mansonella perstans, 76; *see also: Filaria perstans*

Martin, Ranald (1793–1874), 20, 21

medical careers in the tropics, 227–9; women and, 227

medical establishment: major dispute within the, **101–46**

Medical Research Council, 225

Mediterranean fever, 140

Melania libertina, 73

Mepacrine: in management of malaria, 268–9

Metropolitan Asylums Board, 51, 52, 53, 54, 287

Metropolitan Free Hospital: use of zinc phosphate in epilepsy, at, 305

miasmatic theory, of disease transmission, 2, 5, 11, 298

Michelli, James (1853–1935): and 'acrimonious correspondence', 111, 113, 114–5, 120–1, 123, 125, 130–1, 139; and finances of LSTM, 180; and formation of LSTM, 86, 104, 112–3, 147, 192; and LSHTM, 240; Secretary of SHS, 86; and SHS medical staff, 66

Middlesex Hospital Medical School, 218, 247

Ministry of Pensions Tropical Diseases Unit, Roehampton, 285–6

Mond, Alfred (1868–1930); and formation of LSHTM, 243; and future of voluntary hospitals, 254–5

Morehead, Charles (1807–82), 20, 22

Mosquito Day: celebrated by luncheons at LSHTM, 264–6

Mountbatten, Edwina (1901–60), [*43b*]; visit to Devonshire Street building, 280–1

nagana (animal trypanosomiasis), 27

Nairne, Perceval (1841–1921): Chairman of SHS Committee of Management 90, 93, 149, 192; and 'acrimonious correspondence', 122

Napoleonic wars, 33

Nelson, Horatio (1758–1805), 39, 55

Nepomuceno, hospital-ship, 39

Netley, *see* Royal Victoria Hospital, Netley

Newham, Hugh (1874–1959): fourth Director of LSTM, 198–9, 220

Nightingale, Florence (1820–1910), 30, 31, 63, [*14*]

Nuttall, George (1862–1937): lecture to LSTM, 170–1; and LSTM, 162, 199; and Tropical Diseases Research Fund, 197

Old St Pancras, and Hospital for Tropical Diseases, **287–99**; history of, 287–8, 294–6

Osler, William (1849–1919): appointment to Regius Chair of Medicine, Oxford, 78; lecture to LSTM, 172–3; letter on 'malaria in Italy', 182; and opening of LSTM, 149

Paragonimus westermani (Distoma ringeri), 73

Parkes, Edmund (1819–76), 22–23

Passmore Edward's Hospital, Tilbury Docks, 66

Pasteur, Louis (1822–95), 188, 203, 250

pellagra, 222

plague: in Asia, 5; the 'Black Death', 4; in the Caribbean, 14; in England, 1, 4–5; in Europe, 5; in India, 17; in London, 5, 110, 163, 165; and servants of Empire, 85, 119, 186, 222, 230; transmission of, 5, 238

Plasmodium sp: elucidation of mosquito-man transmission, 73, 75, 77, 80, 200–1; *see also*: malaria; *see also*: Ross, Ronald

pneumonia, in tropics, 119

Poor Laws, 287–8

Port of London: and dispensaries, 65; and hospital-ships, 36, 39, 53

Preventive medicine: Post-Graduate Medical Committee, and Athlone, Earl of, 242–3; balance with clinical medicine, xiv; and disease prevalence in nineteenth century, 174; and expatriates in tropical environments, 175–6; role of LSHTM in, 252

primary health care: and LSHTM, 266

Pringle, John (1707–82), 6, 30–1, 250, [*12*]

prostitution, female, in London Docklands, 304

Public Health Act: in Victorian Britain, 12

qualifications in tropical medicine, in 1923, 225–7

Queen Alexandra Memorial Hospital, Marseilles, 66

Queensland Institute of Tropical Medicine, 212–3

Raffles, Stamford (1781–1826), 100

Read, Herbert (1863–1949): Private Secretary to Chamberlain, Joseph 86, 87, 90

Rees, David (1868–1917): first superintendent/medical tutor of LSTM, 198

relapsing fever, 24, 238

Research Memoir series of LSTM, 225

Rhin, hospital-ship, 54

Rhodes, Cecil (1853–1902), 100

Rockefeller Foundation: ancylostoma eradication programme, 242–3; charitable foundation, 222, 240–1, 244, 249; financial support for LSHTM, 241, 242, 245, 249, 266; motto of, 242; role in development of British tropical medicine, 266, 297

Roehampton, *see* Ministry of Pensions Tropical Diseases Unit

Rogers, Leonard (1868–1962), [*51*]; address at Royal Society of Medicine, 223; and foundation of Calcutta Medical College, 216; leprosy research and, 231

Roman Campagna expedition, 200–1; mosquito box used at, [*45*]

Rose, Wickliffe (1862–1931): and foundation of LSHTM, 242–3, 245
'Ross Institute and Hospital for Tropical Diseases', 259–66; appeal for public donations towards, 207–8, 259–61; an expensive failure, 266; founding of, 203, 259–61; incorporation into LSHTM, 261–4; opened by Prince of Wales, 261
Ross, Ronald (1857–1932), [47]; account of foundation of schools of tropical medicine, 159–61; appointed Lecturer in Tropical Medicine at Liverpool School, 154; appointed Physician for Tropical Diseases at King's College Hospital, London, 203; awarded Nobel Prize for medicine, 203, 204; Chadwick lectures given by, 174; commemorated on frieze of LSHTM, 263; death of, 261; early career, 202–3; financial ambitions, 203–4; financial support from the Royal Society 98; and funding of Liverpool School of Tropical Medicine, 161; help received from Manson, Patrick, 207; honours, 203; inaugural lecture at Liverpool School of Tropical Medicine, 159; influence on London School of Tropical Medicine 199, 208–12; Institute of Tropical Hygiene at LSHTM, 261–4; lecture at Royal Colonial Institute, 196; libel action against Manson, Patrick, 204–7; Manson's malaria hypothesis and, 75; pioneer of tropical medicine, 32; plaque commemorating, [48]; report on teaching at LSTM, 209–12; results of malaria research, 75, 92, 152, 183–4, 203, 230; and ward at Endsleigh Gardens Hospital, 263; see also: 'Ross Institute and Hospital for Tropical Diseases'
Royal Army Medical College, Millbank, 20, 87, [30]
Royal Army Medical Corps, 256
Royal College of Physicians of London: Comitia meeting at, 108; meeting of Society of Tropical Medicine and Hygiene at, 217; and origin of

LSTM, 116, 118, 123, 125, 129, 145; tropical medicine, and the, 200
Royal College of Surgeons, 146
Royal Free Hospital; careers for women graduates in the tropics, 227; and education of lady doctors for India, 126; Manson, Patrick appointed lecturer in tropical diseases at, 86; see also: Metropolitan Free Hospital
Royal Naval College, Greenwich, 56; see also: Greenwich Hospital
Royal Naval Hospital, Haslar; and SHS, 36, 147; and training in tropical medicine, 91, 95, 102, 109, 143, 170
Royal Navy, 37, 39; training of medical officers for, 81, 84
Royal Shakespeare Company: and LSHTM site, 245
Royal Society, The: correspondence from Fellows of the, 123; and the Liverpool School of Tropical Medicine, 155–6; and malaria research, 143; and sleeping-sickness research, 173, 201; support for LSTM, 90, 143, 161; tropical medicine, and the, 200
Royal Society of Medicine: meeting on tropical neurasthenia, 233–4
Royal Society of Tropical Medicine and Hygiene: foundation of, 216–7; meeting on tropical medicine teaching, 276–9; Presidential Address by Manson-Bahr, Philip, 280–3
Royal Victoria and Albert Docks, 63, 64, 65, 93
Royal Victoria Hospital, Netley, [29]; and LSTM, 109, 116, 117, 124, 131–2, 140, 143, 147; and Manson, Patrick, 87; and training in tropical medicine, 20, 87, 91, 102, 142

St Bartholomew's Medical School: and course of sanitary law and administration, 247
St George's Hospital: lectures by Manson, Patrick, 76–7, 87, 101, 102
St John of Jerusalem, Order of, 218
St Mary's Hospital, London, 107, 120
St Pancras: and Hospital for Tropical

Diseases, 287–96; Coroner's court, 296, [69]; Hospital, history of, 287–8, 289, [64]; Old Church, and burials at, 294–6, [68]; station, 296; workhouse and infirmary, 287–8, [64, 65]

St Paul's Cathedral, London, 55; memorial service for Manson, Patrick, 79

St Thomas' Hospital, London, and SHS, 67

Salisbury, Third Marquess of [Prime Minister] (1830–1903), 80, 83, 93–4

sanitary conditions in British Army, 31

sanitation: importance in medical practice, xiv, 11; increasing emphasis on, 223; role of LSHTM in, xiv, 252

schistosomiasis: and British Empire, 222, 231, 238; in London, 165

School of Medicine for Women (Royal Free Hospital), 218; see also: Royal Free Hospital

seamen, in London's dockland; chronic diseases in, 33; physical handicaps of, 33

Seamen's Hospital, Amoy, China, 69

Seamen's Hospital, Greenwich: accommodation at, 60–1; administration and finances, 57–8; fire at, 58; funding of, 58–9, 61; medical diagnoses at, 61–3; staffing of, 65–6, 136–7, 139; surgical diagnoses at, 62; and tropical diseases, 104, 108, 136–7, 151; see also: Dreadnought [Seamen's] Hospital, Greenwich

Seamen's Hospital Society, The, 33–67; Anniversary Dinner in 1853, 40–1; beds at Dreadnought Hospital, Greenwich, during Second World War (1939–45), 267; Board of Management of, 90; Branch Hospital of, 64–5, 67, 111, 147, 239; Chamberlain, Joseph writes to, 88; charity dinner at Hotel Cecil, 1899, 97–100; donations to, 300–2; 'foster mother' of tropical medicine, 33, 34; foundation of, 33–4: Founder's Day, 34; funding of, 60; and LSTM, 93, 94,

117, 125; major benefaction to, by Lydekker, John, 38; medical staff of, 65–6; provenance of patients at, 300; recommendations of Committee of Management, 90–1; royal patronage for, 35; and St Thomas' Hospital, 67; terms of reference, 39; title, incorporated hy Act of Parliament, 39; and tropical medicine cases, 89

Second World War (1939–45): increase in tropical medicine cases in London, 267

sexually transmitted diseases: introduced hy colonialists, 25; in sailors at Greenwich, 304

Shakespeare Memorial Committee; and LSHTM site, 245

Simon, John (1816–1904), 12, 250

Singapore, founding of, 100

sleeping-sickness: and the British Empire, 85, 186, 201–2; in the Caribbean, 14; in London, 76, 165; outbreak in Uganda, 201–2; research on, 76, 230–1

Sleeping-Sickness Bureau, 173, 182, 187, 223; see also: Tropical Diseases Bureau

Slessor, Mary (1848–1915), 27, 29, [10]

Sloane, Hans (1660–1753), 14–5; and cure of Jamaican diseases, 14

smallpox: in Amoy, China, 69; in the Caribbean, 14; in England, 6–7; eradication of, 7, [4]; in India, 17; Jenner, Edward and, 6–7; last case of, 7; in the temperate zone, 1, 298, 305; vaccination and, 6–7, 8, 272; variolation and, 6

smallpox hospitals, 51, 52, 54

Snow, John (1813–58), 3–4, 25, 30, [2]

Soane, John (1803–87), grave at Old St Pancras, 295

Society of Tropical Medicine and Hygiene, foundation of, 79, 216–7; see also: Royal Society of Tropical Medicine and Hygiene

Society, The Seamen's Hospital, 33–67; see also: Seamen's Hospital Society

south-east Asian prisoners of war, and persisting *Strongyloides stercoralis* infection, 285–6

sprouw, see sprue, 70

sprue: at Albert Dock Hospital, 165; research into cause of, 70, 224, 274; see also: tropical malabsorption

Strongyloides stercoralis infection in south-east Asian prisoners of war, 285–6

Sydenham, Thomas (1624–89), 2, 250, [*1*]

syphilis, in Barbados, 271; *see also*: venereal diseases

tetanus, inoculation for, 272

tinea imbricata, at Amoy, China, 69

Transactions of The [Royal] Society of Tropical Medicine and Hygiene, 217

tropical Africa: survival of expatriates in, 189

'tropical' disease: and the British pioneers, **13–32**; in England before 1900, **1–12**; research into, 222–5; textbook by Manson, Patrick, 77, 78; *see also*: tropical medicine

Tropical Diseases Bulletin, 223

Tropical Diseases Bureau, 223–4; *see also*: Sleeping-Sickness Bureau

Tropical Diseases Research Fund, 180, 196–7; advisory committee for, 181; inadequacy of Government contributions to, 183; report of advisory committee, 185; setting up of, 180

tropical malabsorption, 15, 70

tropical medicine; and the Albert Dock years, **163–217**; controversial beginning in London, **101–46**; during the Second World War (1939–45), **267–85**; removal to Old St Pancras, **287–96**; as a biological discipline, 298–9; and the British Empire, 298; careers in the tropics in, 227–9; changing emphases in practice of, xiv; clinical courses in, 284–5; 'constructive imperialism' and, 298; continuing importance of in Britain,

292–4; courses held during Second World War, 268; in days of Empire and Raj, xiii–xv; use of Dreadnought Hospital, Greenwich during Second World War (1939–45), 267; emergence as a separate specialty, 298–9; funding for the clinical discipline, 254–5; future of in London at end of Second World War, 273–5; future of the discipline, 255; and Hippocrates, 1; institution of lectureships in, 170; an itinerant specialty, 296–7; lack of effective chemotherapy in early days, 299; lectures on by Manson, Patrick, 76–7; major advances since nineteenth century, 299; modification of course at LSHTM, 257–8; origin of *clinical* discipline in London, xiii; pioneers of, at LSHTM, 250; qualifications in, 268; separation of clinical discipline from LSHTM, 297; teaching of after Second World War, 276–9; teaching in London medical schools, 76–7, 84–5; training of doctors for steam shipping companies and, 169–70; transition from clinical to preventive orientation, 266; *see also*: 'tropical disease'

tropical neurasthenia, 233–4

tropical research, and the Medical Research Council, 225

tropics, health hazards of, 229–39

Trypanosoma gambiense, 25

trypanosomiasis, 1, 182, 237; in Africa, 76, 271; and Bruce, David, 76; and Livingstone, David, 27; and Manson, Patrick, 76; treated with Bayer '205', 224

tsetse fly, 27, 271

tuberculosis: BCG vaccine and, 9; in Caribbean, 14, 271; early descriptions of, 7; in England, 1, 7–9; *Mycobacterium tuberculosis* and, 9; prevention of, 119; pulmonary, 110; sanatoria and, 9; treatment of, 9

Turner, George (1855–1941): 'acrimonious correspondence' regarding foundation of LSTM, and, 107,

110–1, 113–6, 121–3, 134–6, 138–9; resignation from *Dreadnought* Hospital, 144–6; and SHS medical staff, 65

Twining, William (1790–1835), 20, 22

typhoid: at Amoy, China, 69; cause of, 9–11; early descriptions of, 9; and indigenous populations of tropics, 238; inoculation and, 11; mortality rate in England and Wales, 11; in northern Europe, 9, 298; 'typhoid Mary' and, 9–11

typhus: association with houses, 238; Chadwick, Edwin and, 6, 11; 'jail fever' and, 6, 11; in London, 6; Pringle, John and, 6; in the temperate zone, 1

ulcerating granuloma in New Guinea, 224

University College, London, and public health teaching, 247

University College Hospital: and Hospital for Tropical Diseases, 283, 284, 289–91, 299; Medical school, 218

University of Cambridge, and tropical medicine qualifications, 208, 226

University of Liverpool, and tropical medicine qualifications, 226–7

University of London: LSTM admitted to, 177; and Tropical Diseases Research Fund, 185, 196; and tropical medicine qualifications, 226; *see also*: London School of Hygiene and Tropical Medicine

venereal diseases, 14, 304; *see also*: syphilis

Wade, John (17?–18?), 20, 22

Waring, Edward (1819–91), 20, 23

Waterloo, 55

Weil's disease, 224

Wellcome Bureau of Scientific Research, 225; teaching and research museum, 225

West Africa: disease in, 85–6, 103, 146, 155; and the 'white man's grave',

85, 228; *see also*: West African Dependencies

West African Dependencies, British: disease in, 94; health of Europeans in, 89, 142, 189, 298; Lagos, Nigeria, mortality at, 89; Medical Research Institute at Lagos, Nigeria, 182

'West African fever', 144

West African Medical Service, 86, 103

West Indies, 13–17, 173

'white man's grave', 85, 89, 228

Wilberforce, William (1759–1833), 33, 34, 288

Wollstonecraft, Mary, *see* Godwin, Mary Wollstonecraft

women medical practitioners, 28, 227

World War (1914–18), **176–7**

World War (1939–45), **267–9**

Wren, Christopher (1632–1723), 30, 55

Wright, William (1735–1819), 15, 16

Wuchereria bancrofti, 24, 70–3, 75; diurnal variation of, 72–3; migration to lungs of, 72, 73; mosquito-man cycle of, 72; *see also: Filaria bancrofti, Filaria sanguinis hominis*

yaws, 14, 222, 231, 271

yellow fever: in Africa, 25, 85, 237; and British Empire, 186, 230; in Caribbean, 14; and houses, 238; imported to England, 119; transmission of, 1; vaccine for, 26, 272

zoonotic diseases, 153